Evidence-Based Medicine: Reading and Writing Medical Papers

CRASH COURSE

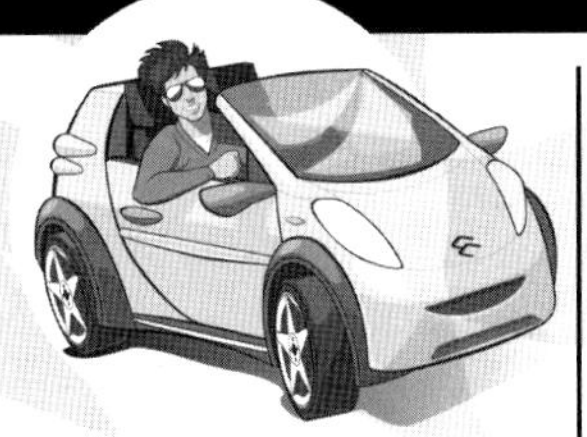

SERIES EDITOR:
Dan Horton-Szar
BSc(Hons) MBBS(Hons) MRCGP
Northgate Medical Practice
Canterbury Kent, UK

FACULTY ADVISOR:
Andrew Polmear
MA MSc FRCP FRCGP
Former Senior Research Fellow Academic Unit
of Primary Care The Trafford Centre for
Medical Education and Research University of Sussex;
Former General Practitioner Brighton and Hove, UK

Evidence-Based Medicine: Reading and Writing Medical Papers

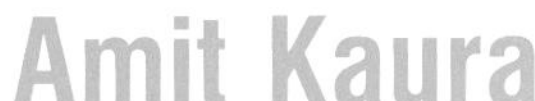

Amit Kaura
BSc(Hons) MB ChB
Core Medical Trainee
King's College Hospital
London, UK

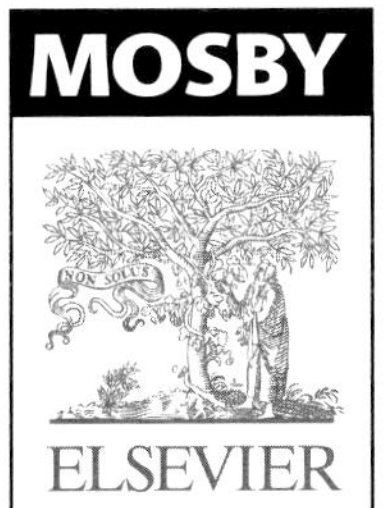

Edinburgh London New York Oxford Philadelphia St Louis Sydney Toronto 2015

ELSEVIER
MOSBY

Commissioning Editor: Jeremy Bowes
Development Editor: Sheila Black
Project Manager: Andrew Riley
Designer: Christian Bilbow
Illustration Manager: Jennifer Rose

Updated First edition 2015

ISBN: 978-0-7234-3869-4

British Library Cataloguing in Publication Data
A catalogue record for this book is available from the British Library

Library of Congress Cataloging in Publication Data
A catalog record for this book is available from the Library of Congress

Notices
Knowledge and best practice in this field are constantly changing. As new research and experience broaden our understanding, changes in research methods, professional practices, or medical treatment may become necessary.

Practitioners and researchers must always rely on their own experience and knowledge in evaluating and using any information, methods, compounds, or experiments described herein. In using such information or methods they should be mindful of their own safety and the safety of others, including parties for whom they have a professional responsibility.

With respect to any drug or pharmaceutical products identified, readers are advised to check the most current information provided (i) on procedures featured or (ii) by the manufacturer of each product to be administered, to verify the recommended dose or formula, the method and duration of administration, and contraindications. It is the responsibility of practitioners, relying on their own experience and knowledge of their patients, to make diagnoses, to determine dosages and the best treatment for each individual patient, and to take all appropriate safety precautions.

To the fullest extent of the law, neither the Publisher nor the authors, contributors, or editors, assume any liability for any injury and/or damage to persons or property as a matter of products liability, negligence or otherwise, or from any use or operation of any methods, products, instructions, or ideas contained in the material herein.

The Publisher's policy is to use **paper manufactured from sustainable forests**

Printed in China

Last digit is the print line: 10 9 8 7 6 5 4 3 2 1

Series editor foreword

The *Crash Course* series first published in 1997 and now, 16 years on, we are still going strong. Medicine never stands still, and the work of keeping this series relevant for today's students is an ongoing process. Along with revising existing titles, now in their fourth editions, we are delighted to add this new title to the series.

Among the changes to our profession over the years, the rise of evidence-based medicine has dramatically improved the quality and consistency of medical care for patients and brings new challenges to doctors and students alike. It is increasingly important for students to be skilled in the critical appraisal of published medical research and the application of evidence to their clinical practice, and to have the ability to use audit to monitor and improve that practice over the years. These skills are now an important and explicit part of the medical curriculum and the examinations you need to pass. This excellent new title presents the foundations of these skills with a clear and practical approach perfectly suited to those embarking on their medical careers.

With this new book, we hold fast to the principles on which we first developed the series. *Crash Course* will always bring you all the information you need to revise in compact, manageable volumes that integrate basic medical science and clinical practice. The books still maintain the balance between clarity and conciseness, and provide sufficient depth for those aiming at distinction. The authors are medical students and junior doctors who have recent experience of the exams you are now facing, and the accuracy of the material is checked by a team of faculty advisors from across the UK.

I wish you all the best for your future careers!

Dr Dan Horton-Szar

Prefaces

Author

Crash Course Evidence-Based Medicine: Reading and Writing Medical Papers is directed at medical students and healthcare professionals at all stages of their training. Due to the ever-increasing rate at which medical knowledge is advancing, it is crucial that all professionals are able to practice evidence-based medicine, which includes being able to critically appraise the medical literature. Over the course of this book, all study types will be discussed using a systematic approach, therefore allowing for easy comparison. In addition to equipping readers with the skills required to critically appraise research evidence, this book covers the key points on how to conduct research and report the findings. This requires an understanding of statistics, which are used throughout all stages of the research process – from designing a study to data collection and analysis. All commonly used statistical methods are explored in a concise manner, using examples from real-life situations to aid understanding. As with the other books in the *Crash Course* series, the material is designed to arm the reader with the essential facts on these subjects, while maintaining a balance between conciseness and clarity. References for further reading are provided where readers wish to explore a topic in greater detail.

The General Medical Council's *Tomorrow's Doctors – guidance for undergraduate medical students* states that student-selected components (SSCs) should account for 10-30% of the standard curriculum. SSCs commonly include clinical audit, literature review, and quantitative or qualitative research. Not only will this book be an invaluable asset for passing the SSC assessments, it will enable students to prepare high-quality reports and therefore improve their chances of publishing papers in peer-reviewed journals. The importance of this extends beyond undergraduate study, as such educational achievements carry weight when applying for Foundation Programme positions and specialist training.

Evidence-based medicine is a vertical theme that runs through all years of undergraduate and postgraduate study and commonly appears in exams. The self-assessment questions, which follow the modern exam format, will help the reader pass that dreaded evidence-based medicine and statistics exam with flying colours!

Amit Kaura

Faculty advisor

For decades three disciplines have been converging slowly to create a new way of practising medicine. Statisticians provide the expertise to ensure that research results are valid; clinicians have developed the science of evidence-based medicine to bring the results of that research into practice; and educators and managers have developed clinical audit to check that practitioners are doing what they think they are doing. Yet the seams still show. Few articles present the statistics in the way most useful to clinicians. If this surprises you, look to see how few articles on therapy give the Number Needed to Treat. Have you ever seen an article on diagnosis give the Number Needed to Test? It is even more rare for an article that proposes a new treatment to suggest a topic for audit.

This book is, to my knowledge, the first that sees these three strands as a single way of practising medicine. It is no coincidence that it took a doctor who qualified in the second decade of the 21st century to bring these strands together. Many doctors who teach have still not mastered the evidence-based approach and some still see audit as something you do to satisfy your managers. Armed with this book, the student can lay a foundation for his or her clinical practice that will inform every consultation over a lifetime in medicine.

Andrew Polmear

Acknowledgements

I would like to express my deep gratitude to:

- Dan Horton-Szar, Jeremy Bowes, Sheila Black and the rest of the team at Elsevier, who granted me this amazing opportunity to teach and inspire the next generation of clinical academics;
- Andrew Polmear, the Faculty Advisor for this project, for his valuable and constructive suggestions during the development of this book;
- Andy Salmon, Consultant in Renal Medicine, a role model providing inspiration that has been a shining light;
- All those who have supported me in my academic career to date including Jonathan Byrne and Narbeh Melikian, Consultant Cardiologists at King's College Hospital, and Sanjay Sharma, Professor of Inherited Cardiac Diseases and Sports Cardiology at St. George's Hospital;
- Rina Patel and Hajeb Kamali, for all their encouragement during the preparation of this book.

Amit Kaura

Dedication

I dedicate this book to my dad, mum, brother, Vinay, and the rest of my family, near and far, for their encouragement, love and support.

Contents

Evidence-based medicine

Objectives

By the end of this chapter you should:

- Understand the importance of evidence-based medicine in healthcare.
- Know how to formulate clinically relevant, answerable questions using the Patient Intervention Comparison Outcome (PICO) framework.
- Be able to systematically perform a literature search to identify relevant evidence.
- Understand the importance of assessing the quality and validity of evidence by critically appraising the literature.
- Know that different study designs provide varying levels of evidence.
- Know how to assess and implement new evidence in clinical practice.
- Understand the importance of regularly evaluating the implementation of new evidence-based practice.
- Understand why clinical recommendations are regularly updated and list the steps involved in creating new clinical practice guidelines.

WHAT IS EVIDENCE-BASED MEDICINE?

- Sackett and colleagues describe evidence-based medicine (a.k.a. 'evidence-based practice') as 'the conscientious, explicit and judicious use of current best evidence in making decisions about the care of individual patients'.
- Considering the vast rate at which medical knowledge is advancing, it is crucial for clinicians and researchers to make sense of the wealth of data (sometimes poor) available.
- Evidence-based medicine involves a number of key principles which will be discussed in turn:
  - Formulate a clinically relevant question
  - Identify relevant evidence
  - Systematically review and appraise the evidence identified
  - Extract the most useful results and determine whether they are important in your clinical practice
  - Synthesise evidence to draw conclusions
  - Use the clinical research findings to generate guideline recommendations which enable clinicians to deliver optimal clinical care to your patients
  - Evaluate the implementation of evidence-based medicine.

HINTS AND TIPS

Evidence-based practice is a systematic process primarily aimed at improving the care of patients.

FORMULATING CLINICAL QUESTIONS

- In order to practise evidence-based medicine, the initial step involves converting a clinical encounter in to a clinical question.
- A useful approach to formatting a clinical (or research) question is using the Patient Intervention Comparison Outcome (PICO) framework (Fig. 1.1). The question is divided in to four key components:
  1. *Patient/Population*: Which patients or population group of patients are you interested in? Is it necessary to consider any subgroups?
  2. *Intervention*: Which intervention/treatment is being evaluated?
  3. *Comparison/Control*: What is/are the main alternative/s compared to the intervention?
  4. *Outcome*: What is the most important outcome for the patient? Outcomes can include short- or long-term measures, intervention complications, social functioning or quality of life, morbidity, mortality or costs.
- Not all research questions ask whether an *intervention* is better than existing interventions or no treatment at all. From a clinical perspective, evidence-based medicine is relevant for three other key domains:
  1. *Aetiology*: Is the exposure a risk factor for developing a certain condition?
  2. *Diagnosis*: How good is the diagnostic test (history taking, physical examination, laboratory

Fig. 1.1 PICO.

Clinical Encounter

John, 31 years old, was diagnosed with heart failure 3 years old and prescribed a beta-blocker which dramatically improved his symptoms. John's 5-year-old daughter, Sarah, has been recently diagnosed with chronic symptomatic congestive heart failure. John asks you, Sarah's paediatrician, whether his daughter should also be prescribed a beta-blocker.

Is there a role for beta-blockers in the management of heart failure in children?

Patient	Children with congestive heart failure
Intervention	Carvedilol
Comparison	No carvedilol
Outcome	Improvement of congestive heart failure symptoms

or pathological tests and imaging) in determining whether a patient has a particular condition? Questions are usually asked about the clinical value or the diagnostic accuracy of using the test (discussed in Chapter 14).
3. *Prognosis*: Are there factors related to the patient that predict a particular outcome (disease progression, survival time after diagnosis of the disease, etc.)? The prognosis is based on the characteristics of the patient ('prognostic factors') (discussed in Chapter 14).

- It is important that the patient experience is taken into account when formulating the clinical question. Understandably, the ('p')atient experience may vary depending on which patient population is being addressed. The following patient views should be determined:
  - The acceptability of the proposed ('i')ntervention being evaluated
  - Preferences for the treatment options already available ('c')
  - What constitutes an appropriate, desired or acceptable ('o')utcome.
- Incorporating the above patient views will ensure the clinical question is patient-centred and therefore clinically relevant.

IDENTIFYING RELEVANT EVIDENCE

Sources of information

- Evidence should be identified using systematic, transparent and reproducible database searches.
- While a number of medical databases exist, the particular source used to identify evidence of clinical effectiveness will depend on the clinical question.
- It is advisable that all core databases (Fig. 1.2) are searched for every clinical question.
- Depending on the subject area of the clinical question, subject-specific databases (Fig. 1.2) and other relevant sources should also be searched.

HINTS AND TIPS

Using Dr 'Google' to perform your entire literature search is not recommended!!!

- It is important to take into account the strengths and weaknesses of each database prior to carrying out a literature search. For example, EMBASE, which is

Fig. 1.2 Types of scientific databases.

Core databases

Cochrane Library
- Cochrane Database of Systematic Reviews – (CDSR; Cochrane Reviews)
- Database of Abstracts of Reviews of Effects (DARE; Other Reviews)
- Cochrane Central Register of Controlled Trials – (CENTRAL; Clinical Trials)

MEDLINE/MEDLINE In-Process
EMBASE
Health Technology Assessment (HTA) database (Technology Assessments)
Cumulative Index to Nursing and Allied Health Literature (CINAHL)

Subject-specific databases

PsycINFO
Education Resources Information Center (ERIC)
Physiotherapy Evidence Database (PEDro)
Allied and Complementary Medicine Database (AMED)

operated by Elsevier Publishing, is considered to have better coverage of European and non-English language publications and topics, such as toxicology, pharmacology, psychiatry and alternative medicine, compared to the MEDLINE database.

- Overlap in the records retrieved from different databases will exist. For example, the overlap between EMBASE and MEDLINE is estimated to be 10 to 87%, depending on the topic.
- Other sources of information may include:
  - Websites (e.g. ClinicalTrials.gov)
  - Registries (e.g. national or regional registers)
  - Conference abstracts
  - Checking reference lists of key publications
  - Personal communication with experts in the field.

HINTS AND TIPS

Different scientific databases cover different time periods and index different types of journals.

The search strategy

- The PICO framework can be used to construct the terms for your search strategy. In other words, the framework can be used to devise the search terms for the population, which can be combined with search terms related to the intervention(s) and comparison(s) (if there are any).
- It is common that outcome terms are not often mentioned in the subject headings or abstracts of database records. Consequently, 'outcome' terms are often omitted from the search strategy.

Search terms

- When you input search terms, you can search for:
  - a specific citation (author and publication detail)
  - 'free-text' (text word) terms within the title and abstract
  - subject headings with which relevant references have been tagged.
- Subject headings can help you identify appropriate search terms and find information on a specific topic without having to carry out further searches under all the synonyms for the preferred subject heading. For example, using the MEDLINE database, the subject heading 'heart failure' would be 'exp Heart Failure', where 'exp' stands for explode; i.e. the function gathers all the different subheadings within the subject heading 'Heart Failure'.
- Free-text searches are carried out to complement the subject heading searches. Free-text terms may include:
  - acronyms, e.g. 'acquired immune deficiency syndrome' versus 'AIDS'
  - synonyms, e.g. 'shortness of breath' versus 'breathlessness'
  - abbreviations, e.g. 'abdominal aortic aneurysm' versus 'AAA'
  - different spellings, e.g. 'paediatric' (UK spelling) versus 'pediatric' (US spelling).
  - lay and medical terminology, e.g. 'indigestion' (lay) versus 'dyspepsia' (medical)
  - brand and generic drug names, e.g. 'septrin' (brand name) versus 'co-trimoxazole' (generic name).
- It is important to identify the text word syntax (symbols) specific for each database in order to expand your results set, e.g. '.tw' used in MEDLINE.
- If entering two text words together, you may decide to use the term 'adj5', which indicates the two words must be adjacent within 5 words of each other, e.g. '(ventricular adj5 dysfunction).tw'.
- A symbol can be added to a word root in order to retrieve variant endings, e.g. 'smok*' or 'smok$' finds citations with the words smoked, smoker, smoke, smokes, smoking and many more.
- Referring to Fig. 1.3:
  - in order to combine terms for the same concept (e.g. synonyms or acronyms), the Boolean operator 'OR' is used.
  - in order to combine sets of terms for different concepts, the Boolean operator 'AND' is used.

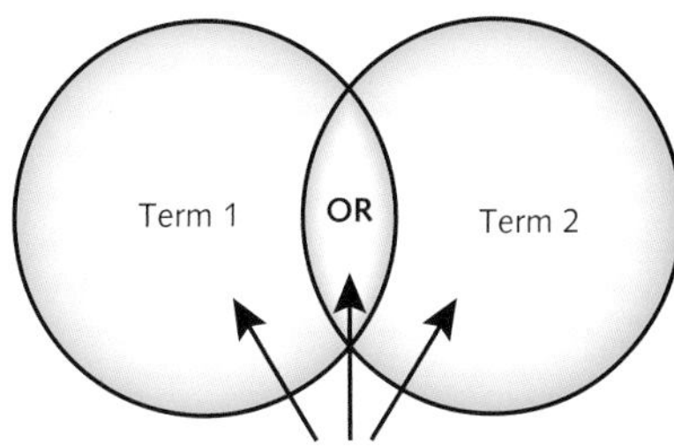
Term 1
OR
Term 2
The Boolean operator 'OR' identifies all the citations that contain EITHER term

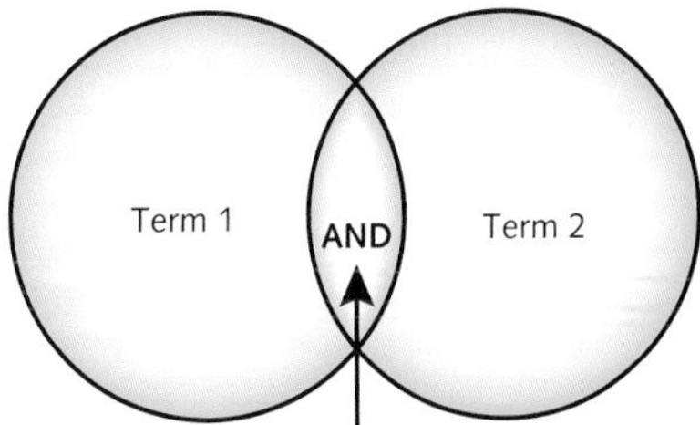
Term 1
AND
Term 2
The Boolean operator 'AND' identifies all the citations that contain BOTH terms

Fig. 1.3 Boolean logic.

HINTS AND TIPS

While subject headings are used to identify the main theme of an article, not all conditions will have a subject heading, so it is important to also search for free-text terms.

Reviewing the search strategy

Expanding your results

If there are too few references following your original search you should consider the following:

- Add symbols ($ or *) to the word root in order to retrieve variant endings.
- Ensure the text word spellings are correct.
- Ensure that you have combined your search terms using the correct Boolean logic concept (AND, OR).
- Consider reducing the number and type of limits applied to the search.
- Ensure you have searched for related words, i.e. synonyms, acronyms.
- Search for terms that are broader for the topic of interest.

Limiting your results

If there are too many references following your original search you should consider the following:

- Depending on the review question, you may consider limiting the search:
  - to particular study designs (e.g. searching for systematic reviews for review questions on the effectiveness of interventions)
  - by age (limiting searches by sex is not usually recommended)
  - to studies reported only in English
  - to studies involving only humans and not animals.
- Consider adding another Boolean logic concept (AND).
- Ensure you have searched for appropriate text words; otherwise, it may be appropriate to only search for subject headings.

Documentation of the search strategy

- An audit trail should be documented to ensure that the strategy used for identifying the evidence is reproducible and transparent. The following information should be documented:
  1. The names (and host systems) of the databases, e.g. MEDLINE (Ovid)
  2. The coverage dates of the database, e.g. MEDLINE (Ovid) <1950 to week 24, 2012>
  3. The date on which the search was conducted
  4. The search strategy
  5. The limits that were applied to the search
  6. The number of records retrieved at each step of your search.
- The search strategy used for the clinical question described above (Fig. 1.1) is shown in Fig. 1.4.

CRITICALLY APPRAISING THE EVIDENCE

- Once all the possible studies have been identified with the literature search, each study needs to be assessed for eligibility against objective criteria for inclusion or exclusion of studies.
- Having identified those studies that meet the inclusion criteria, they are subsequently assessed for methodological quality using a critical appraisal framework.
- Despite satisfying the inclusion criteria, studies appraised as being poor in quality should also be excluded.

Critical appraisal

- Critical appraisal is the process of systematically examining the available evidence to judge its *validity*, and *relevance* in a particular context.
- The appraiser should make an objective assessment of the study quality and potential for bias.
- It is important to determine both the internal validity and external validity of the study:
  - *External validity*: The extent to which the study findings are generalisable beyond the limits of the study to the study's target population.
  - *Internal validity*: Ensuring that the study was run carefully (research design, how variables were measured, etc.) and the extent to which the observed effect(s) were produced solely by the intervention being assessed (and not by another factor).
- The three main threats to internal validity (confounding, bias and causality) are discussed in turn for each of the key study designs in their respective chapters.
- Methodological checklists for critically appraising the key study designs covered in this book are provided in Chapter 19.

1) MEDLINE (Ovid)

2) <1950 to week 24 2012>

3) Search conducted on 14/06/12

4 – 6) Underneath:

	History	Results
1	exp Heart Failure	77,457
2	exp Ventricular Dysfunction	22,530
3	cardiac failure.tw.	9098
4	heart failure.tw.	88,104
5	(ventric$ adj5 dysfunction$).tw	16,759
6	(ventric$ adj5 function$).tw	38,132
7	1 or 2 or 3 or 4	166,646
8	carvedilol.tw.	2049
9	7 and 8	1103
10	child$.tw	852,930
11	infant$.tw	270,114
12	paediatr$.tw	32,804
13	pediatr$.tw	148,202
14	adolesc$.tw	140,587
15	10 or 11 or 12 or 13 or 14	1,197,954
16	9 and 15	41
17	limit 9 to "all child (0 to 18 years)"	71
18	16 or 17	74
19	**limit 18 to English language**	**66**
20	**limit 19 to humans**	**66**

Fig. 1.4 Documenting the search strategy.

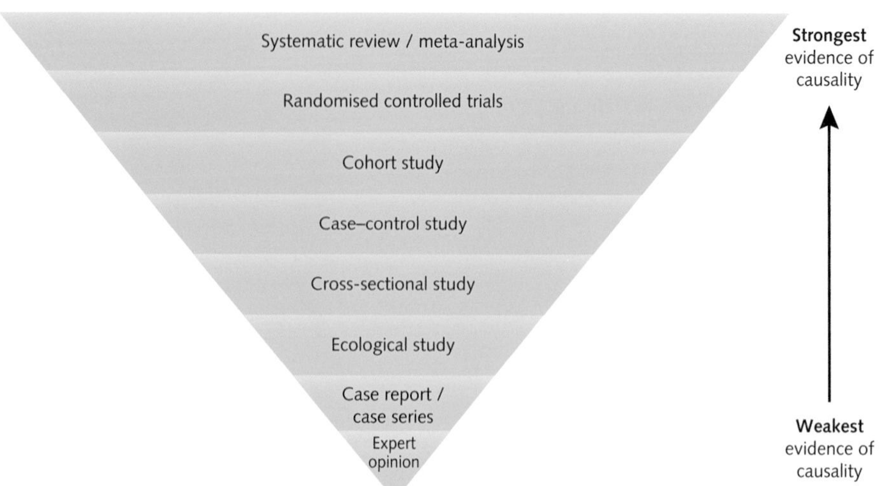

Fig. 1.5 Hierarchy of evidence.

Hierarchy of evidence

- Different study designs provide varying levels of evidence of causality (Fig. 1.5).
- The rank of a study in the hierarchy of evidence is based on its potential for bias, i.e. a systematic review provides the strongest evidence for a causal relationship between an intervention and outcome.

HINTS AND TIPS

Practising medicine using unreliable evidence could lead to patient harm or limited resources being wasted – hence the importance of critical appraisal.

ASSESSING THE RESULTS

Of the remaining studies, the reported results are extracted on to a data extraction form which may include the following points:

- Does the main outcome variable measured in the study relate to the outcome variable stated in the PICO question?
- How large is the effect of interest?
- How precise is the effect of interest?/Have confidence intervals been provided? (Narrower confidence intervals indicate higher precision.)
- If the lower limit of the confidence interval represents the true value of the effect, would you consider the observed effect to be clinically significant?
- Would it be clinically significant if the upper limit of the confidence interval represented the true value of the effect?

IMPLEMENTING THE RESULTS

Having already critically appraised the evidence, extracted the most useful results and determined whether they are important, you must decide whether this evidence can be applied to your individual patient or population. It is important to determine whether:

- your patient has similar characteristics to those subjects enrolled in the studies from which the evidence was obtained
- the outcomes considered in the evidence are clinically important to your patient
- the study results are applicable to your patient
- the evidence regarding risks is available
- the intervention is available in your healthcare setting
- an economic analysis has been performed.

The evidence regarding both efficacy and risks should be discussed with the patient in order to make an informed decision about their care.

EVALUATING PERFORMANCE

Having implemented the key evidence-based medicine principles discussed above, it is important to:

- integrate the evidence into clinical practice.
- audit your performance to demonstrate whether this approach is improving patient care (discussed in Chapter 16).
- evaluate your approach at regular intervals to determine whether there is scope for improvement in any stage of the process.

CREATING GUIDELINE RECOMMENDATIONS

- The evidence-based medicine approach may be used to develop clinical practice guidelines.
- Clinical guidelines are recommendations based on the best available evidence.
- They are developed taking into account the views of those affected by the recommendations in the guideline, i.e. healthcare professionals, patients, their families and carers, NHS trusts, the public and government bodies. These stakeholders play an integral part in the development of a clinical guideline and are involved in all key stages (Fig. 1.6).
- Topics for national clinical guideline development are highlighted by the Department of Health, based on recommendations from panels considering topic selection. Local guidelines may be commissioned by a hospital or primary care trust.
- The commissioning body identifies the key areas which need to be covered, which are subsequently translated into the scope for the clinical guideline.
- As highlighted by the National Institute for Health and Clinical Excellence (NICE), clinical guidelines can be used to:
    - educate and train healthcare professionals
    - develop standards for assessing current clinical practice
    - help patients make informed decisions
    - improve communication between healthcare professionals and patients.
- Healthcare providers and organisations should implement the recommendations with use of slide sets, audit support and other tools tailored to need.
- It is important that healthcare professionals take clinical guidelines into account when making clinical decisions. However, guidelines are intended to be flexible, and clinical judgement should also be based on clinical circumstances and patient preferences.

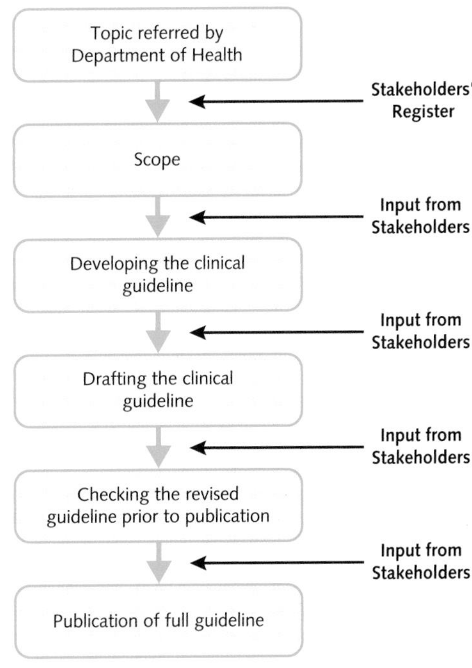

Fig. 1.6 Key stages of clinical guideline development.

HINTS AND TIPS

The goal of a clinical guideline is to improve the quality of clinical care delivered by healthcare professionals and to ensure that the resources used are not only efficient but also cost-effective.

Handling data 2

Objectives

By the end of this chapter you should:

- Know how to differentiate between the four types of variables used in medical statistics: nominal, ordinal, interval, ratio.
- Understand the difference between continuous and discrete data.
- Know how to display the distribution of a single variable.
- Know how to display the association between two variables.
- Be able to use measures for central tendency or variability to describe the frequency distribution of a variable.
- Know how to define probability distributions and understand the basic rules of probability.
- Be able to recognise and describe the normal distribution.
- Be able to calculate and interpret the reference range.
- Understand that skewed distributions can sometimes be transformed to follow a normal distribution.

TYPES OF VARIABLES

- The data collected from the studies we conduct or critique comprise observations on one or more variables.
- A variable is a quantity that varies and can take any one of a specified set of values. For example, when collecting information on patient demographics, variables of interest may include gender, race or age.
- As described by the psychologist Stanley Stevens in 1946, research data usually falls into one of the following four types of variables:
  1. Nominal
  2. Ordinal
  3. Interval
  4. Ratio.

Nominal variable

- Variables assessed on a nominal scale are called categorical variables.
- The order of the categories is meaningless.
- The categories are mutually exclusive and simply have names.
- A special type of nominal variable is a dichotomous variable, which can take only one of two values, for example gender (male or female). The data collected are therefore binomial.
- If there are three or more categories for a variable, the data collected are multinomial. For example, for marital status, the categories may be single, married, divorced or widowed.
- Data collected for nominal variables are usually presented in the form of contingency tables (e.g. 2 × 2 tables).

HINTS AND TIPS

In nominal measurements, the categories of variables differ from one another in name only.

Ordinal variable

- An ordinal variable is another type of categorical variable. When a 'rank-ordered' logical relationship exists among the categories, the variable is only then known as an ordinal variable.
- The categories may be ranked in order of magnitude. For example, there may be ranked categories for disease staging (none, mild, moderate, severe) or for a rating scale for pain, whereby response categories are assigned numbers in the following manner:
  1. (no pain)
  2. (mild pain)
  3. (moderate pain)
  4. (severe pain)
  5. (unbearable pain).
- The distance or interval between the categories is not known. Referring to our example above, you do not know whether the distance between 1 (no pain) and 2 (mild pain) is the same as the distance between 3 (moderate pain) and 4 (severe pain). It is possible that respondents falling into categories 1, 2 and 3

Fig. 2.1 Ordinal measurement of pain score.

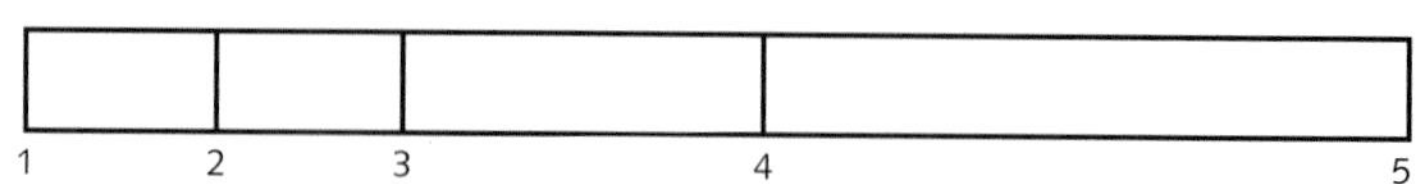

are actually very similar to each other, while those falling into pain category 4 and 5 are very different from the rest (Fig. 2.1).

HINTS AND TIPS

While a rank order in the categories of an ordinal variable exists, the distance between the categories is not equal.

Interval variable

- In addition to having all the characteristics of nominal and ordinal variables, an interval variable is one where the distance (or interval) between any two categories is the same and constant.
- Examples of interval variables include:
  - temperature, i.e. the difference between 80 and 70°F is the same as the difference between 70 and 60°F.
  - dates, i.e. the difference between the beginning of day 1 and that of day 2 is 24 hours, just as it is between the beginning of day 2 and that of day 3.
- Interval variables do not have a natural zero point. For example, in the temperature variable, there is no natural zero, so we cannot say that 40°F is twice as warm as 20°F.
- On some occasions, zero points are chosen arbitrarily.

Ratio variable

- In addition to having all the characteristics of interval variables, a ratio variable also has a natural zero point.
- Examples of ratio variables include:
  - height
  - weight
  - incidence or prevalence of disease.
- Figure 2.2 demonstrates the number of children in a family as a ratio scale. We can make the following statements about the ratio scale:
  - The distance between any two measurements is the same.
  - A family with 2 children is different from a family with 3 children (as is true for a nominal variable).
  - A family with 3 children has more children than a family with 2 children (as is true for an ordinal variable).
  - You can say one family has had 3 more children than another family (as is true for an interval variable).
  - You can say one family with 6 children has had twice as many children as a family with 3 children (as is true for a ratio variable, which has a true zero point).

Quantitative (numerical) data

When a variable takes a numerical value, it is either discrete or continuous.

Discrete variable

- A variable is discrete if its categories can only take a finite number of whole values.
- Examples include number of asthma attacks in a month, number of children in a family and number of sexual partners in a month.

Continuous variable

- A variable is continuous if its categories can take an infinite number of values.
- Examples include weight, height and systolic blood pressure.

Qualitative (categorical) data

- Nominal and ordinal variables are types of categorical variables as each individual can only fit into one of a number of distinct categories of the variable.
- For quantitative variables, the range of numerical values can be subdivided into categories, e.g. column 1 of the table presented in Fig. 2.3 demonstrates what categories may be used to group weight data. A numerical variable can therefore be turned into a categorical variable.
- The categories chosen for grouping continuous data should be:
  - exhaustive, i.e. the categories cover all the numerical values of the variable.
  - exclusive, i.e. there is no overlap between the categories.

Fig. 2.2 Ratio measurement of number of children in a family.

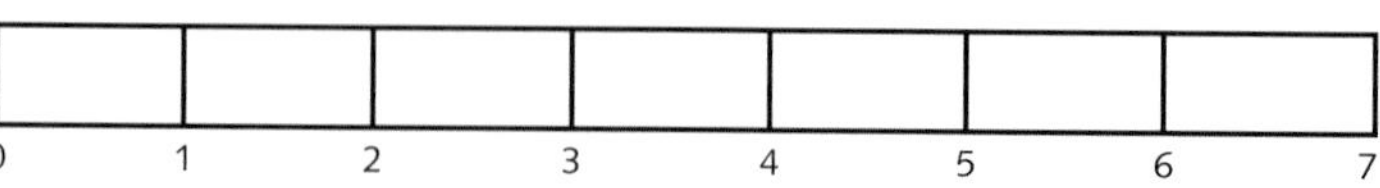

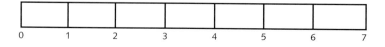

Fig. 2.3 The frequency distribution of the weights of a sample of medical students.

Weight (kg)	Frequency	Relative frequency (%)	Cumulative frequency	Relative cumulative frequency (%)
40–49.99	1	1.16	1	1.16
50–59.99	3	3.49	4	4.65
60–69.99	11	12.79	15	17.44
70–79.99	20	23.26	35	40.70
80–89.99	30	34.88	65	75.58
90–99.99	15	17.44	80	93.02
100–109.99	6	6.98	86	100.00
TOTAL	86	100.00	86	100.00

DISPLAYING THE DISTRIBUTION OF A SINGLE VARIABLE

- Having undertaken a piece of research, producing graphs and charts is a useful way of summarising the data obtained so it can be read and interpreted with ease.
- Prior to displaying the data using appropriate charts or graphs, it is important to use frequency distributions to tabulate the data collected.

Frequency distributions

- Frequency tables should first be used to display the distribution of a variable.
- An empirical frequency distribution of a variable summarises the observed frequency of occurrence of each category.
- The frequencies are expressed as an absolute number or as a relative frequency (the percentage of the total frequency).
- Using relative frequencies allows us to compare frequency distributions in two or more groups of individuals.
- Calculating the running total of the absolute frequencies (or relative frequencies) from lower to higher categories gives us the cumulative frequency (or relative cumulative frequencies) (Fig. 2.3).

HINTS AND TIPS

Frequency tables can be used to display the distribution of:

- nominal categorical variables
- ordinal categorical variables
- some discrete numerical variables
- *grouped* continuous numerical variables

Displaying frequency distributions

- Once the frequencies for your data have been obtained, the next step is to display the data graphically.
- The type of variable you are trying to display will influence which graph or chart is best suited for your data (Fig. 2.4).

Bar chart

- Frequencies or relative frequencies for categorical variables can be displayed as a bar chart.
- The length of each bar (either horizontal or vertical) is proportional to the frequency for the category of the variable.
- There are usually gaps between the bars to indicate that the categories are separate from each other.
- Bar charts are useful when we want to compare the frequency of each category relative to others.
- It is also possible to present the frequencies or relative frequencies in each category in two (or more) different groups.
- The grouped bar chart displayed in Fig. 2.5 shows:
  - the categories (ethnic groups) along the horizontal axis (x-axis)
  - the number of admissions to the cardiology ward (over one month) along the vertical axis (y-axis)
  - the number of admissions according to ethnic group which correspond to the length of the vertical bars
  - two bars for each ethnic group, which represent gender (male and female).
- We can see that most people admitted on to the cardiology ward were:
  - of male gender (regardless of ethnicity)
  - from South Asia (especially Indian in ethnicity).

Fig. 2.4 Displaying single variables graphically.

Type of variable	Display method
Categorical (nominal, ordinal, some discrete)	Bar chart Pie chart
Grouped continuous (interval and ratio)	Histogram

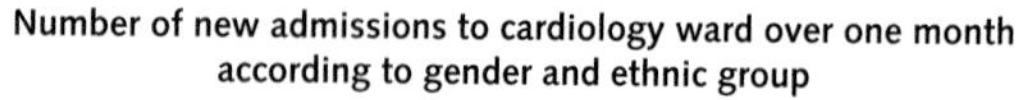

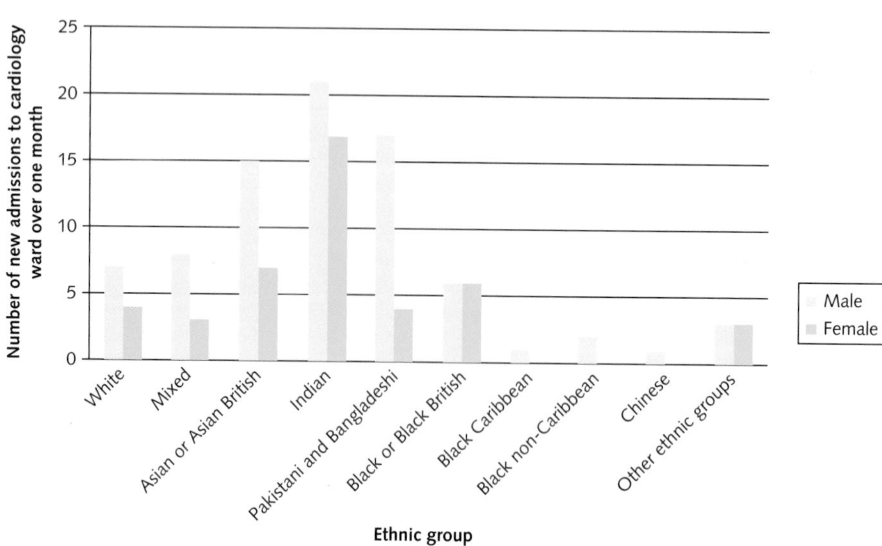

Fig. 2.5 Grouped bar chart.

- Alternatively, a stacked bar chart could be used to display the data above (Fig. 2.6). The stacked bars represent the different groups (male and female) on top of each other. The length of the resulting bar shows the combined frequency of the groups.

Pie chart

- The Frequencies or relative frequencies of a categorical variable can also be displayed graphically using a pie chart.
- Pie charts are useful for displaying the relative proportions of a few categories.
- The area of each sector (or category) is proportional to its frequency
- The pie chart displayed in Fig. 2.7 shows the various intrinsic factors that were found to cause inpatient falls over one month on a geriatric ward. It is evident that having cognitive impairment was by far the most common intrinsic factor responsible for causing inpatient falls.

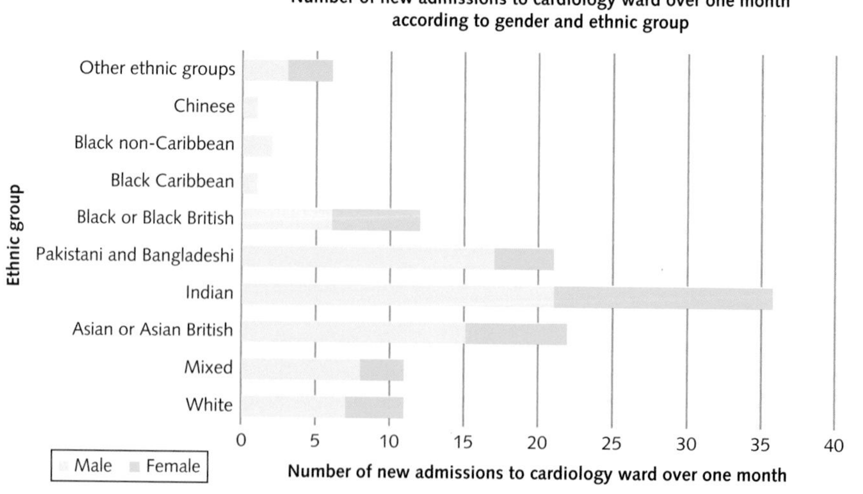

Fig. 2.6 Stacked bar chart.

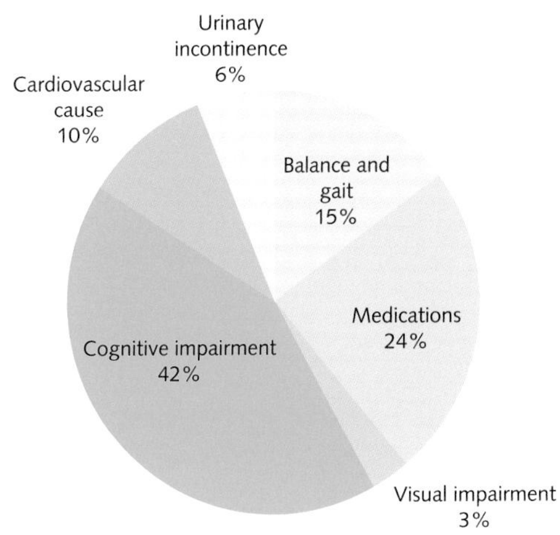

Fig. 2.7 Pie chart.

> **HINTS AND TIPS**
>
> Pie charts are useful for:
> - Displaying the relative sizes of the sectors that make up the whole.
> - Providing a visual representation of the data when the categories show some variation in size.

Histogram

- Grouped continuous numerical data are often displayed using a histogram.
- Although histograms are made up of bars, there are some key differences between bar charts and histograms (Fig. 2.8).
- The horizontal axis consists of intervals ordered from lowest to highest.
- The width of the bars is determined by the width of the categories chosen for the frequency distribution, as shown in Fig. 2.3.
- The area of each bar is proportional to the number of cases (frequency) per unit interval.
- There are no gaps between the bars as the data represented by the histogram are not only exclusive, but also continuous.
- For example, a histogram of the weight data shown in Fig. 2.3 is presented in Fig. 2.9. As the grouping intervals of the categories are all equal in size, the histogram looks very similar to a corresponding bar chart. However, if one of the categories has a different width than the others, it is important to take this into account:
    - For example, if we combine the two highest weight categories, the frequency for this combined group (90–109.99 kg) is 21.
    - As the bar area represents frequency, it would be incorrect to draw a bar of height 21 from 90 to 109.99 kg.
    - The correct approach would be to halve the total frequency for this combined category as the group interval is twice as wide as the others.
    - The correct height is therefore 10.5, as demonstrated by the dotted line in Fig. 2.9.

> **HINTS AND TIPS**
>
> The vertical axis of a histogram doesn't always show the absolute numbers for each category. An alternative is to show percentages (proportions) on the vertical axis. The length of each bar is the percentage of the total that each category represents. In this case, the total area of all the bars is equal to 1.

DISPLAYING THE DISTRIBUTION OF TWO VARIABLES

Selecting an appropriate graph or chart to display the association between two variables depends on the types of variables you are dealing with (Fig. 2.10).

Fig. 2.8 Bar chart versus histogram.

	Bar chart	Histogram
Type of variable displayed	Categorical	Grouped continuous
Purpose	Compare frequencies of each category within a variable	Display the frequency distribution of a variable
Width of bars	Similar	Different
Gap between bars	Yes (However, not strictly true)	No (Unless there are no values within a given interval)
What is the frequency represented by?	Length of bar	Area of bar

Fig. 2.9 Histogram.

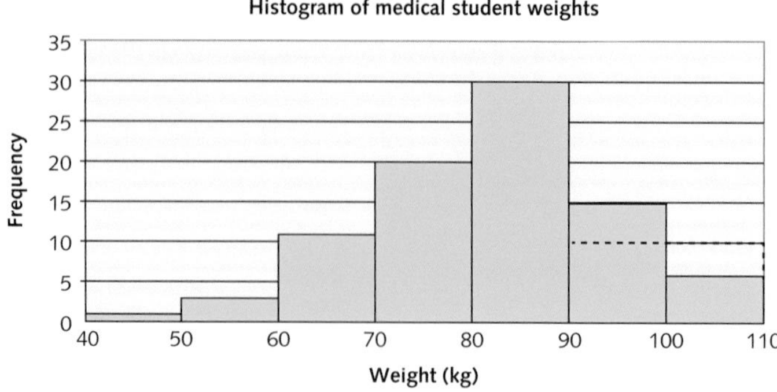

Fig. 2.10 Displaying the association between two variables graphically.

Type of variables	Display method
Numerical vs numerical	Scatter plot
Categorical vs categorical	Contingency table
Numerical vs categorical	Box and whisker plot Bar chart Dot plot

Numerical versus numerical variables

- If both the variables are numerical (or ordinal), the association between them can be illustrated using a scatter plot.
- If investigating the effect of an exposure on a particular outcome, it is conventional to plot the exposure variable on the horizontal axis and the outcome variable on the vertical axis.
- The extent of association between the two variables can be quantified using correlation and/or regression (discussed in Chapter 15).

Categorical versus categorical variables

- If both variables are categorical, a contingency table should be used.
- Conventionally, the rows should represent the exposure variable and the columns should represent the outcome variable.
- Simple contingency tables are 2 × 2 tables where both the exposure and outcome variables are dichotomous. For example, is there an association between smoking status (smoker versus non-smoker) and heart attacks (heart attack versus no heart attack)?
- The two variables can be compared and a *P*-value generated using a chi-squared test or Fisher's exact test (discussed in Chapter 15).

Numerical versus categorical variables

Box and whisker plot

- A box and whisker plot displays the following information (the numbers underneath correspond to the numbers labelled in Fig. 2.11):
  [1] The sample maximum (largest observation) – top end of whisker above box
  [2] The upper quartile – top of box
  [3] The median – line inside box
  [4] The lower quartile – bottom of box
  [5] The sample minimum (smallest observation) – bottom end of whisker below box
  [6] Which observations, if any, are considered as outliers.
- The central 50% of the distribution of the numerical variable is contained within the box. Consequently, 25% of obsrervations lie above the top of the box and 25% below the bottom of the box.
- The spacings between the different parts of the box indicate the degree of spread and skewness of the data (discussed underneath).

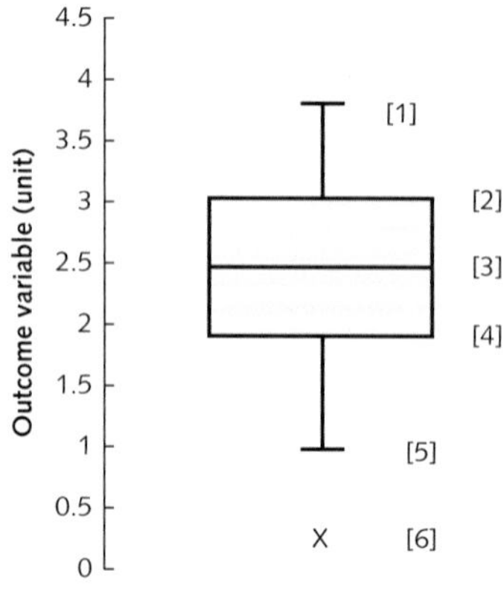

Fig. 2.11 Box and whisker plot.

- A box and whisker plot can be used to compare the distribution of a numerical outcome variable in two or more exposure groups, i.e. if comparing two exposure groups, a box and whisker plot would be constructed for each group. For example, if comparing the frequency distribution of haemoglobin level in three separate sample groups (i.e. in smokers, ex-smokers and non-smokers), a separate box and whisker plot would be drawn for each group.

HINTS AND TIPS

Other than representing the maximum and minimum sample observations, the ends of the whiskers may signify other measures, such as 1.96 standard deviations above and below the mean of the data. This range (known as the reference interval or reference range) contains the central 95% of the observations. A definition of what the whiskers represent should, therefore, always be given.

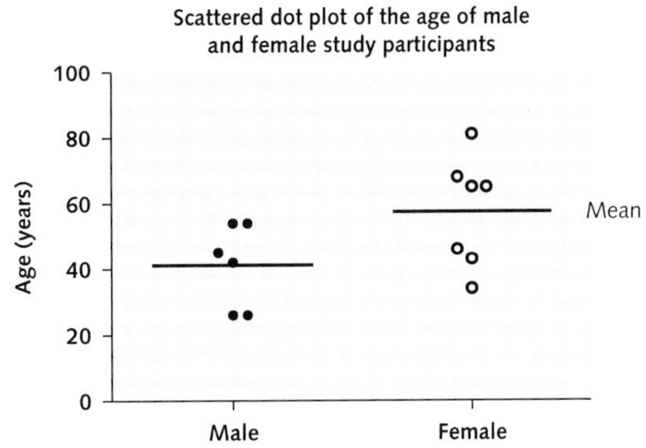

Fig. 2.12 Scattered dot plot.

- In addition to summarising the data obtained using a graphical display, a frequency distribution can also be summarised using measures of:
  - central tendency ('location')
  - variability ('spread').

Bar chart

- In a bar chart, the horizontal axis represents the different groups being compared and the vertical axis represents the numerical variable measured for each group.
- Each bar usually represents the sample mean for that particular group.
- The bars sometimes have an error bar (extended line) protruding from the end of the bar, which represents either the standard deviation or standard error of the mean (please refer to Chapter 3 for a discussion on how to interpret errors bars).
- A bar chart comparing the mean systolic blood pressure between two different groups is presented in Fig. 3.9.
- Please refer to Fig. 2.8 for a comparison between histograms and bar charts.

Dot plot

- Rather than using a bar to represent the sample mean, each observation can be represented as one dot on a single vertical (or horizontal) line. This is known as an aligned dot plot.
- However, sometimes there are two or more observations that have the same value. In this situation, a scattered dot plot should be used to ensure the dots plotted do not overlap (Fig. 2.12).
- While dot plots are simple to draw, it can be very cumbersome with large data sets.
- As demonstrated in Fig. 2.12, a summary measure of the data, such as the mean or median, is usually shown on the diagram.

DESCRIBING THE FREQUENCY DISTRIBUTION: CENTRAL TENDENCY

There are three key measures of central tendency (or location):

1. The arithmetic mean
2. The mode
3. The median.

The arithmetic mean

- The arithmetic mean is the most commonly used average.
- 'Mu' (μ) is often used to denote the population mean, while x-bar ($\bar{x}$) refers to the mean of a sample.
- It is calculated by adding up all the values in a set of observations and dividing this by the number of values in that set.
- This description of the mean can be summarised using the following algebraic formula:

$$\bar{x} = \frac{x_1 + x_2 + x_3 + \cdots + x_n}{n}$$

$$\bar{x} = \frac{\sum_{i=1}^{n} x_i}{n}$$

where

- x = variable
- $\bar{x}$ (x-bar) = mean of the variable x

Fig. 2.13 Raw data: weights (kg) of a sample of 86 medical students.

Lowest value	66.32	74.23	79.12	83.76	88.24	90.01	98.54
42.34	66.56	74.34	79.43	84.32	88.43	90.43	98.65
51.56	67.33	75.32	79.76	84.87	88.54	91.23	99.35
53.54	68.92	75.43	80.03	85.33	88.65	92.46	99.75
58.49	69.12	75.78	81.23	85.55	88.65	94.56	100.54
60.32	70.33	76.78	81.24	85.63	88.67	95.43	104.23
60.94	71.23	77.65	81.34	85.78	88.75	95.45	106.45
61.44	71.28	77.67	82.34	85.78	89.46	96.45	107.35
62.55	72.35	77.96	82.43	86.43	89.55	96.54	107.52
64.32	73.43	78.45	83.45	87.54	89.64	97.45	109.35
65.87	73.65	78.54	83.45	87.56	89.89	97.46	Highest value

  - n = number of observations of the variable
  - Σ (sigma) = the sum of the observations of the variable
  - Sub- and superscripts on the Σ = sum of the observations from $i = 1$ to n.
- For example, let's look at the raw data of weights from a sample of 86 medical students, ordered from the lowest to the highest value (Fig. 2.13). In this case, as x represents the student's weight, x_1 is the weight of the first individual in the sample and x_i is the weight of the ith individual in the sample. Therefore,

$$\text{Mean}(x) = \frac{42.34 + 51.56 + 53.54 + \cdots + 107.35 + 107.52 + 109.35}{86}$$

$$= 82.3033$$

Therefore, the mean weight of the 86 medical students sampled is 82.3 kg.

The mode

- The mode is the most frequently occurring value in a data set.
- For data that are continuous, the data are usually grouped and the modal group subsequently calculated.
- If there is a single mode, the distribution of the data is described as being unimodal. For example, returning to the data on weights of medical students (Fig. 2.13), the nature of which is continuous, the first step in calculating the mode is to group the data as shown in Fig. 2.3.
- The modal group is the one associated with the largest frequency. In other words, it is the group with the largest peak when the frequency distribution is displayed using a histogram (Fig. 2.9). In this instance, the modal group is 80 to 89.99 kg.
- If there is more than one mode (or peak), the distribution is either bimodal (for two peaks) or multimodal (for more than two peaks).

The median

- The median is the middle value when the data are arranged in ascending order of size, starting with the lowest value and ending with the highest value.
- If there are an odd number of observations, n, there will be an equal number of values both above and below the median value. This middle value is therefore the $[(n+1)/2]$th value when the data are arranged in ascending order of size.
- If there are an even number of observations, there will be two middle values. In this case, the median is calculated as the arithmetic mean of the two middle values ($[(n/2)]$th and $[(n/2)+1]$th values) when the data are arranged in ascending order of size. For example, returning to the data on weights of medical students (Fig. 2.13), the sample consists of 86 observations. The median will therefore be the arithmetic mean of the 43rd $[(86/2)]$ and 44th $[(86/2)+1]$ values when the data are arranged in ascending order of size. These two values are highlighted in the data set (Fig. 2.13). Therefore, the median weight of the 86 medical students sampled is 83.61 kg $[(83.45+83.76)/2]$.

DESCRIBING THE FREQUENCY DISTRIBUTION: VARIABILITY

- The variability of the data indicates the extent to which the values of a variable in a distribution are spread a short or long way away from the centre of the data.

- There are three key measures of variability (or spread):
  1. The range
  2. The inter-quartile range
  3. The standard deviation.

The range

- The range is the difference between the highest and lowest values in the data set.
- Rather than presenting the actual difference between the two extremes, the highest and lowest values are usually quoted. The reason for this is because the actual difference may be misleading if there are outliers. For example, returning to the data on weights of medical students (Fig. 2.13), the range is 42.34 to 109.35 kg.

HINTS AND TIPS

Outliers are observations that are numerically different from the main body of the data. While outliers can occur by chance in a distribution, they are often indicative of either:

- measurement error or
- that the population has a frequency distribution with a heavy tail (discussed below).

The inter-quartile range

- The inter-quartile range:
  - is the range of values that includes the middle 50% of values when the data are arranged in ascending order of size
  - is bounded by the lower and upper quartiles (25% of the values lie below the lower limit and 25% lie above the upper limit)
  - is the difference between the upper quartile and the lower quartile.

Percentiles

- A percentile (or centile) is the value of a variable below which a certain per cent of observations fall. For example, the median (which is the 50th centile) is the value below which 50 per cent of the observations may be found. The median and quartiles are both examples of percentiles.
- Although the median, upper quartile and lower quartile are the most common percentiles that we use in practice, any centile can in fact be calculated from continuous data.
- A particular centile can be calculated using the formula $q(n+1)$, where q is a decimal between 0 and 1, and n is the number of values in the data set. For example, returning to the data on weights of medical students, which consists of 86 observations (Fig. 2.13):
  - the calculation for the lower quartile is $0.25 \times (86+1) = 21.75$; therefore the 25th centile lies between the 21st and 22nd values when the data are arranged in ascending order of size.
  - the 21st value is 73.65 and the 22nd value is 74.23; therefore the lower quartile is 74.085:

$$73.65 + [(74.23 - 73.65) \times 0.75] = 74.085.$$

The standard deviation

Population standard deviation

- The standard deviation (denoted by the Greek letter sigma, σ) is a measure of the spread (or scatter) of observations about the mean.
- The standard deviation is the *square root of the variance*, which is based on the extent to which each observation deviates from the arithmetic mean value.
- The deviations are squared to remove the effect of their sign, i.e. negative or positive deviations.
- The mean of these squared deviations is known as the variance.
- This description of the population variance (usually denoted by σ^2) can be summarised using the following algebraic formula:

$$\sigma^2 = \frac{\sum (x_i - \bar{x})^2}{n}$$

where

- σ^2 = population variance
- x = variable
- $\bar{x}$ (x-bar) = mean of the variable x
- x_i = individual observation
- n = number of observations of the variable
- Σ (sigma) = the sum of (the squared differences of the individual observations from the mean).

- The population standard deviation is equal to the square root of the population variance:

$$\sigma = \sqrt{\sigma^2}$$

Sample standard deviation

- When we have data for the entire population, the variance is equal to the sum of the squared deviations, divided by n (number of observations of the variable).
- When handling data from a sample the divisor for the formula is $(n - 1)$ rather than n.
- The formula for the sample variance (usually denoted by s^2) is:

$$s^2 = \frac{\sum (x_i - \bar{x})^2}{n - 1}$$

- The sample standard deviation is equal to the square root of the sample variance:

$$s = \sqrt{s^2}$$

- For example, returning to the data on weights of medical students (Fig. 2.13), the variance is

$$s^2 = \frac{(42.34 - 82.303)^2 + (51.56 - 82.303)^2 + \ldots + (109.35 - 82.303)^2}{86 - 1}$$

$$= \frac{15\,252.123}{85} = 179.437 \text{ kg}^2$$

The standard deviation is

$$s = \sqrt{179.437} = 13.395 \text{ kg}$$

- As the standard deviation has the same units as the original data, it is easier to interpret than the variance.

THEORETICAL DISTRIBUTIONS

Probability distributions

- Earlier in this chapter we explained that the observed data of a variable can be expressed in the form of an empirical frequency distribution.
- When the empirical distribution of our data is approximately the same as a particular probability distribution (which is described by a mathematical model), we can use our theoretical knowledge of that probability distribution to answer questions about our data. These questions usually involve evaluating probabilities.

The rules of probability

- A probability measures the chance of an event occurring.
- It is described by a numerical measure that lies between 0 and 1:
  - If an event has a probability of 0, it cannot occur.
  - If an event has a probability of 1, it must occur.

Mutually exclusive events

- If two events (A and B) are mutually exclusive (both events cannot happen at the same time), then the probability of event A happening OR the probability of event B happening is equal to the sum of their probabilities.

$$\text{Probability(A or B)} = \text{P(A)} + \text{P(B)}.$$

- For example, Fig. 2.14 shows the probabilities of the range of grades achievable for Paper 1 on 'Study Design' and Paper 2 on 'Statistical Techniques' of the Evidence-Based Medicine exam. The probability of a student passing Paper 1 is (0.60 + 0.20 + 0.10) = 0.90.

Fig. 2.14 Probabilities of grades for evidence-based medicine exam.

	Paper 1 (study design)	Paper 2 (statistical techniques)
Fail	0.10	0.20
Pass	0.60	0.50
Pass with merit	0.20	0.25
Pass with distinction	0.10	0.05
Total probability	1	1

Independent events

- If two events (A and B) are independent (the occurrence of one event makes it neither more nor less probable that the other occurs), then the probability of both events A AND B occurring is equal to the product of their respective probabilities:

$$\text{Probability(A and B)} = \text{P(A)} \times \text{P(B)}.$$

- For example, referring to Fig. 2.14, the probability of a student passing both Paper 1 and Paper 2 is:

$$[(0.60 + 0.20 + 0.10) \times (0.50 + 0.25 + 0.05)] = 0.90 \times 0.80 = 0.72$$

Defining probability distributions

- If the values of a random variable are mutually exclusive, the probabilities of all the possible values of the variable can be illustrated using a probability distribution.
- Probability distributions are theoretical and can be expressed mathematically.
- Each type of distribution is characterised by certain parameters such as the mean and variance.
- In order to make inferences about our data, we must first determine whether the mean and variance of the frequency distribution of our data corresponds to the mean and variance of a particular probability distribution.
- The probability distribution is based on either continuous or discrete random variables.

Continuous probability distributions

- As the data are continuous, there are an infinite number of values of the random variable, x. Consequently, we can only derive probabilities corresponding to a certain range of values of the random variable.

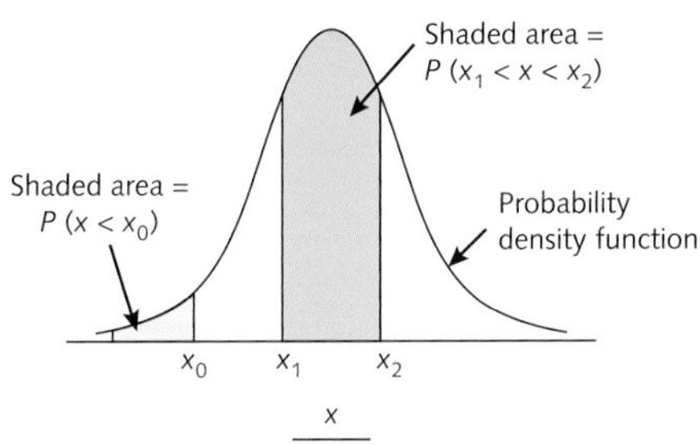

Fig. 2.15 The probability density function of a variable (x).

- If the horizontal x-axis represents the range of values of x, the equation of the distribution can be plotted. The resulting curve resembles an empirical frequency distribution and is known as the probability density function.
- The area under the curve represents the probabilities of all possible values of x and those probabilities (which represent the total area under the curve) always summate to 1.
- Applying the rules of probability described previously, the probability that a value of x lies between two limits is equal to the sum of the probabilities of all the values between these limits. In other words, the probability is equal to the area under the curve between the two limits (Fig. 2.15).
- The following distributions are based on continuous random variables.

The normal (Gaussian) distribution

- In practice, the normal distribution is the most commonly used probability distribution in medical statistics. It is also referred to as the Gaussian distribution or as a bell-shaped curve.
- The probability density function of the normal distribution:
  - is defined by two key parameters: the mean (μ) and the variance (σ^2)
  - is symmetrical about the mean and is bell-shaped (unimodal) (Fig. 2.16A)
  - shifts to the left if the mean decreases (μ_1)and shifts to the right if the mean increases (μ_2), provided that the variance (σ^2) (and therefore the standard deviation) remains constant (Fig. 2.16B)
  - becomes more peaked (curve is tall and narrow) as the variance decreases (σ_1^2) and flattens (curve is short and wide) as the variance increases (σ_2^2), provided that the mean (μ) remains fixed (Fig. 2.16C).
- The mean, median and mode of the distribution are identical and define the location of the curve.

HINTS AND TIPS

It is worth noting that there is no relation between the term 'normal' used in a statistical context and that used in a clinical context.

Reference range

- We can use the mean and standard deviation of the normal distribution to determine what proportion of the data lies between two particular values.
- For a normally distributed random variable, x, with mean, μ, and standard deviation, σ:
  - 68% of the values of x lie within 1 standard deviation of the mean ($\mu - \sigma$ to $\mu + \sigma$). In other words, the probability that a normally distributed random variable lies between ($\mu - \sigma$) and ($\mu + \sigma$) is 0.68.
  - 95% of the values of x lie within 1.96 standard deviations of the mean ($\mu - 1.96\sigma$ to $\mu + 1.96\sigma$). In other words, the probability that a normally distributed random variable lies between ($\mu - 1.96\sigma$) and ($\mu + 1.96\sigma$) is 0.95.
  - 99% of the values of x lie within 2.58 standard deviations of the mean ($\mu - 2.58\sigma$ to $\mu + 2.58\sigma$). In other words, the probability that a normally distributed random variable lies between ($\mu - 2.58\sigma$) and ($\mu + 2.58\sigma$) is 0.99.
- These intervals can be used to define an additional measure of spread in a set of observations: the reference range. For example, if the data are normally distributed, the 95% reference range is defined as follows ($\mu - 1.96\sigma$) to ($\mu + 1.96\sigma$); 95% of the data lies within the 95% reference range (Fig. 2.17). The 68% and 99% reference ranges can be defined using a similar approach.

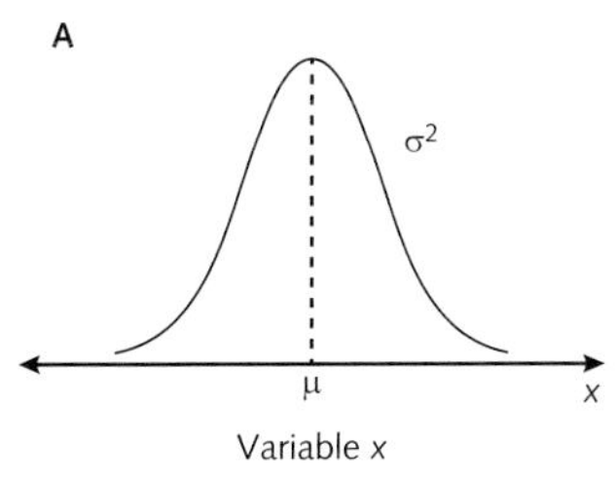

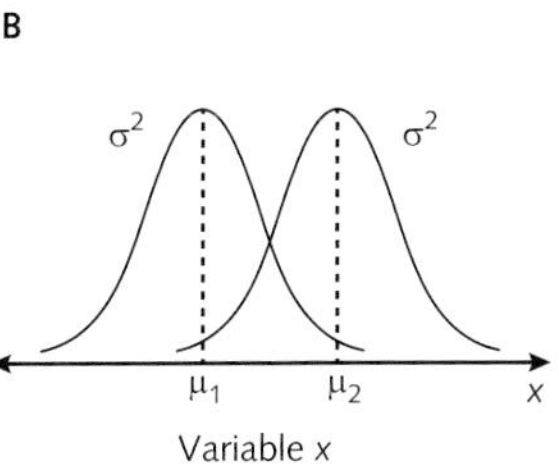

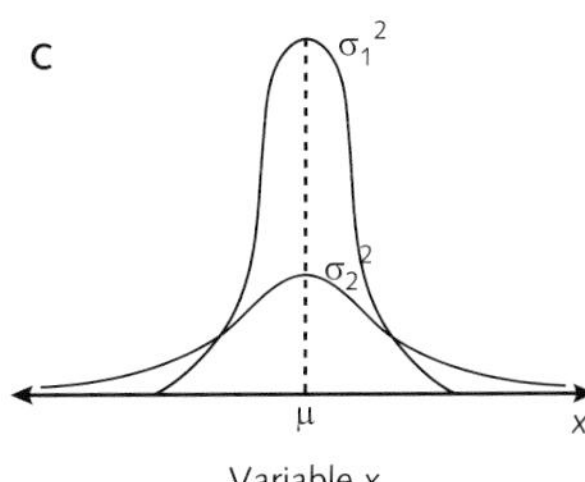

Fig. 2.16 Shifting the probability density function of a variable (x) by varying the mean (μ) or variance (σ^2).

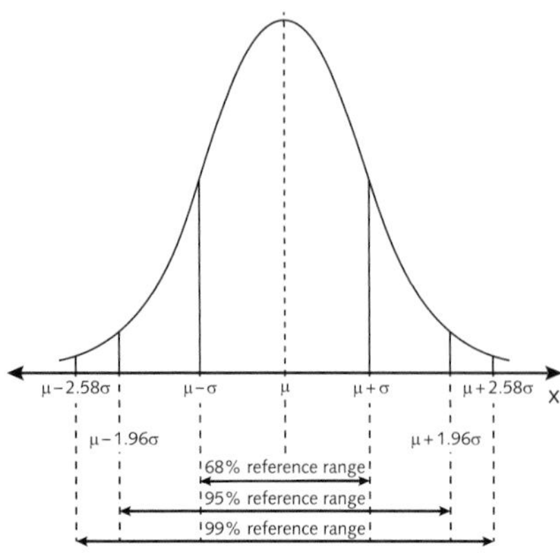

Fig. 2.17 Reference range.

- Considering the normal distribution is symmetrical, we can also say that:
  - 16% of the values of x lie above $(\mu+\sigma)$ and 16% of the values of x lie below $(\mu-\sigma)$
  - 2.5% of the values of x lie above $(\mu+1.96\sigma)$ and 2.5% of the values of x lie below $(\mu-1.96\sigma)$
  - 0.5% of the values of x lie above $(\mu+2.58\sigma)$ and 0.5% of the values of x lie below $(\mu-2.58\sigma)$.

'Standard' normal distribution

- As you may be thinking, there are an infinite number of normal distributions depending on the values of the mean and the standard deviation.
- A normal distribution can be transformed (or standardised) to make a 'standard' normal distribution, which has a mean of 0 and a variance of 1. The standard normal distribution allows us to compare distributions and perform statistical tests on our data.

Other continuous probability distributions

- On some occasions, the normal distribution may not be the most appropriate distribution to use for your data.
  - The chi-squared distribution is used for analysing categorical data.
  - The t-distribution is used under similar circumstances as those for the normal distribution, but when the sample size is small and the population standard deviation is unknown. If the sample size is large enough ($n > 30$), the t-distribution has a shape similar to that of the standard normal distribution.
  - The F-distribution is the distribution of the ratio of two estimates of variance. It is used to compare probability values in the analysis of variance (ANOVA) (discussed in Chapter 15).

Discrete probability distributions

- As the data are discrete, we can derive probabilities corresponding to every possible value of the random variable, x.
- The sum of the probabilities of all possible mutually exclusive events is 1.
- The main discrete probability distributions used in medical statistics are as follows:
  - The Poisson distribution is used when the variable is a count of the number of random events that occur independently in space or time, at an average rate, i.e. the number of new cases of a disease in the population.
  - The binomial distribution is used when there are only two outcomes, e.g. having a particular disease or not having the disease.

Skewed distributions

A frequency distribution is not always symmetrical about the mean. It may be markedly skewed with a long tail to the right (positively skewed) or the left (negatively skewed).

Positively skewed distributions

- For positively skewed distributions (Fig. 2.18A), e.g. the F-distribution:
  - the mass of the distribution is concentrated on the left.
  - there is a long tail to the right.
  - the mode is lower than the median, which in turn is lower than the mean (mode < median < mean).

Negatively skewed distributions

- For negatively skewed distributions (Fig. 2.18B):
  - the mass of the distribution is concentrated on the right.
  - there is a long tail to the left.
  - the mean is lower than the median, which in turn is lower than the mode (mean < median < mode).

TRANSFORMATIONS

- If the observations of a variable are not normally distributed, it is often possible to transform the values so that the transformed data are approximately normal.
- Transforming the values to create a normal distribution is beneficial, as it allows you to use statistical tests based on the normal distribution (discussed in Chapter 15).

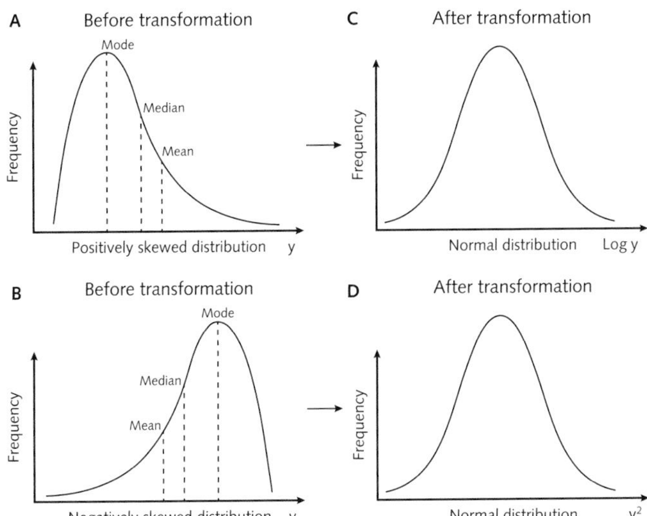

Fig. 2.18 Skewed distribution.

- When a transformation is used, all analyses, including calculating the mean or 95% confidence interval (discussed in Chapter 3), should be carried out on the transformed data. However, the results are back-transformed into their original units when interpreting the estimates.
- Note: *P*-values (discussed in Chapter 3) are not back-transformed.

The logarithmic transformation

- The logarithmic transformation:
  - is the most common choice of transformation used in medical statistics
  - is used where continuous data are not normally distributed and are highly skewed to the right
  - stretches the lower end of the original scale and compresses the upper end, thus making positively skewed data more symmetrical (Fig. 2.18C).
- Log transformed variables are said to have a lognormal distribution.
- When log transforming data, we can choose to take logs to any base, but the most commonly used are to the base 10 ($\log_{10} y$, the 'common' log) or to the base e ($\log_e y = \ln y$, the 'natural' log).
- Following log transformation of the data, calculations are carried out on the log scale. For example, we can calculate the mean using log-transformed data.

The geometric mean

- The mean calculated using log-transformed data is known as the geometric mean. For example, let's look at a few values from the data set of 500 triglyceride level measurements, which have a positively skewed distribution (Fig. 2.19). The triglyceride level values are first log-transformed to the base *e*. The mean of all 500 transformed values is:

$$= \frac{0.2624 + 0.4055 + (-0.9163) + 0.8329 + (-0.5108) + \ldots + 1.4586}{500}$$

$$= \frac{177.4283}{500} = 0.3549$$

The geometric mean is the anti-log of the mean of the log-transformed data:

$$= \exp(0.3549) = e^{0.3549} = 1.43 \text{ mM}$$

- Similarly, in order to derive the confidence interval for the geometric mean, all calculations are performed on the log scale and the two limits back-transformed at the end.

Fig. 2.19 Logarithmic transformation of positively skewed data.

Measurement	Triglyceride level (mM)	$\log_e$(triglyceride level)
1	1.3	0.2624
2	1.5	0.4055
3	0.4	−0.9163
4	2.3	0.8329
5	0.6	−0.5108
...	...	...
500	4.3	1.4586

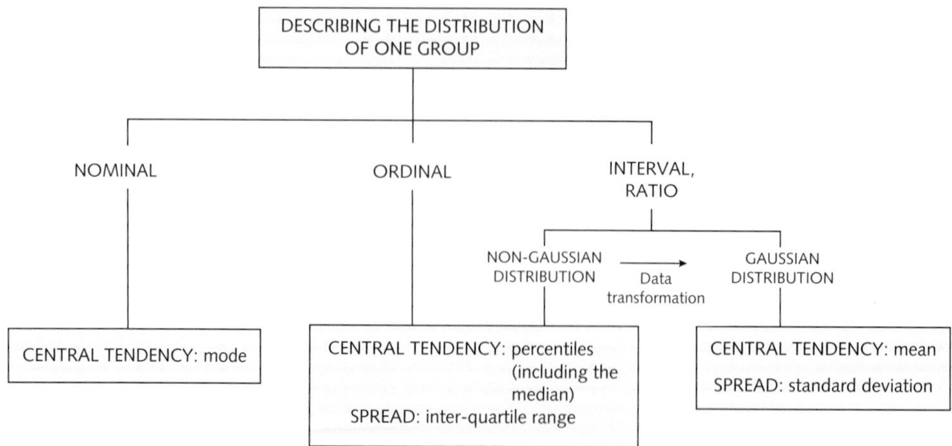

Fig. 2.20 Choosing the correct summary measure.

HINTS AND TIPS

It is impossible to log-transform negative values and the log of 0 is $-\infty$. If there are negative values in your data, it is possible to add a small constant to each value prior to transforming the data. Following back-transformation of your results, this constant needs to be subtracted from the final value. For example, if you add 4 units to each value prior to log-transforming your data, you must remember to minus 4 units from the calculated geometric mean.

Calculating the anti-log

- As any base can be used to log-transform your data, it is important that you understand some basic rules when working with logs.

Rule 1: Don't worry ... It's actually quite easy!

Rule 2: You can log transform your value using the formula:

$$\log_a x = y$$

where

- a = the 'base'
- x = the value you are transforming
- y = the result of the transformation.

Rule 3: You can back-transform (anti-log) your result, y, using the formula:

$$a^y = x$$

For example, if $\log_e 4 = \ln 4 = 1.3863$, then $e^{1.3863} = 4$.

The square transformation

- The square transformation is used where continuous data are not normally distributed and are highly skewed to the left. It achieves the reverse of the log transformation.
- Referring to Fig. 2.18B, if the variable y is skewed to the left, the distribution of y^2 is often approximately normal (Fig. 2.18D).

CHOOSING THE CORRECT SUMMARY MEASURE

- The measure used to describe the centre and spread of the distribution of your data depends on the type of variable you are dealing with (Fig. 2.20).
- In addition to the information summarised in Fig. 2.20, there are three key points:
  1. A frequency distribution can be used for all four types of variables: nominal, ordinal, interval and ratio.
  2. As previously discussed, a positively skewed distribution can sometimes be transformed to follow a normal distribution. In this situation, the central tendency is usually described using the geometric mean. However, the standard deviation cannot be back-transformed correctly. In this case, the untransformed standard deviation or another measure of spread, such as the inter-quartile range, can be given.
  3. For continuous data with a skewed distribution, the median, range and/or quartiles are used to describe the data. However, if the analyses planned are based on using means, it would be sensible to give the standard deviations. Furthermore, the use of the reference range holds even for skewed data.

Investigating hypotheses

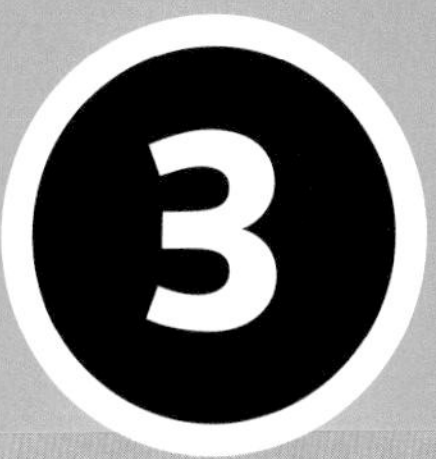

Objectives

By the end of this chapter you should:

- Understand the steps involved in hypothesis testing.
- Understand the reasons why study subjects are randomly sampled.
- Know the difference between the terms accuracy and precision.
- Know the difference between standard errors and standard deviations.
- Be able to calculate and interpret confidence intervals for means and proportions.
- Be able to interpret *P*-values for differences in means and proportions.
- Know the definitions of statistical significance and statistical power.
- Recognise how incorrect conclusions can be made when using the *P*-value to interpret the null hypothesis of a study.

HYPOTHESIS TESTING

As described in Chapter 1, the aim of a study may involve examining the association between an 'intervention' or 'exposure' and an 'outcome'. We must first state a specific hypothesis for a potential association.

The null and alternative hypotheses

- A hypothesis test uses sample data to assess the degree of evidence there is against a hypothesis about a population. We must always define two mutually exclusive hypotheses:
  - *Null hypothesis* (H_0): there is *no* difference/association between the two variables in the population.
  - *Alternative hypothesis* (H_A): there is a difference/association between the two variables in the population.
- For example, we may test the null hypothesis that there is no association between an exposure and outcome.
- In 1988 the Physicians' Health Study research group reported the results of a 5-year trial to determine whether taking aspirin reduces the risk of a heart attack. Patients had been randomly assigned to either aspirin or a placebo. The hypotheses for this study can be stated as follows:
  - Null hypothesis (H_0): There is *no* association between taking aspirin and the risk of a heart attack in the population. This is equivalent to saying:

$$H_0 : \text{(risk of heart attack in group treated with aspirin)} - \text{(risk of heart attack in group treated with placebo)} = 0$$

  - Alternative hypothesis (H_A): There is an association between taking aspirin and the risk of a heart attack in the population. The difference in the risk of a heart attack between the aspirin and placebo groups does *not equal* 0.
- Having defined the hypotheses, an appropriate statistical test is used to compute the *P*-value from the sample data. The *P*-value provides a measure of the evidence for or against the null hypothesis. If the *P*-value shows evidence against the null hypothesis being tested, then the alternative hypothesis must be true.

HINTS AND TIPS

There are four basic steps involved in hypothesis testing:

1. Specify the null hypothesis and the alternative hypothesis.
2. Collect the data and determine what statistical test is appropriate for data analysis.
3. Perform the statistical test to compute the *P*-value
4. Use the *P*-value to make a decision in favour of the null or alternative hypothesis.

CHOOSING A SAMPLE

The basic principle of statistics is simple: Using limited amounts of data (your 'sample'), we wish to make the strongest possible conclusions about the wider population. For these conclusions to be valid, we must consider the precision and accuracy of the analyses.

Accuracy versus precision

Distinguishing between accuracy and precision is an important but difficult concept to understand. Imagine playing darts where the bull's-eye in the centre of the dartboard represents the population statistic we are trying to estimate and each dart represents a statistic calculated from a study sample. If we throw nine darts at the dartboard, we see one of four patterns regarding the accuracy and precision of the sample estimates (darts) relative to the population statistic (bulls-eye) (Fig. 3.1).

Accuracy

The study sample is accurate if it is representative of the population from which it was chosen (Figs. 3.1A and 3.1B). This can be achieved if:

- each individual of the population has an equal chance of being selected (random sampling).
- the selection is completely independent of individual characteristics such as age, sex or ethnic origin.

The methods used in practice to ensure randomisation are discussed in Chapter 6. If samples were not randomly selected (systematic bias), on average, any sample estimate will differ from the population statistic. As a result, the study sample will be inaccurate (Figs. 3.1C and 3.1D).

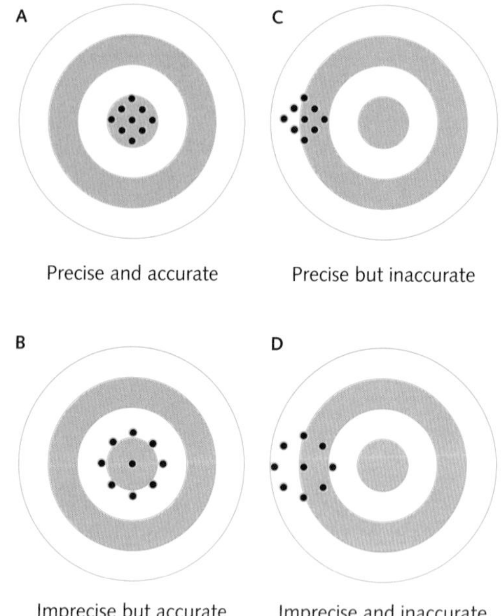

Fig. 3.1 Precision versus accuracy. (A) Precise and accurate. (B) Precise but inaccurate. (C) Imprecise but accurate. (D) Imprecise and inaccurate.

Precision

The amount of variation between the sample estimates determines the precision of the study sample.

- If there is little variability between the sample estimates, i.e. the estimates themselves are similar to each other, the study sample statistics are more precise (Figs. 3.1A and 3.1C).
- The less precise the sample statistics (Figs. 3.1B and 3.1D), the less we are able to narrow down the likely values of the population statistic.

HINTS AND TIPS

When choosing between accurate and precise study samples, it is more important to be accurate because, on average, the study sample estimates will be closer to the true population value.

EXTRAPOLATING FROM 'SAMPLE' TO 'POPULATION'

Having chosen an appropriate study sample, the rules of probability are applied to make inferences about the overall population from which the sample was drawn (Fig. 3.2). The following steps are followed:

1. Choose a random sample from population.
2. Take measurements for each subject, denoted x.
3. Calculate the mean value of the sample data, denoted $\bar{x}$.
4. As estimates vary from sample to sample, calculate the standard error and the confidence interval of the mean to take this imprecision into account.

Standard error of the mean

When we choose only one sample for a study, the sample mean will not necessarily be the same as the true population mean. Due to sampling variation, different samples selected from the same population will give different sample means. Therefore, if we calculate the mean from all the possible samples in the population, we would have a *distribution* of the sample mean. This distribution has the following properties:

- If the sample is large enough, the sampling distribution of the mean will follow a Gaussian distribution (even if the population is not Gaussian!) because of the central limit theorem. What sample size should be used? In general, this depends on how far the population distribution differs from a Gaussian (normal) distribution.

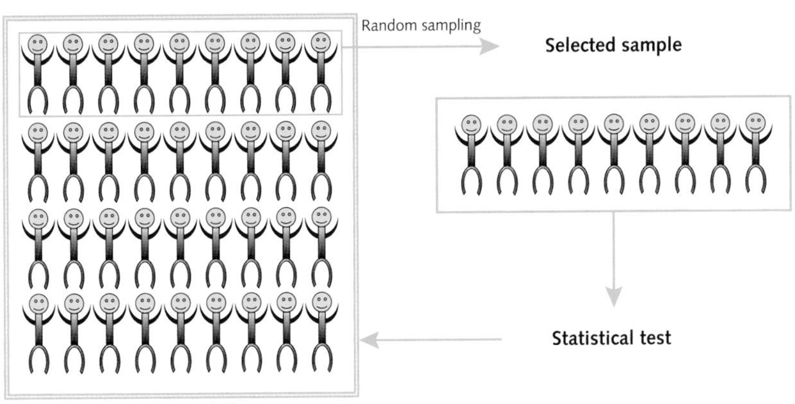

Fig. 3.2 Hypothesis testing.

- The mean of the distribution is equal to the population mean.
- The standard deviation of the sampling distribution of a mean is known as the standard error of the mean (SEM), which quantifies the precision of the mean. The SEM has the same units as the data:

$$\text{Standard error of the sample mean} = \frac{\text{standard deviation}}{\sqrt{\text{sample size}}} = \frac{SD}{\sqrt{n}}$$

- As the sample size increases, the standard error of the sample mean decreases; therefore, the average difference between the sample mean and the population mean decreases.

HINTS AND TIPS

The standard error of the mean (SEM) is a measure of how far the sample mean is likely to be from the true population mean. The larger the sample size, the greater the precision of the sample mean as an estimate of the population mean.

Standard error versus standard deviation

What is the difference between the standard deviation and the standard error of the mean? Figure 3.3 highlights the key differences.

Confidence interval for the mean

- With large samples, as the distribution of the sample mean is normally distributed, we can use the properties of a Gaussian distribution, as described in Chapter 2, to state that 95% of individual sample means would be expected to lie within 1.96 standard errors of the distribution mean, i.e. the true population mean (95% confidence interval). In other words, on 95% of occasions (95% probability), the true population mean is within 1.96 standard errors of the observed sample mean.
- If the sample is large, the 95% confidence interval for a mean can be calculated using the formula:

  mean − [1.96 × standard error (mean)] to
  mean + [1.96 × standard error (mean)]

- 95% is the most commonly used percentage for confidence intervals.

Fig. 3.3 Standard error versus standard deviation.

Standard error	Standard deviation
Quantifies how accurately you know the true population mean; measures the precision of the sample mean as an estimate of the population mean. It takes into account the sample size and the value of the standard deviation.	Quantifies scatter; measures the amount of variability in the population. Informs us how far an individual observation is likely to be from the true population mean.
Always smaller than the standard deviation.	Always larger than the standard error.
As the sample size increases, the standard error gets smaller; the mean of a large sample is likely to be closer to the true population mean. You'll know the value of the mean with a lot more precision even if the data are very scattered.	As the sample size increases, the standard deviation of the population can be assessed with more precision. However, the standard deviation does not change predictably as the sample size increases; it can be bigger or smaller as the sample size increases.

- The multiplier of 1.96 in the formula above is based on the assumption that the sample means follow a Gaussian distribution. This assumption is accepted if the sample is large enough.
- If the sample size is too small:
  - we use an alternative multiplier, t', which is derived from the t-distribution.
  - the 95% confidence interval for a mean can be calculated using the formula:

$$\text{mean} - [t' \times \text{standard error (mean)}] \text{ to}$$
$$\text{mean} + [t' \times \text{standard error (mean)}]$$

- As the sample size decreases:
  - the standard error of the mean increases.
  - the multiplier, t', increases.
- Consequently, plugging these changes into the above formula, the smaller the sample size, the wider the confidence interval.

HINTS AND TIPS

By tradition, confidence intervals are usually expressed with 95% confidence. However, other percentages can be used such as 90% or 99%:

- Ninety per cent of the sample means would be expected to lie within 1.64 standard errors of the population mean (90% confidence interval).
- Ninety-nine per cent of the sample means would be expected to lie within 2.58 standard errors of the population mean (99% confidence interval).

Confidence interval versus reference range

- The 95% reference range, defined in Chapter 2, is commonly confused with the 95% confidence interval. Figure 3.4 highlights the key differences between these two measures.
- Let's use some sample data from a hypothetical study on systolic blood pressure measurements in foundation year 1 (FY1) doctors to demonstrate how to interpret the 95% confidence interval and 95% reference range: stress is a normal part of life. However, chronic stress has been shown to increase blood pressure, making the heart work harder to produce the blood flow needed for normal bodily functions. From a total population of 8000 FY1 doctors, suppose we randomly select a study sample of 2012 FYIs and calculate their mean blood pressure:

$$\text{Mean systolic blood pressure} = 134 \text{ mmHg}$$
$$\text{Standard deviation} = 14.7 \text{ mmHg}$$

- The 95% confidence interval is:

$$\text{mean} - [1.96\ \text{SE(mean)}] \text{ to mean} + [1.96\ \text{SE(mean)}]$$
$$= 134 - \left(1.96 \times \frac{14.7}{\sqrt{2012}}\right) \text{ to } 134 + \left(1.96 \times \frac{14.7}{\sqrt{2012}}\right)$$
$$= 133.4 \text{ to } 134.6 \text{ mmHg}$$

- We are therefore 95% confident that the mean systolic blood pressure in the target population lies between 133.4 and 134.6 mmHg.
- The 95% reference range is:

$$\text{mean} - [1.96\ \text{SD(mean)}] \text{ to mean} + [1.96\ \text{SD(mean)}]$$
$$= 134 - (1.96 \times 14.7) \text{ to } 134 + (1.96 \times 14.7)$$
$$= 105.2 \text{ to } 162.8 \text{ mmHg}$$

- We therefore expect 95% of FY1 doctors in the population to have a systolic blood pressure between 105.2 and 162.8 mmHg.

Confidence interval for a proportion

- So far we have only focused on estimating the true population mean. However, it is also possible to quantify the uncertainty in a *proportion* that has been measured from a sample of the population.
- The confidence interval gives a range of values within which we are confident the true population proportion will lie.
- The sampling distribution of a proportion follows a binomial distribution (discussed in Chapter 2). However, as the sample size increases, the sampling distribution of the proportion becomes approximately normal about the mean π.

Fig. 3.4 Confidence interval versus reference range.

Confidence interval	Reference range
mean – [1.96 × standard **error** (mean)] to mean + [1.96 × standard **error** (mean)]	mean – [1.96 × standard **deviation** (mean)] to mean + [1.96 × standard **deviation** (mean)]
Shows how precise an estimate the sample mean is of the true population mean.	Shows how much variation there is between the individual observations in the sample.
The standard error is always smaller than the standard deviation so the confidence interval is narrower than the reference range.	The reference range is wider than the confidence interval.

- The population mean is estimated by calculating the proportion in the sample, p, using the formula:

$$p = r/n$$

where,
  - p=population proportion
  - r=number of individuals in the sample with the characteristic of interest
  - n=sample size.
- The standard error of the population proportion can be calculated using the formula:

$$\text{SE}(p) = \sqrt{\frac{p \times (1-p)}{n}}$$

- If the sample is large, the 95% confidence interval for a proportion can be calculated using the formula:

proportion − [1.96 × standard error (proportion)] to proportion + [1.96 × standard error (proportion)]

- If the sample size is small, the binomial distribution is used to calculate the confidence intervals.
- Let's use some sample data from a study on the effect of simvastatin on stroke risk to demonstrate how to calculate and interpret the 95% confidence interval of a proportion.

The effect of simvastatin on stroke risk

It is well documented that increased blood cholesterol levels are associated with a higher risk of cardiovascular disease. A randomised placebo-controlled trial in the UK investigated the effect of the cholesterol-lowering drug simvastatin on cardiovascular disease risk. A total of 20,536 adults (aged 40–80 years) with diabetes, coronary disease or other occlusive arterial disease were randomly allocated to receive either the drug simvastatin (40 mg each evening) or a matching placebo (an inactive substance). The mean duration of follow-up was 5 years, during which time the number of ischaemic, haemorrhagic and unclassified strokes were recorded. Figure 3.5 shows the number and percentage of strokes in the placebo and simvastatin groups.

Fig. 3.5 Placebo versus simvastatin.

Stroke	Placebo	Simvastatin	Total
No	9682 (94.3%)	9825 (95.7%)	19,507 (95.0%)
Yes	585 (5.7%)	444 (4.3%)	1029 (5.0%)
Total	10,267	10,269	20,536

Data from Heart Protection Study Collaborative Group, 2002. Lancet 360: 7–22.

- The standard error of the percentage (proportion) of strokes in the placebo group is:

$$\text{SE}(p) = \sqrt{\frac{p \times (1-p)}{n}} = \sqrt{\frac{0.057 \times (0.943)}{10,267}} = 0.00229$$
$$= 0.229\%$$

- Therefore, the 95% confidence interval of the proportion of strokes in the placebo group is:

proportion − [1.96 × standard error (proportion)] to proportion + [1.96 × standard error (proportion)]

$$= 5.7 - (1.96 \times 0.229) \text{ to } 5.7 + (1.96 \times 0.229)$$
$$= 5.25 \text{ to } 6.15\%$$

- We are therefore 95% confident that the true population incidence risk (proportion) of first stroke in individuals not on simvastatin is between 5.25 and 6.15% over 5 years.
- We can use a similar approach to calculate the standard error of the percentage of strokes in the simvastatin group:

$$\text{SE}(p) = \sqrt{\frac{p \times (1-p)}{n}} = \sqrt{\frac{0.043 \times (0.957)}{10,269}} = 0.00200$$
$$= 0.2\%$$

- The 95% confidence interval is therefore:

proportion − [1.96 × standard error (proportion)] to proportion + [1.96 × standard error (proportion)]

$$= 4.3 - (1.96 \times 0.2) \text{ to } 4.3 + (1.96 \times 0.2)$$
$$= 3.91 \text{ to } 4.69\%$$

- We are therefore 95% confident that the true population incidence risk (proportion) of first stroke in individuals on simvastatin is between 3.91 and 4.69% over 5 years.
- In the next section we will calculate the 95% confidence interval for the difference in proportions between the two groups (placebo versus simvastatin).

Online calculators

You can use online calculators to assist you in calculating the confidence interval for a mean or proportion. One example accessible online is http://www.mccallum-layton.co.uk/stats/ConfidenceIntervalCalc.aspx to calculate the confidence interval for a mean, and http://www.mccallum-layton.co.uk/stats/ConfidenceIntervalCalcProportions.aspx to calculate the confidence interval for a proportion.

HINTS AND TIPS

Interpreting the 95% confidence interval for a proportion

We have 95% *confidence* that the true value of the proportion in the target population (from which the sample was taken) lies within the range of values calculated (the interval).

In other words, the 95% confidence interval for a proportion is the range of values which have 95% *probability* of containing the true population proportion.

What is a large sample?

The distribution of a sample mean tends to have a normal distribution as the size of the sample increases, even if the underlying distribution is not normal. However, what is considered to be a large sample when calculating the confidence interval for means or proportions (Fig. 3.6)?

COMPARING MEANS AND PROPORTIONS: CONFIDENCE INTERVALS

In the first part of this chapter we showed how to calculate the 95% confidence interval for a single sample mean or proportion. However, in practice, it is more common that we compare the means or proportions in different groups. The formulae discussed in this section are only valid for large samples.

Confidence interval for the difference between two independent means

Using the example discussed previously, let's investigate whether the mean systolic blood pressure differs between FY1 and foundation year two (FY2) doctors. The mean systolic blood pressure, the standard deviation and the 95% confidence intervals for each group are shown in Fig. 3.7. There is very little overlap between the 95% confidence intervals for the two groups, suggesting there might be a difference in mean systolic blood pressure between FY1 and FY2 doctors. Whether there is a statistically significant difference in mean systolic blood pressure between the two groups will require an understanding of the *P*-value, which will be discussed later in this chapter. However, for the meantime, the main question we are interested in answering is: How big is the difference in mean systolic blood pressure between the two groups in the target population?

The difference in mean systolic blood pressure comparing FY1with FY2 doctors in our sample (the sample difference) is:

$$(\bar{x}_1) - (\bar{x}_0) = 133 - 134 = -1 \text{ mmHg}$$

Due to sampling variation, the true difference between the two groups in the population will not be exactly the same as the difference calculated in our sample. We therefore need to calculate the 95% confidence interval for the difference between the means. Let's start by

Fig. 3.6 What is a large sample?

	Mean	Proportion
Large sample	$n = 100$ Use the multiplier 1.96 to calculate the confidence interval	r and $(n - r)$ are both >5 Use the multiplier 1.96 to calculate the confidence interval
Small sample	$n < 100$ Use the *t*-distribution to calculate the confidence interval	r and $(n - r)$ are both <5 Use the binomial distribution to calculate the confidence interval

Fig. 3.7 Mean systolic blood pressure measurements in two independent groups.

	Group	Sample size (n)	Mean systolic blood pressure ($\bar{x}$)	Standard deviation	Standard error (mean)	95% confidence interval
0	FY1 doctors	2012 n_0	134 $(\bar{x}_0)$	14.7	0.3277	133.4 to 134.6 mmHg
1	FY2 doctors	2012 n_1	133 $(\bar{x}_1)$	15.1	0.3366	132.3 to 133.7 mmHg

calculating the standard error (SE) of the difference between the means ($\bar{x}_1 - \bar{x}_0$):

$$\begin{aligned} SE(\bar{x}_1 - \bar{x}_0) &= \sqrt{[SE(\bar{x}_1)]^2 + [SE(\bar{x}_0)]^2} \\ &= \sqrt{\left[\frac{SD(\bar{x}_1)}{\sqrt{n_1}}\right]^2 + \left[\frac{SD(\bar{x}_0)}{\sqrt{n_0}}\right]^2} \\ &= \sqrt{\left[\frac{15.1}{\sqrt{2012}}\right]^2 + \left[\frac{14.7}{\sqrt{2012}}\right]^2} \\ &= \sqrt{0.3366^2 + 0.3277^2} \\ &= 0.4698 \end{aligned}$$

The next step is to use the standard error to calculate the 95% confidence interval (CI) for the difference between the means:

$$\begin{aligned} 95\%\ CI\ \text{for}\ (\bar{x}_1 - \bar{x}_0) &= (\bar{x}_1 - \bar{x}_0) - [1.96 \times SE(\bar{x}_1 - \bar{x}_0)]\ \text{to} \\ &\quad (\bar{x}_1 - \bar{x}_0) + [1.96 \times SE(\bar{x}_1 - \bar{x}_0)] \\ &= [(-1) - (1.96 \times 0.4698)]\ \text{to} \\ &\quad [(-1) + (1.96 \times 0.4698)] \\ &= -1.921\ \text{to}\ -0.0791 \end{aligned}$$

Therefore, with 95% confidence, the mean systolic blood pressure is between 0.079 and 1.92 mmHg *lower* in FY2 doctors than in FY1 doctors. How can we interpret this finding? Is it that FY2 doctors are less stressed (hence have a lower blood pressure) than FY1 doctors as they actually know what they're doing ☺

HINTS AND TIPS

In Fig. 3.7, the FY1 group was labelled '0' and the FY2 group was labelled '1'. However, what would happen to the results if the groups were labelled with the opposing number. The 95% confidence interval for the difference between the means would be positive 0.0791 to positive 1.921. This interval can be interpreted in exactly the same way as described in the main text. However, you could also say that with 95% confidence, the mean systolic blood pressure is between 0.079 and 1.92 mmHg *higher* in FY1 doctors than in FY2 doctors.

Confidence interval for the difference between paired means

- In some studies, you are interested in the difference in a measure made on the same individuals on two separate occasions.
- Leading on from the example used in the previous section, Fig. 3.8 shows the data from a hypothetical observational study in which blood pressure measurements were recorded from a sample of 200 FY1 doctors and then repeated one year later on the same sample. Figure 3.8 shows data from the study for the first 5 subjects. As the data are paired, we are more interested in the differences between the measurements for each subject. The differences calculated can be treated as a single sample of observations. The mean of the differences, denoted $\bar{d}$, is 6 mmHg. As you may have noted, the standard deviation of the differences is relatively smaller than the standard deviation of the measurements taken during either FY1 or FY2 years of training. The reason for this is because the between-subject variability in blood pressure has been excluded. As we are treating the differences as a single sample of observations, the standard error of the differences, denoted $SE(\bar{d})$, can be calculated in the usual way:

Fig. 3.8 Systolic blood pressure measurements in two paired groups.

Subject ($n = 200$)	**Systolic blood pressure (mmHg)**		**Difference (d)**
	FY1 doctors	**FY2 doctors**	
1	134	130	4
2	125	120	5
3	140	150	−10
4	135	130	5
5	120	118	2
⋮	⋮	⋮	⋮
Mean	128	122	$(\bar{d}) = 6$
SD	8.3	10.2	$SD(d) = 3.5$

$$\begin{aligned} SE(\bar{d}) &= \frac{SD(d)}{\sqrt{n}} \\ &= \frac{3.5}{\sqrt{200}} \\ &= 0.2475 \end{aligned}$$

- The 95% confidence interval for the population mean difference is therefore:

$$\begin{aligned} 95\%\ CI &= \bar{d} - [1.96 \times SE(\bar{d})]\ \text{to}\ \bar{d} + [1.96 \times SE(\bar{d})] \\ &= [6 - (1.96 \times 0.2475)]\ \text{to}\ [6 + (1.96 \times 0.2475)] \\ &= 5.515\ \text{to}\ 6.485 \end{aligned}$$

- Therefore, with 95% confidence, the true population *reduction* in mean blood pressure after one year of working as a FY1 doctor is between 5.52 and 6.49 mmHg.

HINTS AND TIPS

- If outcome measurements are repeated on the *same* study sample at two separate time points, we can say that there is a *change*, i.e. increase or decrease (or *no change*), in the mean outcome measure over time.
- On the other hand, when comparing two independent means, we can only say that one group mean is *higher* or *lower* (or the *same*) than the other group mean.

Confidence interval for the difference between two independent proportions

- In some studies, you are interested in comparing the proportion of observations with a particular characteristic in two or more groups.
- Using the example discussed previously (Fig. 3.5), let's investigate the effect of simvastatin on stroke risk in individuals with a high risk of cardiovascular disease. As previously calculated:
  - The 95% confidence interval for the incidence risk of first stroke following randomisation to a placebo is 5.25 to 6.15% over 5 years.
  - The 95% confidence interval for the incidence risk of first stroke following randomisation to simvastatin is 3.91 to 4.69% over 5 years.
- The fact that these two confidence intervals do not overlap suggests that the population proportion of first stroke may be reduced among individuals on simvastatin. Whether this difference is statistically significant requires an understanding of the *P*-value, which will be discussed in the next section. However, in the meantime, the main question we are interested in answering is: How big is the difference in the incidence risk of first stroke between the simvastatin and placebo groups in the target population? The difference in proportion of the incidence risk of stroke in the simvastatin group (group 1) compared to the placebo group (group 0) is:

$$p_1 - p_0 = 0.043 - 0.057 = -0.014 \text{ or } -1.4\%$$

- The next step is to calculate the standard error of this difference. This involves combining the standard errors of the proportions in the two groups:

$$\mathrm{SE}(p_1 - p_0) = \sqrt{\mathrm{SE}(p_1)^2 + \mathrm{SE}(p_0)^2} = \sqrt{\frac{p_1(1-p_1)}{n_1} + \frac{p_0(1-p_0)}{n_0}}$$

- In our study, the standard error for the difference in proportions:

$$= \sqrt{\frac{0.043 \times 0.957}{10{,}269} + \frac{0.057 \times 0.943}{10{,}267}} = 0.00304 \text{ or } 0.304\%$$

- The 95% confidence interval for a difference in proportions is calculated in the usual way:

$$\begin{aligned} 95\%\ \mathrm{CI} &= (p_1 - p_0) - [1.96 \times \mathrm{SE}(p_1 - p_0)] \text{ to } (p_1 - p_0) + [1.96 \times \mathrm{SE}(p_1 - p_0)] \\ &= [-0.014 - (1.96 \times 0.00304)] \text{ to } [-0.014 + (1.96 \times 0.00304)] \\ &= -0.01996 \text{ to } -0.008042 \\ &= -2.0 \text{ to } -0.8\% \end{aligned}$$

- With 95% confidence, the true population reduction in the 5-year incidence risk of stroke in the simvastatin group compared to the placebo group lies between 0.8 and 2.0%. It therefore appears that simvastatin lowers the risk of stroke in individuals with a high risk of cardiovascular disease.
- It is also possible to compare proportions by calculating a risk ratio (discussed in Chapter 7).

Plotting error bars

- Having undertaken a piece of research, producing graphs and charts are a useful way of summarising the data obtained so it can be read and interpreted with ease (discussed in Chapter 2).
- If you decide to create a graph with error bars, you need to decide whether to display the standard deviation, the standard error of the mean or the 95% confidence interval of the mean:
  - If there is a lot of scatter (due to biological variation) in your data, display the standard deviation.
  - If you feel the scatter in your data is due to imprecision in the study design (and not due to biological variation), you may prefer to focus on the mean and how precisely it has been determined by displaying:
    - the 95% confidence interval of the mean, or
    - the standard error of the mean.
  - If you are unsure about what type of error bar you wish to use, displaying the standard deviation is usually the preferred option.
- If using errors bars to summarise your data, remember to state exactly what measure the error bars are displaying either in the main text or in the figure legend. To highlight the importance of this, the data summarised in Fig. 3.8 have been graphically displayed using different types of error bars:
  - Figure 3.9A – Error bars displaying the standard deviation.
  - Figure 3.9B – Error bars displaying the 95% confidence interval of the mean.

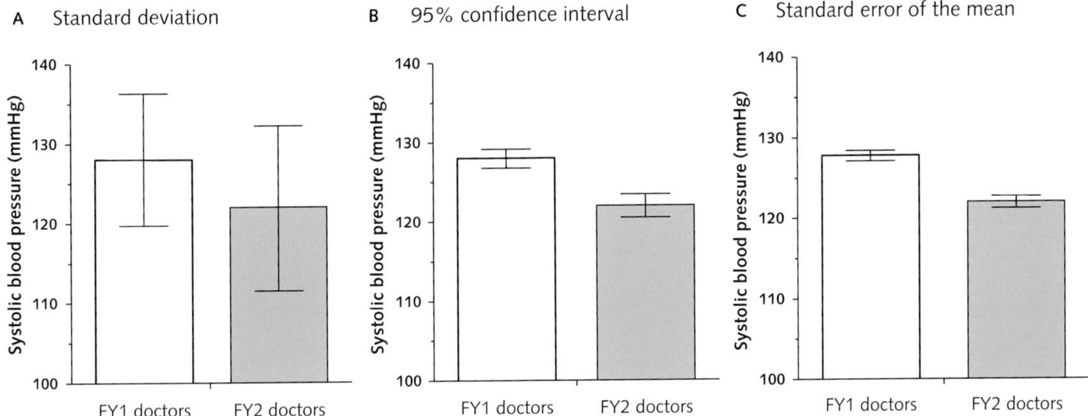

Fig. 3.9 Error bars. (A) Standard deviation. (B) 95% confidence interval. (C) Standard error of the mean.

 - Figure 3.9C – Error bars displaying the standard error of the mean.
- Comparing all three graphs in Fig. 3.9 (which all have the same scale on the vertical axis), the lengths of the error bars differ depending on the type of measure displayed. Therefore, always explain exactly what the error bars are displaying!

HINTS AND TIPS

Error bars: displaying confidence intervals or standard errors?

Which measure you use to display how precisely the mean has been determined is not too important. Confidence intervals are a more straightforward measure to interpret. However, showing the error bars as standard errors is sometimes conventional in many research groups.

THE *P*-VALUE

Statistical hypothesis testing

- In the previous section we used confidence intervals to make statistical inferences about the size of the difference in the incidence risk of first stroke between individuals randomised to either simvastatin or a placebo. Simvastatin lowered the 5-year incidence risk of stroke by 1.4% (CI 0.8 to 2.0%). However, observing different proportions between the simvastatin and placebo groups is not enough to convince you to conclude that the populations have different proportions. It is possible that the two populations (simvastatin and placebo) have the same proportion (i.e. simvastatin does not lower the 5-year incidence risk of stroke) and that the difference observed between the sample proportions occurred only by chance. The only way to determine whether the difference you observed reflects a true difference or whether it occurred due to random sampling is to use the rules of probability.
- As discussed in the section headed 'Hypothesis testing' at the start of this chapter, there are four basic steps involved in hypothesis testing.
- The first step is to specify the hypothesis and the alternative hypothesis:
    - Null hypothesis (H_0): There is *no* association between simvastatin and the risk of stroke in individuals with a high risk of cardiovascular disease.
    - Alternative hypothesis (H_A): There is an association between simvastatin and the risk of stroke in individuals with a high risk of cardiovascular disease.
- The second step is to collect the data (Fig. 3.5) and determine what statistical test is appropriate for data analysis (discussed in Chapter 15).
    - As we are comparing nominal data in two unpaired groups, with $n > 5$ in each cell (Fig. 3.5), the statistical test most appropriate for analysing these data is the chi-squared test (please refer to Fig. 15.3).
- The final two steps are to calculate and then interpret the *P*-value.

Calculating the *P*-value

- The *P*-value:
    - is calculated using a statistical test that is testing the null hypothesis.

- is derived from the test statistic, which is dependent on the standard error of the difference between means or proportions.
- is a probability, with a value ranging between 0 and 1.
- represents the weight of evidence there is in favour of or against the null hypothesis.

- Specifically, the *P*-value is the probability that the difference between the two groups would be as big or bigger than that observed in the current study, if the null hypothesis was true.
- A total of 0.05 or 5% is traditionally used as the cut-off.
  - If the observed *P*-value is less than 0.05 ($P<0.05$), there is good evidence that the null hypothesis is not true. This is related to the type 1 error rate (discussed later in this chapter).
  - $P<0.05$ is described as statistically significant.
  - $P\geq0.05$ is described as not statistically significant.
- For example, let's assume that you compared two means and obtained a *P*-value of 0.02. This means:
  - there is a 2% chance of observing a difference between the two groups at least as large as that observed even if the null hypothesis is true (i.e. even if the two population means are identical).
  - random sampling from similar populations would lead to a difference between the two groups smaller than that observed in 98% of occasions, and at least as large as that observed in 2% of occasions.

One-tail versus two-tail *P*-values

- When comparing two groups, you will either calculate a one-tail or two-tail *P*-value. Both types of *P*-values are based on the same null hypothesis.
- The two-tail *P*-value answers the following question:
  - Assuming that the null hypothesis is true, what is the chance that random samples from the same population would have means (or proportions) at least as far apart as those observed in the current study, with *either* group having the larger mean (or proportion)?
- For example, using the chi-squared test for our data on simvastatin and stroke risk, the two-tail *P*-value was calculated. With a two-tail *P*-value of <0.0001, we have extremely significant evidence against the null hypothesis.
- The one-tail *P*-value answers the following question:
  - Assuming that the null hypothesis is true, what is the chance that random samples from the same population would have means (or proportions) at least as far apart as observed in the current study, with the *specified group* having the larger mean (or proportion)?
- A one-tail *P*-value is used when we can predict which group will have the larger mean (or proportion) even prior to collecting any data. Common sense or prior data may inform us that a potential difference can only go in one direction. Therefore, if the other group ends up with the larger mean (or proportion), we should attribute that outcome to chance, even if the difference is relatively large.
- If you are unsure whether to choose a one- or two-tail *P*-value, it is advisable to choose the latter.

STATISTICAL SIGNIFICANCE AND CLINICAL SIGNIFICANCE

- The aim of this section is to highlight that:
  - a statistically significant result does not necessarily imply that the differences observed are clinically significant.
  - a non-statistically significant result does not necessarily imply that the differences observed are clinically *in*significant, merely that the differences may have occurred due to chance.
- Inferences about the target population can be made from the sample using the 95% confidence interval and the *P*-value (Fig. 3.10).
- Considering both *P*-values and confidence intervals are derived from the size of the difference in means (or proportions) between two groups and the standard error of this difference, the two measures are closely related.

Interpreting small *P*-values ($P<0.05$)

- If the *P*-value is small ($P<0.05$), the difference observed is unlikely to be due to chance.
- As previously discussed, a small *P*-value suggests we have evidence against the null hypothesis, i.e. there truly is a difference. However, you must consider

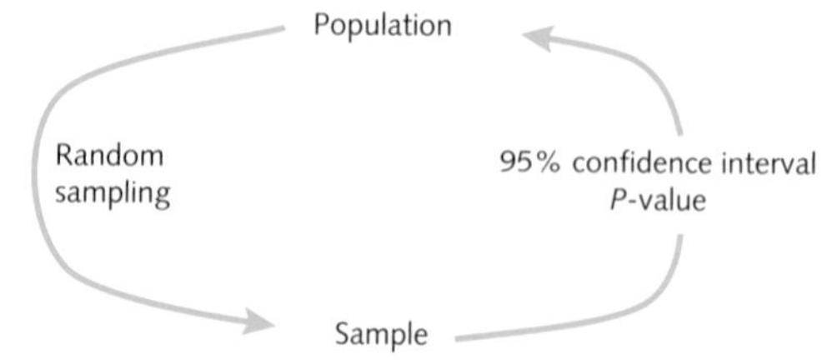

Fig. 3.10 Extrapolating from sample to population using statistical methods.

whether this difference is large enough to be clinically significant? Therefore, based on scientific judgement, statistical significance may not equate to clinical significance.

Using confidence intervals

- When comparing two means, the 95% confidence interval will not contain 0 if the *P*-value is less than 0.05.
- It is important to interpret the clinical significance of both ends of the confidence interval of the difference between means. For example,
  - the confidence interval may include differences that are all considered to be clinically significant. In this case, even the lower end of the confidence interval represents a difference that is large enough to be clinically important.
  - the confidence interval may only include differences that are relatively small and insignificant. In other words, even though the 95% confidence interval does not include a difference of 0 (remember, the *P*-value is <0.05), the treatment effect is too small to be considered as being clinically significant. Therefore, the treatment has an effect, but a relatively small one.
  - sometimes you're stuck in the middle! The confidence interval may range from a clinically unimportant difference to one considered as being clinically significant. Even though you can be 95% confident that the true difference is not 0, you can't reach a solid conclusion.

Interpreting large *P*-values ($P \geq 0.05$)

- If the *P*-value is large ($P \geq 0.05$), the difference observed may be due to random sampling.
- As previously discussed, a large *P*-value suggests we don't have enough evidence against the null hypothesis, i.e. the true means do not differ. This is not implying that the true means are the same.
- If the true means were equal, finding a difference between the means as large as the one observed in the current study would be due to chance.

Using confidence intervals

- When comparing two means, the 95% confidence interval will range from a negative number to a positive number if the *P*-value is less than 0.05.
- It is important to interpret the clinical significance of both ends of the confidence interval of the difference between means. For example,
  - the confidence interval may range from a negative number, which has no clinical importance, to a positive number that actually has clinical significance. In this case, with 95% confidence, the difference in means is either 0, small and unimportant or large enough to be clinically significant. No solid conclusion can be made. You would reach the same conclusion even if both ends of the confidence interval included clinically significant differences.
  - the confidence interval may only include differences that are relatively small and insignificant. Therefore, with 95% confidence, the difference in means is either 0 or small enough to be considered as being clinically unimportant. In conclusion, the results seem to confirm the negative findings.

P-values and study design

On some occasions, due to poor study design, e.g., having a small sample size, you may calculate a *P*-value that should be interpreted with caution. For example, a potentially clinically significant difference may be observed in a small study; however, the *P*-value is ≥ 0.05. Therefore the results are statistically non-significant. Such a scenario can be avoided if statistical power is considered during the design phase of a study.

STATISTICAL POWER

Type I and type II errors

When we test a hypothesis, we make a conclusion about whether an effect is statistically significant (or not). However, when we decide to either reject or fail to reject the null hypothesis, due to random sampling, our decision can be wrong in two ways. We can:

1. incorrectly reject the null hypothesis when it is true (type I error).
2. incorrectly fail to reject the null hypothesis when it is false (type II error).

Type I error

- When random sampling causes your data to show a statistically significant association/difference, but there really is no effect, a *type I error* has been made.
- Your conclusion that the sample means of the two groups are really associated/different is incorrect.
- Type I error is also our alpha (α) level in our hypothesis test, which represents the level of error we are willing to accept in our study.

Type II error

- When random sampling causes your data to *not* show a statistically significant association/difference, but there really is an effect, a *type II error* has been made.
- Your conclusion that the sample means of the two groups are *not* really associated/different is incorrect.
- We use the letter beta (β) to represent type II error.

The different types of error are displayed in Fig. 3.11.

Definitions of power and beta

Due to the statistical nature of hypothesis testing, statistical error must always be considered when making a conclusion about whether an effect is statistically significant. For example, even though a treatment is known to have an effect on the measured variable, a statistically significant difference might not be obtained in your study. *Due to chance*, your sample data may yield a *P*-value greater than your predefined cut-off for α, most commonly 0.05, as discussed above. Let's illustrate this point by looking at a study investigating the effect of amitopril on systolic blood pressure.

Statistical power: the effect of amitopril on systolic blood pressure

- A hypothetical phase II clinical trial (clinical trial phases are discussed in Chapter 5) has shown that a new (made-up) angiotensin-converting-enzyme inhibitor (ACEi; anti-hypertensive drug), 'amitopril', at a dose of 10 mg daily for 12 weeks, can reduce the systolic blood pressure by more than the gold standard ACEi used in clinical practice, ramipril.
- Considering that one tablet of amitopril costs a staggering 8 times as much as one tablet of ramipril, a cost-effectiveness analysis (discussed in Chapter 18) was carried out. Based on this economic review, the Department of Health issued a statement saying that amitopril could only be approved for use in clinical practice if it reduced the systolic blood pressure by more than 30 mmHg compared to the reduction in systolic blood pressure caused by ramipril.
- You decide to carry out a phase III clinical trial by randomising young, non-smoking, white males, with newly diagnosed hypertension, to either amitopril or ramipril for 12 weeks, measuring the systolic blood pressure before and after treatment.
- Taking the above into account, let's specify the null and alternative hypotheses:
  - The null hypothesis (H_0): Mean change in systolic blood pressure caused by amitopril *minus* mean change in systolic blood pressure caused by ramipril is $\leq$ 30 mmHg.
  - The alternative hypothesis (H_A): Mean change in systolic blood pressure caused by amitopril *minus* mean change in systolic blood pressure caused by ramipril is $>$ 30 mmHg.
- The sampling distributions for the null and alternative hypotheses are presented in Fig. 3.12.
- We sample 5000 patients and compare our sample mean to the null hypothesis. Referring to Fig. 3.12, the sample mean from our study has been plotted on the null hypothesis sampling distribution. With α set at 0.05, our mean of 36.2 mmHg falls within our rejection region so we can reject the null hypothesis.
- As shown on the graph, the probability that our study will yield a 'non-statistically significant' result is defined by beta (β). Correctly rejecting a false null hypothesis is therefore represented by the (1 – β) area of the distribution. Remember that the area under the curve represents the probability or relative frequency. We can therefore calculate the statistical power by calculating the probability that our sample mean falls into the (1 – β) area under the distribution curve.

If we perform many similar studies with the same sample size, we can deduce the following:

- Due to chance, some studies will yield a statistically significant finding with a *P*-value less than α.
- In other studies, the mean change in systolic blood pressure caused by amitopril minus the mean

Fig. 3.11 Hypothesis testing outcomes.

		Null hypothesis	
		True	*False*
Null hypothesis test decision	*Reject*	*Type I error* False positive **Alpha (α)**	*Correct outcome* True positive **Power (1 – β)**
	Fail to reject	*Correct outcome* True negative **(1 – α)**	*Type II error* False negative **Beta (β)**

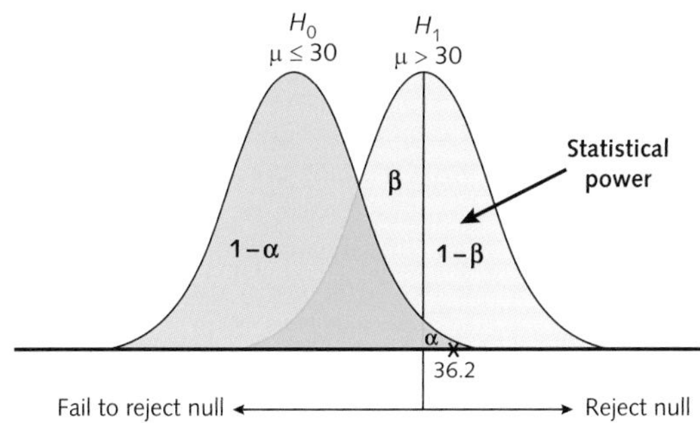

Fig. 3.12 Statistical power.

change in systolic blood pressure caused by ramipril will be less than 30 mmHg, and will not be statistically significant.

- If there is a high chance that our study will yield a statistically significant result, the study design has high power.
- As amitopril really causes a difference in blood pressure, the probability that our study will yield a 'not statistically significant' result is defined by β, which represents type II error, as discussed above.
- β is therefore equal to 1.0 minus power (or 100% minus power (%)).

HINTS AND TIPS

Even if there is a real numerical difference between group means, a statistically significant difference won't always be found in every study. The power of the study predicts the fraction of studies that are expected to yield a *P*-value that is statistically significant.

Interpreting non-significant results

If your results fail to show a statistically significant association/difference, we can use confidence intervals and power analyses to interpret the negative data. These approaches allow two different ways of analysing the data using the same assumptions.

Confidence interval

- The confidence interval (discussed above) approach shows *how precisely* you have determined the differences of interest.
- It combines the variability (standard deviation) and sample size to generate a confidence interval for the population mean.
- Having calculated the confidence interval, it is up to you to put the result in a scientific context.

Power analysis

- A power analysis can assist you in putting your results in perspective. This approach helps you plan or criticise other similar studies.
- Having failed to reject the null hypothesis, statistical power calculations firstly involve estimating a value for the sample mean for the alternative hypothesis. We usually estimate this value from previously published studies on the same topic or from a small pilot study.
- Having established this value, you then ask what is the probability that a study (with the same sample size) would have resulted in a statistically significant difference if your alternative hypothesis was true.

HINTS AND TIPS

The statistical power should be addressed:
1. when we fail to reject the null hypothesis
2. when we are planning a study.

To demonstrate the steps involved in interpreting non-significant results, let's look at a study investigating whether alterations of receptor numbers can affect the force of contraction in chronic heart failure.

Confidence interval versus power analysis: receptor numbers in chronic heart failure

Catecholamines, such as noradrenaline, have positive inotropic effects in the human heart via their actions through β_1- and β_2-adrenergic receptor binding. Despite having identified other receptor systems in the heart that also mediate these positive inotropic effects, the cardiac β-adrenergic receptor pathway is the most powerful mechanism to influence cardiac contractility.

Since nearly all β-adrenergic cardiac receptors are required to induce maximal inotropic effects on the heart, any reduction in the number of β-adrenergic receptors will consequently lead to a reduced inotropic response to receptor stimulation. Due to the enhanced sympathetic drive to the heart in chronic heart failure, there are reasons to believe that β-adrenergic receptors are reduced in these patients. Theoretical results are shown in Fig. 3.13.

- Assuming that the values follow a Gaussian distribution, an unpaired *t*-test (please refer to Fig. 15.3) was used to compare the means of the two unmatched groups.

Fig. 3.13 Receptor numbers/cardiac cell.

Variable	Chronic heart failure	Control
Number of subjects	20	19
Mean beta-adrenergic receptor number per cardiac cell	143	137
Standard deviation	33.8	58.2

- The mean receptor number per heart cell was very similar in the two patient groups and the *t*-test yielded a very high *P*-value.
- We can therefore conclude that the cardiac cells of people with chronic heart failure do not have an altered number of β-adrenergic receptors.
- Let's use the confidence interval of the difference in mean receptor number between the groups and also carry out a power analysis to assist us in interpreting the results.

Using confidence intervals

- The difference in mean receptor number between the two groups is 6 receptors per cardiac cell.
- The 95% confidence interval for the difference between the group means = −25 to 37 receptors/cardiac cell. Therefore, the true increase in mean receptor number per cardiac cell in subjects with chronic heart failure is 6 receptors/cell (95% CI −25 to 37). We can be 95% sure that this interval contains the true difference between the mean receptor number in the two subject groups.
- If the average number of β-adrenergic receptors per cardiac cell is 140, the confidence interval includes possibilities of an 18% decrease or 26% increase in receptor number. In other words, there could be a relatively big increase/decrease or no change in receptor number in people with chronic heart failure.
- To put this into a scientific perspective, as the majority of β-adrenergic receptors in the normal human heart are needed to cause a maximal inotropic effect, an 18% decrease in receptor number seems scientifically important.
- On the other hand, the 26% increase in receptor number is biologically trivial as even in the normal human heart there are still a few spare receptors when maximal inotropic effects have been reached.

Using power analysis

- If there truly is a change in cardiac β-adrenergic receptor number in people with chronic heart failure, what was the power of the study to find this change? This depends on how large the difference in mean receptor number between normal and chronic heart failure subjects actually is. This is denoted by the term delta, as shown in the power curve in Fig. 3.14.
- Considering the majority of β-adrenergic receptors in the normal human heart are needed to cause a maximal inotropic effect, any decrease in receptor number is biologically significant. For this reason, even if the difference in receptor number was only by 10%, we would want to conduct follow-up studies.
- As the mean number of receptors per cardiac cell is 140, we would want to find a difference of approximately 14 receptors per cell (delta = 14). Reading this value off the power curve below, we can conclude that the power of this study to find a difference of 16 receptors per cardiac cell was only about 15%. In other words, even if the difference really was this large, this study had only a 15% chance of finding a statistically significant result. With such low power to detect a biologically significant finding, we are unable to make any confident conclusions from the study results.

HINTS AND TIPS

Interpreting the power graph depends on what value for the difference in the mean between the two groups being compared (the delta value) is thought to be scientifically (or clinically) significant.

Sample size calculations

When comparing means or proportions between two groups in a study, it is important to choose a sample size

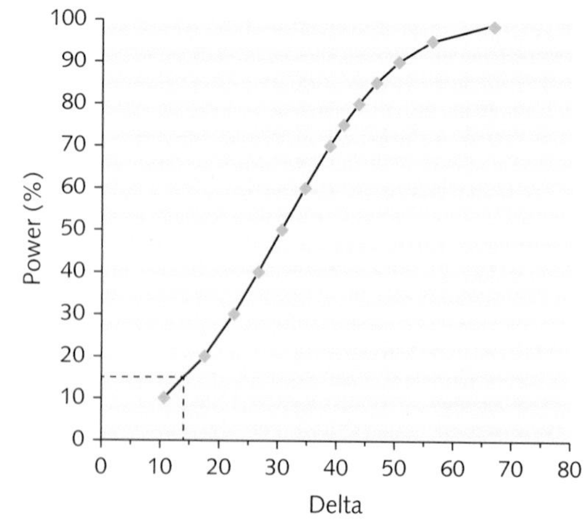

Fig. 3.14 The power curve.

that gives a high probability of detecting a given effect size (if it exists). Power analysis can be used to calculate the sample size we need for a future study using the following information:

- The power of the test (1 – β): More subjects will be needed if a higher power is chosen.
- The significance level (α): More subjects will be needed if a smaller significance level is chosen.
- The standard deviation (SD): More subjects will be needed if the data have a high SD. The SD is estimated from previous data or pilot studies. If different SDs are expected in the two groups, the average is used.
- The minimum difference (*d*) that is clinically important: More subjects will be needed if you want to detect a smaller difference.
- The value for *K*: This is a multiplier that depends on the significance level and the power of the study, and is derived from the normal distribution. Figure 3.15 shows a table with common values of *K* used for studies comparing two proportions or two means.

The number of subjects required in each group depends on whether we are comparing two means or comparing two proportions (Fig. 3.16).

HINTS AND TIPS

If you're still not sure how to calculate the sample size for a study comparing two means or two proportions, try using a statistical package, such as StatMate, which walks you through the basic steps. StatMate can also be used to determine the power of a completed study.

Determining acceptable statistical power levels

How much power is required?

- Referring to the power graph in Fig. 3.14, the rate of increase in power starts to reduce dramatically at around 80% as we increase the power of the study further. Several investigators therefore choose a sample size to obtain an 80% power in their study.
- As power is equal to (1 – β), your choice of an acceptable level of power for your study should ideally be influenced by the consequence of making a type II error.

Fig. 3.15 Multipliers (*K*) for studies comparing two proportions or two means.

Power (1 – β)	Significance level (α)		
	0.05	0.01	0.001
80%	7.8	11.7	17.1
90%	10.5	14.9	20.9
95%	13.0	17.8	24.3
99%	18.4	24.1	31.6

Fig. 3.16 Sample size calculations using power analysis.

(i) Sample size – comparing two means	(ii) Sample size – comparing two proportions
$n = \frac{2K(SD^2)}{d^2}$	$n = \frac{K[P_1(1-P_1)+P_2(1-P_2)]}{(P_1-P_2)^2}$

K = A multiplier calculated from the power (1 – β) and the significance level (α)
SD = The standard deviation expected
d = Minimum difference clinically important
P_1 = The expected population proportion in group A
P_2 = The expected population proportion in group B

How to get more power?

There are four main factors that influence statistical power:

1. The significance level
2. The sample size
3. The effect size
4. One-tail versus two-tail tests.

The significance level

Referring to Fig. 3.17A, we can see that there is a direct relationship between:

1. our significance level (α), which is our type I error
2. β, which is our type II error
3. the statistical power (1 – β).

When we increase the significance level, α, we decrease β and increase the statistical power of the study (1 – β) to find a real difference (Fig. 3.17B). However, this approach also increases the chance of falsely finding a 'significant' difference.

The sample size

- The sample size also has a direct influence on the level of statistical power.
- When we increase the sample size, we get a more accurate estimate for the population parameter. In other words, the standard deviation of the sampling distribution (standard error) is smaller.
- The distributions for the null and alternative hypotheses therefore become more leptokurtic, with a more acute peak around the mean and thinner, longer tails. This decreases our type II error (β), and increases the statistical power of the study (Fig. 3.17C).

Fig. 3.17 Factors influencing statistical power. (A) Original distributions. (B) Increased significance (α) level. (C) Increased sample size. (D) Increased effect size.

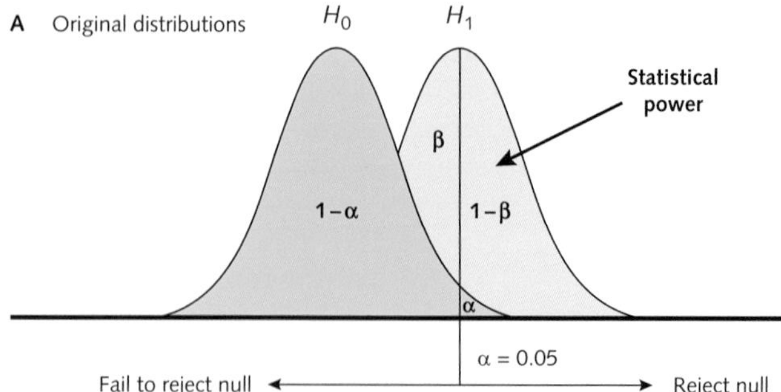

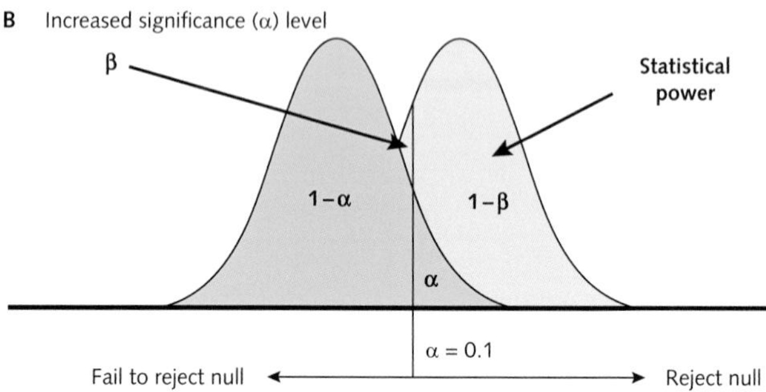

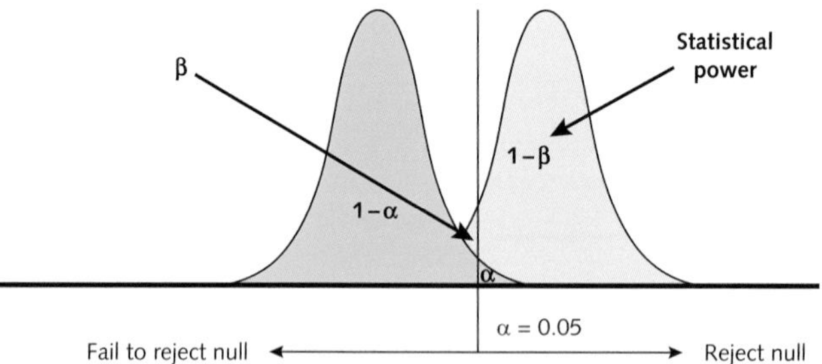

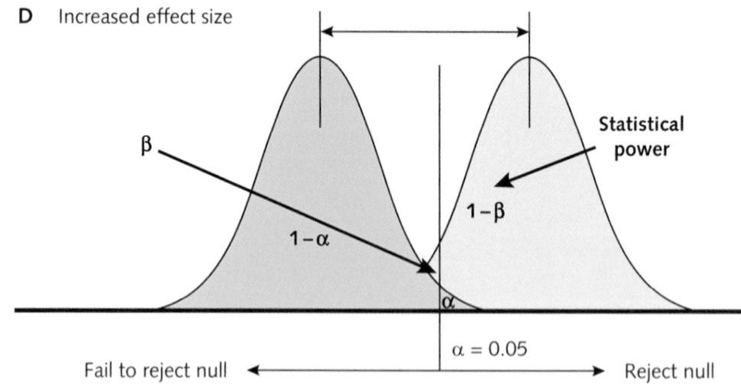

The effect size

- The degree of distance between the alternative hypothesis and null hypothesis distributions denotes the effect size.
- We estimate the anticipated difference between the alternative and null hypotheses from the literature.
- The larger the effect size, the smaller the type II error (β) and consequently the larger the statistical power ($1 - \beta$) (Fig. 3.17D). Understandably, the investigator has no control over the effect size.
- All studies have higher power to detect a large difference between groups than to detect a small one.

One-tail versus two-tail tests

- One-tail (directional) tests have more power than two-tail (non-directional) tests. This topic has been discussed earlier in this chapter.

HINTS AND TIPS

When conducting a study, it is important to have enough statistical power to have a high likelihood of capturing the effect of interest (if it exists). We can increase the power by altering several variables. We can:

1. increase the sample size.
2. increase the significance level, alpha (α).
3. use a one-tailed statistical test (if appropriate).
4. only care about a large difference in effect size between the groups being compared.

Systematic review and meta-analysis

Objectives

By the end of this chapter you should:

- Be familiar with the rationale for systematic reviews.
- Understand the steps involved in conducting a systematic review.
- Be able to explain what meta-analyses are and why they are conducted.
- Recognise the appropriate use of fixed-effects and random-effects meta-analysis procedures.
- Be able to interpret the results of a meta-analysis.
- Be able to explain what is meant by heterogeneity and know how to interpret the I^2 statistic and the Q statistic.
- Know the difference between subgroup and sensitivity analyses and be able to interpret their results.
- Be able to explain the main characteristics of a forest plot.
- Understand the common sources of bias implicated in systematic reviews.
- Be able to list the advantages and disadvantages of systematic reviews.

A methodological checklist on how to critically appraise systematic reviews and meta-analyses is provided in Chapter 19.

WHY DO WE NEED SYSTEMATIC REVIEWS?

Rationale for systematic reviews

- With the introduction of online access to medical, nursing and allied healthcare professional articles, there is a lot of information out there! Furthermore, we only really want to use high-quality evidence when making decisions about the provision of healthcare interventions.
- Due to busy clinical workloads, there is simply too much information around for people to keep up to date. Decision-makers therefore require reviews of the evidence available.
- Although often very useful background reading, traditional (narrative) reviews (discussed underneath) have their limitations. Systematic reviews use a peer-reviewed protocol in an attempt to provide an unbiased summary of the best available evidence.

The role of systematic reviews in healthcare

Systematic reviews are:

1. required to establish the clinical benefit and cost-effectiveness of an intervention.
2. used by the National Institute for Health and Clinical Excellence to appraise single or multiple interventions.
3. crucial when there is an important, potentially life-saving, question which has been addressed by a number of primary randomised controlled trials but there is still uncertainty about the answer.

Traditional reviews

- Traditional reviews:
  - may also be called narrative reviews, commentaries or literature reviews.
  - involve reviewing and summarising the existing knowledge on a particular topic.
  - are influential but have the following disadvantages:
    - Considering they are not based on a peer-reviewed protocol, the findings are often non-reproducible.
    - Bias is likely to be an issue if the collection, appraisal or summarising of information stages of the review are influenced by personal beliefs on the particular topic.
- The lack of rigour involved in writing a traditional review meant that different reviewers often reached different conclusions about the same topic. The need for a systematic approach to reviewing the research evidence was emphasised in 1992 with the publication of two landmark papers by Joseph Lau, Elliot Antman and their colleagues (please refer to the 'Reference' section at the end of this book).

Principles and conduct of systematic reviews

- In 1972, Archie Cochrane published his influential book titled *Effectiveness and Efficiency: Random Reflections on Health Services*.
- He highlighted the importance of using evidence from randomised controlled trials to make healthcare decisions, rather than from studies lower down in the hierarchy of evidence (Fig. 1.5).
- In 1979, he wrote, 'It is surely a great criticism of our profession that we have not organised a critical summary, by specialty or subspecialty, adapted periodically, of all relevant randomised controlled trials'.
- His ideas led to the development of the Cochrane Library database of systematic reviews.
- Developing a systematic review involves a number of steps, which are based on the key principles of evidence-based medicine discussed in Chapter 1:
  1. Formulate and define an appropriate healthcare question.
  2. Identify studies that address this question.
  3. Select relevant studies and critically appraise the evidence.
  4. Combine the results (and conduct a meta-analysis, if appropriate).
  5. Interpret the findings, taking bias into account.

Developing a systematic review: steps 1–3

- The first three steps are discussed in detail in Chapter 1. However, in relation to meta-analyses:
  - The meta-analysis should have a clear and appropriate healthcare question.
  - Once all the possible studies have been identified with a literature search, each study needs to be assessed for eligibility against objective criteria for inclusion or exclusion of studies.
  - Having identified those studies that meet the inclusion criteria, they are subsequently assessed for methodological quality using a critical appraisal framework.
  - A scale should be used for assessing the quality of the individual studies.
  - Despite satisfying the inclusion criteria, studies appraised as having a low-quality score are excluded.
  - The impact of excluding these studies can be assessed by carrying out a sensitivity analysis (discussed underneath).
- The remainder of this chapter will focus on the final two steps involved in developing a systematic review.

EVIDENCE SYNTHESIS

- Of the remaining studies, data (e.g. effect sizes, standard errors) should be extracted onto a purpose-designed data extraction form.

Fig. 4.1 Type of evidence synthesis.

Data type	Type of evidence synthesis
Qualitative	Meta-synthesis
Quantitative	Meta-analysis

- Aggregating the findings from the individual studies identified is known as evidence synthesis.
- The type of evidence synthesis depends on the type of data being reviewed (Fig. 4.1).
- Focusing on quantitative data, a meta-analysis provides a statistical estimate of net benefit aggregated over all the included studies.

META-ANALYSIS

Why do a meta-analysis?

Meta-analyses are conducted to:

- pool all the results on a topic, resolving controversies if individual study findings disagree.
- improve the estimates of the 'effect size' of the intervention.
- increase the overall sample size and therefore the statistical power of the pooled results.

Combining estimates in a meta-analysis

In order to illustrate the methods used to combine the results from different studies for meta-analysis, the example formulated in Chapter 1 on the role of beta-blockers in the management of heart failure in children will be used (Fig. 1.1). Having developed a clear strategy (Fig. 1.4) and reviewed a number of sources, 72 studies satisfied the inclusion criteria. After excluding those studies appraised as having a low-quality score, only 13 studies remained.

In order to make an overall assessment of the effect of carvedilol on congestive heart failure in children, the next step is to combine the results from these 13 studies into a single summary estimate of the exposure effect, together with a measure of reliability of that estimate, the confidence interval. When combining the results, the following points should be considered:

- Study participants treated with carvedilol should only be compared with control participants from the same study, since the selected sample used in the other studies may have different demographic features, especially if different entry criteria were used.
- Combining the results may not be appropriate if there are considerable differences in the study participants, interventions or outcomes.

- Even if the entry criteria are mostly comparable between the studies, the observed treatment effects of carvedilol will vary due to sampling error.
- It is important to take the relative size of each study into account when combining the results.
- Depending on the presence of statistical heterogeneity (discussed underneath), the fixed-effects or random-effects model may be used when carrying out the meta-analysis.

HINTS AND TIPS

A meta-analysis does not simply add together the results from different studies and calculate an overall summary statistic. It looks at the results within each study deemed comparable and then calculates a weighted average.

Heterogeneity

- The presence of observed variability between study estimates, i.e. beyond that expected by chance, indicates there is statistical heterogeneity.

Tests for evidence of heterogeneity

- Based on the chi-squared (χ^2) distribution (discussed in Chapter 15), a statistical test can be used to assess for statistical evidence of heterogeneity.
- The test statistic, Q, follows a χ^2 distribution with $n - 1$ degrees of freedom, where n is the number of study estimates included in the meta-analysis. It tests the null hypothesis that all studies are providing estimates of a single true exposure effect.
- The test often has limited statistical power, such that a non-significant result does not confirm the absence of heterogeneity. Consequently, in some reviews, a cut-off of $P < 0.10$ is commonly taken as evidence against the null hypothesis rather than $P < 0.05$.
- The Q statistic does not provide an estimate of the magnitude of heterogeneity (see below).

HINTS AND TIPS

Heterogeneity suggests the treatment/exposure effects are context-dependent.

Estimating the degree of heterogeneity

- The I^2 statistic provides an estimate of the proportion of the total variation in effect estimates that is due to heterogeneity between studies. In other words, it indicates the percentage of the observed variation in effect estimates that is due to real differences in effect size.
- The I^2 statistic is based on the Q statistic (discussed above) and ranges from 0% to 100%.
- The more heterogeneity, the larger the I^2 statistic.

Investigating sources of heterogeneity

- If statistical heterogeneity is demonstrated, it is important to determine what the source of this heterogeneity might be.
- Heterogeneity can result from clinical or methodological diversity, or both:

Clinical sources of heterogeneity include factors such as:

- Age and sex of study participants
- Diagnosis and disease severity of study participants
- Treatment differences in randomised controlled trials, e.g. dose or intensity of the intervention
- Location and setting of the study
- Outcome definition.

Methodological sources of heterogeneity include factors such as:

- Crossover versus parallel group design for randomised controlled trials
- Randomised by individuals or clusters (e.g. by school or by family)
- Case–control versus cohort for observational studies
- Different approaches to analysing the results
- Differences in the extent to which bias was controlled, e.g. allocation concealment, measurement bias, etc.

Calculating the pooled estimate in the absence of heterogeneity

The calculation method used depends on whether there is statistical heterogeneity.

Fixed-effects meta-analysis

- It is used when there is no evidence of (statistical) heterogeneity between the studies.
- The analysis:
  - assumes that the different studies are estimating the *same* true population exposure effects.
  - assumes that there is a single underlying 'true' effect that each study is estimating.
  - assumes that the only reason for the variation in estimates between the studies is due to sampling error (within-study variability).
  - gives more weight to the bigger studies.

- calculates the weight using the inverse of the variance of the exposure effect estimate (variance = (standard error)^2).
- Names of fixed effect methods include:
  - Inverse variance
  - Mantel–Haenszel
  - Peto.

Dealing with heterogeneity

If heterogeneity is identified, there are three main options available:

1. Not performing a meta-analysis
2. Random-effects meta-analysis
3. Subgroup analysis.

Not performing a meta-analysis

- Carrying out a meta-analysis, despite having a high degree of statistical heterogeneity, can lead to misleading and invalid conclusions.
- In this case, it may be more appropriate to avoid carrying out a meta-analysis and instead use a more qualitative approach to combining the results as part of a systematic review.

Random-effects meta-analysis

- It is used when there is evidence of (statistical) heterogeneity between the studies, but pooling of all the studies is still considered appropriate.
- This approach is used when there are two sources of variability:
  1. True variation between study effects in different studies (between-study variability).
  2. Variation between study participants within a study, due to sampling error (within-study variability).

  The analysis:
- assumes that different studies are estimating *different* true population exposure effects.
- assumes there is no single 'true' exposure effect, rather a distribution of effects, with a central value (mean) and some degree of variability (standard deviation).
- learns about this distribution of effects across the different studies.
- uses both sources of variability to derive the weights for each study.
- weights the studies more equally compared to the fixed-effects meta-analysis.
- uses the variance of the estimated effect in each study to estimate the within-study variability.
- uses the DerSimonian and Laird method (based on the *Q* statistic) to estimate the between-study variability.

HINTS AND TIPS

A random-effects meta-analysis is used when it cannot be assumed that all studies are estimating the same exposure effect value.

Subgroup analysis

- Subgroup analyses are meta-analyses on subgroups of the studies.
- To demonstrate how a subgroup analysis works, consider the following example:
  - Does taking a course in evidence-based medicine at medical school improve your chances of getting a paper published?
- Having carried out a literature search and critically appraised the evidence, suppose we have 18 trials looking at teaching versus no teaching in evidence-based medicine at medical school. Of the 18 trials, 8 of them used a problem-based learning approach while the others used a lecture-based approach.
- As the learning method may have had an impact on whether (or not) the students went on to publish a paper, clinical heterogeneity may exist and it may therefore be inappropriate to combine the trials which used different learning approaches. With this in mind, it will be necessary to carry out a separate meta-analysis for each subgroup (problem-based versus lecture-based learning):
  - Subgroup 1 (problem-based learning) summary estimate from 8 trials:
    - Risk ratio: 1.8
    - Confidence interval of risk ratio: 1.11 to 2.57.
  - Subgroup 2 (lecture-based learning) summary estimate from 10 trials:
    - Risk ratio: 1.71
    - Confidence interval of risk ratio: 1.06 to 2.87.
  - Comparing the summary estimates from the two subgroups:
    - P-value = 0.81.
  - Therefore, there is no evidence of a difference between the estimates. However, with an I^2 value of 60% for subgroup 1 and 52% for subgroup 2, heterogeneity still exists across both groups.
- It is important to pre-specify and restrict the number of subgroup analyses to a minimum in order to limit the number of spurious significant findings due to chance variation.
- All subgroup analyses should be based on scientific rationale.

Fixed-effects versus random-effects meta-analysis

- The key differences between the fixed-effects and random-effects models for meta-analysis are highlighted in Fig. 4.2.
- As the random-effects method takes into account the estimated between-study variance, this approach will, in general, be more conservative than its fixed-effect counterpart. This reflects the greater uncertainty inherent in the random-effects meta-analysis model.
- If the between-study variation is estimated to be 0, then the summary estimate for the fixed-effects and random-effects meta-analyses will be identical.

Sensitivity analysis

- A sensitivity analysis determines whether the findings of the meta-analysis are robust to the methodology used to obtain them.
- It involves comparing the results of two or more meta-analyses, which are calculated using different assumptions. These assumptions may include:
  - omitting low-quality studies.
  - omitting studies with questionable eligibility for the systematic review.
  - omitting studies which appear to be outliers.
  - omitting a particular trial, which you feel is driving the result, i.e. the largest trial.
  - using several alternative imputed values where there is missing data for one of the trials. This may be an issue when including cluster randomised trials or cross-over trials.

Fig. 4.2 Fixed-effects versus random-effects meta-analysis.

	Fixed effects	Random effects
True effect	Assumes that the true effect is the same in each study.	Assumes there is no single 'true' exposure effect but a distribution of effects.
Variation in estimates between studies	Due to sampling error.	Due to sampling error *and* between-study variation.
Influence of study size	Large and small studies provide the same estimates; thus much less weight is given to the inferior information from smaller studies.	Large and small studies provide distinct information; thus information from small studies is down-weighted, but to a lesser extent than in the fixed-effects method.
Confidence interval for the summary estimate	Narrower	Wider
P-value	Smaller	Larger

HINTS AND TIPS

A sensitivity analysis may involve carrying out a meta-analysis with and without an assumption, and subsequently comparing the two results for statistical significance.

PRESENTING META-ANALYSES

- The results of meta-analyses are often presented in a standard way known as a 'forest plot' (Fig. 4.3).
- In a forest plot:
  - the individual study results are represented by a circle or a square to indicate the study estimate.
  - the size of the circle or square is proportional to the weight for that individual study in the meta-analysis.
  - the horizontal line running through the circle or square corresponds to the 95% confidence interval for that particular study estimate.
  - the centre of the diamond (and broken vertical line) represents the summary effect estimate of the meta-analysis.
  - the 95% confidence interval for the summary effect estimate corresponds to the width of the diamond.
  - the unbroken vertical line is at the null value (1).
  - the studies are often displayed in chronological order.

EVALUATING META-ANALYSES

Interpreting the results

- If the confidence interval of the summary effect estimate (width of diamond) crosses the null value (solid vertical line), this is equivalent to saying that there is no statistically significant difference in the effects in the exposure and control groups.
- When interpreting the results it is important to consider the following questions:

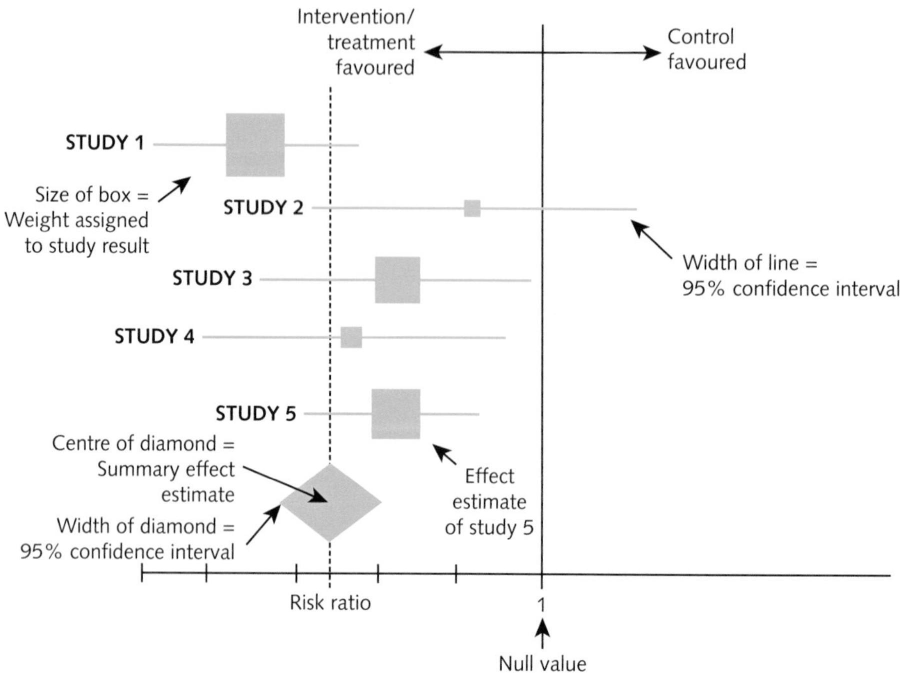

Fig. 4.3 Understanding forest plots.

- Is there strong evidence for an exposure effect?
- Is there unexplained variation in the exposure effect across individual studies?
- Are the results applicable to your patient?
- Are there any implications for future research?
- Are there any potential sources of bias?

Bias in meta-analyses

Production of evidence

- It is crucial that threats to the internal validity of a study (confounding, bias and causality) are reviewed for all studies included in the systematic review.
- The three main threats to internal validity are discussed in turn for each of the key study designs in their respective chapters.
- Methodological checklists for critically appraising the key study designs covered in this book are provided in Chapter 19.

Dissemination of evidence

- While systematic reviews aim to include *all* high-quality studies that address the review question, finding all relevant studies may not be possible.
- Failure to include all relevant studies in a meta-analysis may lead to the exposure effect being under- or overestimated.
- The analyses reported in a published article are more likely to show a statistically significant finding between the competing groups than a non-significant finding. All outcomes should be included in the final research report so as to avoid outcome-reporting bias.
- In general, those studies with significant, positive results are more likely to be:
  - considered worthy of publication (publication bias)
  - published in English (language bias)
  - published quickly (time lag bias)
  - published in more than one journal (multiple publication bias)
  - cited in subsequent journals (citation bias).
- Reporting bias incorporates all of these types of bias.
- The over-representation of studies in systematic reviews that have positive findings may lead to reviews being biased towards a positive exposure effect.

HINTS AND TIPS

Null or non-significant findings are less likely to be published than statistically significant, positive findings.

Publication bias

Detecting publication bias

- Publication bias in meta-analyses is usually explored graphically using 'funnel plots'. These are scatter plots, with:
  - the relative measure of exposure effect (risk ratio or odds ratio) on the horizontal axis. The exposure effects are usually plotted on a logarithmic scale to ensure that effects of the same magnitude but in opposite directions, such as odds ratios of 0.3 and 3, are equidistant from the null value.
  - the standard error of the exposure effect (which represents the study size) on the vertical axis.
- As the sample size of a study increases, there is an increase in the precision (and a reduction in the standard error) of the study in being able to estimate the underlying exposure effect. Furthermore, we would expect more precise studies (with larger sample sizes) to be less affected by the play of chance. In summary:
  - large studies have more precision (i.e. low standard error) and the exposure estimates are expected to be closer to the pooled estimate.
  - small studies have less precision (i.e. high standard error) and the exposure estimates are expected to be more variable (more widely scattered) about the pooled estimate.
- In the absence of publication bias, the plot will resemble a symmetrical inverted funnel (Fig. 4.4A).
- If there is publication bias, where smaller studies showing no statistically significant effect remain unpublished, the funnel plot will have an asymmetrical appearance with the lower right- (or left-, depending on the research question) hand corner of the plot missing (Fig. 4.4B).
- As demonstrated in Fig. 4.4B, publication bias will lead to an overestimation of the treatment effect.

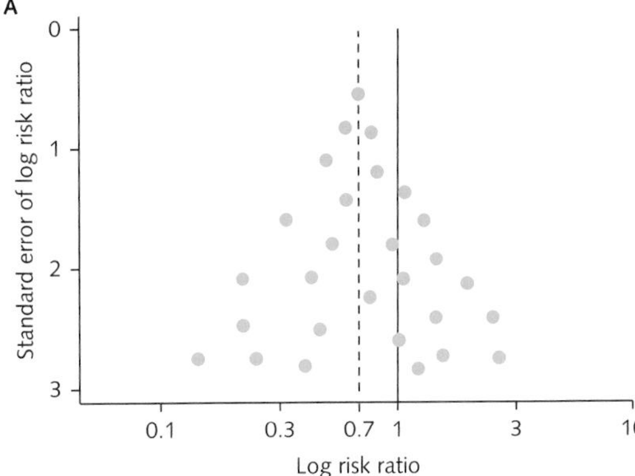

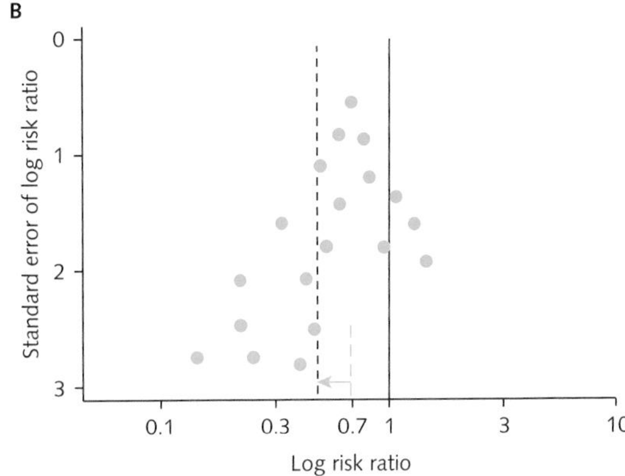

Fig. 4.4 Understanding funnel plots.

HINTS AND TIPS

The standard error measurement increases as you go down the vertical axis. More precise studies are therefore plotted further up on the vertical axis.

Other causes of funnel plot asymmetry

- Publication bias is not the only cause of funnel plot asymmetry.
- Smaller studies of lower methodological quality may produce more extreme treatment effects.
- Differences in study methodologies, such as recruiting only high-risk patients, may lead to larger or smaller true treatment effects. This is usually the case in smaller studies, as fewer participants are required to detect a given effect if there is an increased event rate amongst the high-risk individuals.
- The true treatment effect may also differ according to the intensity of the exposure/intervention.
- Sometimes asymmetry cannot even be assessed as there are too few studies!

HINTS AND TIPS

Funnel plots should be used to identify whether there is a tendency for smaller studies in a meta-analysis to have larger exposure effect estimates. In other words, funnel plots indicate whether 'small study effects' are present.

Preventing publication bias

- One solution has been to put all ongoing established trials on a register.
- Some journals will no longer consider trials for publication unless they are registered from the start.

- It has also been suggested that journals should consider studies for publication based only on the literature review and study methodology. The reviewers are therefore 'blind' to the actual results of the study.
- Importantly, a study should have sufficient power to detect a clinically significant effect (if one exists); therefore trials that have a small sample size (and therefore a low power to detect an exposure effect) should be discouraged.

ADVANTAGES AND DISADVANTAGES

What are the advantages and disadvantages of systematic reviews (Fig. 4.5)?

KEY EXAMPLE OF A META-ANALYSIS

- In 1995, Joseph Lau and his colleagues performed a meta-analysis of controlled trials assessing the effects of prophylactic antibiotics on mortality rates following colorectal surgery, i.e. the perioperative mortality.
- There were 21 trials carried out between 1969 and 1987 that compared the effect of an antibiotic prophylaxis regimen on perioperative mortality rates after colorectal surgery.
- The meta-analysis of these trials is presented in Fig. 4.6A as a forest plot.
- *Interpretation of Fig. 4.6A*:
    - The odds ratio and 95% confidence intervals are shown on a logarithmic scale, with the pooled treatment effect estimate at the bottom of the forest plot.
    - Compared to an inactive treatment, antibiotic prophylaxis was shown to reduce the number of perioperative deaths following colorectal surgery in 17 of the 21 trials, i.e. the odds ratio was less than the null value (1) in 17 trials.
    - However, none of these 17 trials had a statistically significant finding, i.e. the 95% confidence interval of the treatment effect estimate crossed the null value (1) in all 17 trials.
    - Despite this, the pooled treatment effect odds ratio estimate of all 21 trials was in favour of using antibiotic prophylaxis to reduce the number of perioperative deaths following colorectal surgery, i.e. the P value was <0.05.
- If a new meta-analysis had been performed each time the results of a new trial were reported, would we have realised the beneficial effects of antibiotic

Fig. 4.5 Advantages and disadvantages of systematic reviews.

Advantages	Disadvantages
Appear at the top of the 'hierarchy of evidence' that informs evidence-based practice, thus giving us the best possible estimate of any true effect.	Require considerably more effort than traditional reviews.
Can shorten the time lag between research practice and the implementation of new findings into clinical practice.	The clinical questions posed are often too narrow, thus reducing the applicability of the findings to your patient.
Relatively quicker and less costly to perform than a new study.	Sometimes the interventions reviewed do not reflect current practice.
Large amounts of information are critically appraised and synthesised in order to reduce errors (including bias) and improve the accuracy and reliability of the findings.	There may be an insufficient number of high-quality studies available for review.
Compared to a single study, the results can often be generalised to a broader population across a wide range of settings.	The underlying physiological effects of an intervention are not considered.
If the studies included in the review give consistent results, it provides evidence that the phenomenon is robust and transferrable.	Systematic reviews rarely consider the fact that some interventions are delivered as part of a larger package of care.
If the studies included in the review give *in*consistent results, any sources of variation can be studied.	
A meta-analysis has high power to detect exposure effects and estimate these effects with greater precision than single studies.	

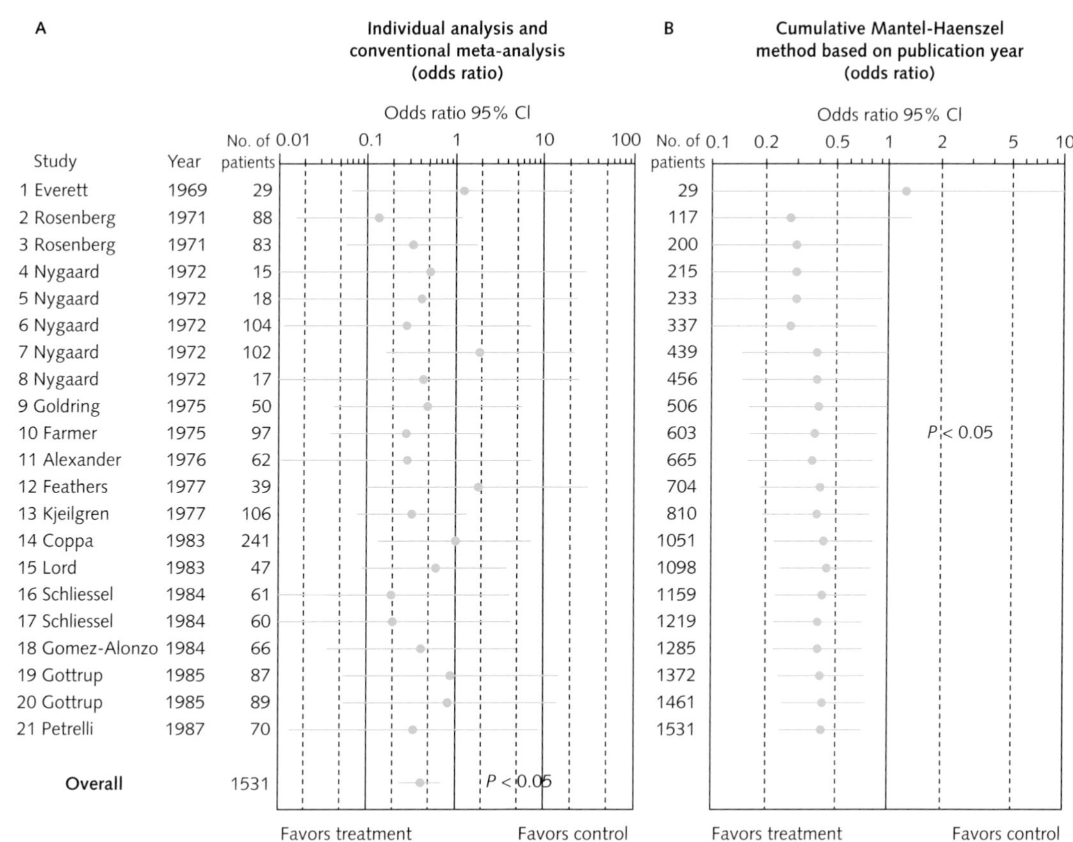

Fig. 4.6 (A) Conventional and (B) cumulative meta-analyses of 21 trials on the effect of prophylactic antibiotics on perioperative mortality rates following colorectal surgery. (Lau, J. et al., 1995. J. Clin. Epidemiol. 48: 45–57. Reproduced with permission.)

prophylaxis prior to 1987 (when the 21st trial was published)? The answer is given by the cumulative meta-analysis presented in Fig. 4.6B.

- *Interpretation of Fig. 4.6B*:
  - There was a statistically significant reduction in perioperative mortality rates by 1975, after only 10 trials, involving a cumulative number of 603 patients.
  - The treatment effect estimates of the 11 subsequent trials, which collectively enrolled an additional 928 patients, had little effect on the odds ratio in terms of establishing treatment efficacy, but increased the power of the analysis (thus slightly narrowing the 95% confidence interval).
- In summary, if the original data from the trials that studied the effects of using antibiotic prophylaxis on perioperative mortality rates following colorectal surgery had been systematically reviewed (each time the results of a new trial were reported), the benefits of using prophylactic antibiotics would have been evident by the mid-1970s. However, reports of trials involving comparison groups given no active treatment continued to appear throughout the 1980s! Ethical? I think not!

REPORTING A SYSTEMATIC REVIEW

- An international group of experienced authors have published guidance for authors to assist them in the reporting of systematic reviews and meta-analyses. This guidance, known as the PRISMA (Preferred Reporting Items for Systematic reviews and Meta-Analyses) statement, consists of a 27-item checklist and a four-phase flow diagram.
- The checklist includes items deemed essential for transparent reporting of a systematic review, thus providing enough information to allow critical appraisal (Fig. 4.7).

Fig. 4.7 Checklist of items to include when reporting a systematic review or meta-analysis.

Section/topic	Item number	Checklist item
Title		
Title	1	Identify the report as a systematic review, meta-analysis, or both.
Abstract		
Structured summary	2	Provide a structured summary including, as applicable, background, objectives, data sources, study eligibility criteria, participants, interventions, study appraisal and synthesis methods, results, limitations, conclusions and implications of key findings, systematic review registration number.
Introduction		
Rationale	3	Describe the rationale for the review in the context of what is already known.
Objectives	4	Provide an explicit statement of questions being addressed with reference to participants, interventions, comparisons, outcomes and study design (PICOS).
Methods		
Protocol and registration	5	Indicate if a review protocol exists, if and where it can be accessed (such as web address), and, if available, provide registration information including registration number.
Eligibility criteria	6	Specify study characteristics (such as PICOS, length of follow-up) and report characteristics (such as years considered, language, publication status) used as criteria for eligibility, giving rationale.
Information sources	7	Describe all information sources (such as databases with dates of coverage, contact with study authors to identify additional studies) in the search and date last searched.
Search	8	Present full electronic search strategy for at least one database, including any limits used, such that it could be repeated.
Study selection	9	State the process for selecting studies (that is, screening, eligibility, included in systematic review, and, if applicable, included in the meta-analysis).
Data collection process	10	Describe method of data extraction from reports (such as piloted forms, independently, in duplicate) and any processes for obtaining and confirming data from investigators.
Data items	11	List and define all variables for which data were sought (such as PICOS, funding sources) and any assumptions and simplifications made.
Risk of bias in individual studies	12	Describe methods used for assessing risk of bias of individual studies (including specification of whether this was done at the study or outcome level), and how this information is to be used in any data synthesis.
Summary measures	13	State the principal summary measures (such as risk ratio, difference in means).
Synthesis of results	14	Describe the methods of handling data and combining results of studies, if done, including measures of consistency (such as I^2 statistic) for each meta-analysis.
Risk of bias across studies	15	Specify any assessment of risk of bias that may affect the cumulative evidence (such as publication bias, selective reporting within studies).
Additional analyses	16	Describe methods of additional analyses (such as sensitivity or subgroup analyses, meta-regression), if done, indicating which were pre-specified.
Results		
Study selection	17	Give numbers of studies screened, assessed for eligibility and included in the review, with reasons for exclusions at each stage, ideally with a flow diagram.
Study characteristics	18	For each study, present characteristics for which data were extracted (such as study size, PICOS, follow-up period) and provide the citations.

Fig. 4.7 Checklist of items to include when reporting a systematic review or meta-analysis—cont'd.

Section/topic	Item number	Checklist item
Risk of bias within studies	19	Present data on risk of bias of each study and, if available, any outcome-level assessment (see item 12).
Results of individual studies	20	For all outcomes considered (benefits or harms), present for each study (a) simple summary data for each intervention group and (b) effect estimates and confidence intervals, ideally with a forest plot.
Synthesis of results	21	Present results of each meta-analysis done, including confidence intervals and measures of consistency.
Risk of bias across studies	22	Present results of any assessment of risk of bias across studies (see item 15).
Additional analysis	23	Give results of additional analyses, if done (such as sensitivity or subgroup analyses, meta-regression) (see item 16).
Discussion		
Summary of evidence	24	Summarise the main findings including the strength of evidence for each main outcome; consider their relevance to key groups (such as healthcare providers, users and policy-makers).
Limitations	25	Discuss limitations at study and outcome level (such as risk of bias), and at review level (such as incomplete retrieval of identified research, reporting bias).
Conclusions	26	Provide a general interpretation of the results in the context of other evidence, and implications for future research.
Funding		
Funding	27	Describe sources of funding for the systematic review and other support (such as supply of data) and role of funders for the systematic review.

Reproduced with permission: Moher D et al. BMJ 2009;339:bmj.b2535

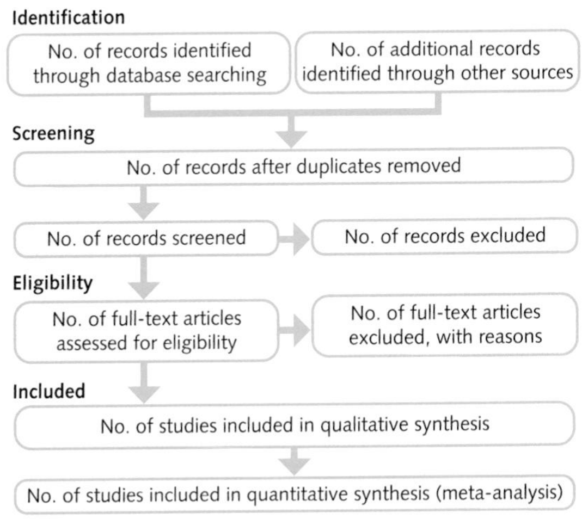

Fig. 4.8 Flow of information through the different phases of a systematic review. (Reproduced with permission: Moher D et al. BMJ 2009;339:bmj.b2535)

- The flow diagram provides guidance on how to summarise the study selection process (Fig. 4.8).
- All sources of information referred to in the systematic review should be acknowledged.
- The Harvard Referencing System is a collection of rules that standardises the format in which common types of material (e.g. books, journal articles, websites, etc.) are referenced (discussed in Chapter 5).

Research design

Objectives

By the end of this chapter you should:

- Understand the steps involved in obtaining data to answer a research question.
- Be able to explain the differences between an interventional and an observational study design.
- Know the definition of a clinical trial and the differences between the various clinical trial phases.
- Understand the differences between association and causality.
- Know the steps involved in assessing whether there is a causal relationship between an exposure and an outcome.
- Be able to discuss the factors that determine when a particular study design is indicated.
- Understand the steps involved in writing up a research study and be able to apply this knowledge to your own work.

OBTAINING DATA

- Before even thinking about how to summarise, display or analyse your data, you must first decide on how you are going to collect your data!
- It is crucial to choose the best study design to investigate your research question.
- Poorly designed studies may yield misleading results, wasting time, money and resources in the process.
- There may be a number of possible study designs for any research question.
- Over the next few chapters you will learn about the major epidemiological study designs currently being used in evidence-based practice today.
- Research studies can be classified into two types:
  1. Interventional studies (or experimental studies)
  2. Observational studies.
- The flowchart presented in Fig. 5.1 summarises the different types of interventional and observational study designs.
- Figure 5.2 uses a timeline to illustrate the time points at which exposure and outcome data are collected for some of the common types of study designs.
- Qualitative research can be carried out on its own or incorporated into a quantitative study design.
- Each study design will be discussed in extensive detail in their respective chapters.

INTERVENTIONAL STUDIES

- An interventional (or experimental) study is when the investigator tests whether intervening in some way leads to a measurable variation in the outcome.
- Interventional studies underpin clinical trials that compare two or more treatments (see below).
- A laboratory study is another type of interventional study and may involve carrying out research using animal models.
- Interventional studies provide data with a high degree of internal validity (discussed in Chapter 1), as it is generally possible to control for factors that may affect the outcome.
- A high level of validity may be needed for studying an intervention that is expected to have a small effect on the outcome. This small effect is usually defined as a difference of up to 20% between the two intervention groups.
- When the difference between the two groups is relatively small, confounding or bias may produce invalid findings, i.e. mask or create an effect.
- However, interventional studies are not always feasible, for example, due to high running costs, patients' reluctance to participate or ethical issues.
- The different types of interventional studies that will be reviewed in this book are:
  - Parallel randomised controlled trials (RCTs)
  - Crossover RCTs
  - Factorial RCTs
  - Cluster RCTs
  - Superiority RCTs
  - Equivalence RCTs
  - Non-inferiority RCTs
- In RCTs, only the play of chance (randomisation) determines the intervention that is allocated to a particular subject. Consequently, large, well-designed

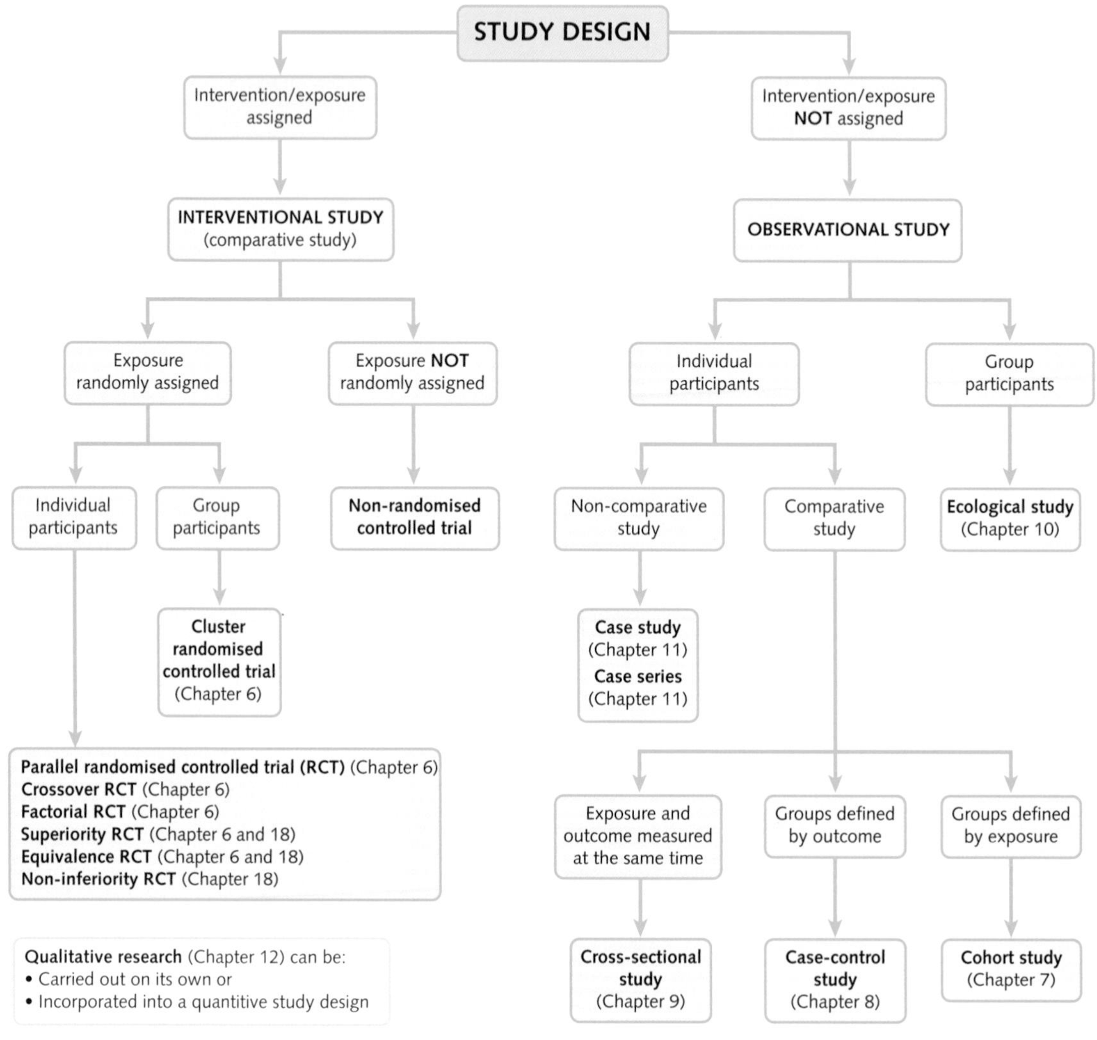

Fig. 5.1 Flowchart of different types of study design.

RCTs provide strong evidence that an association between an intervention and outcome is causal. We will discuss this concept in greater detail in Chapter 6.

OBSERVATIONAL STUDIES

- An observational study is when the investigator collects data on exposures and outcomes without attempting to alter a subject's exposure status.
- Patterns and associations between exposures and outcomes are identified using naturally occurring variation in the population.
- Compared to interventional studies, observational studies can be used to study the effect of a wider range of exposures, including studying the natural history, prevention and treatment of a disease. Consequently, there is a role for observational studies in clinical trials (see below).
- Investigating the natural history of a disease may involve collecting data on:
  - the causes of disease incidence
  - the determinants of disease progression.
- Understanding the natural history of a disease can allow us to predict the future healthcare needs of a population.
- However, observational studies have lower internal validity than interventional studies. This is because the investigator has no control over factors that may affect the outcome.

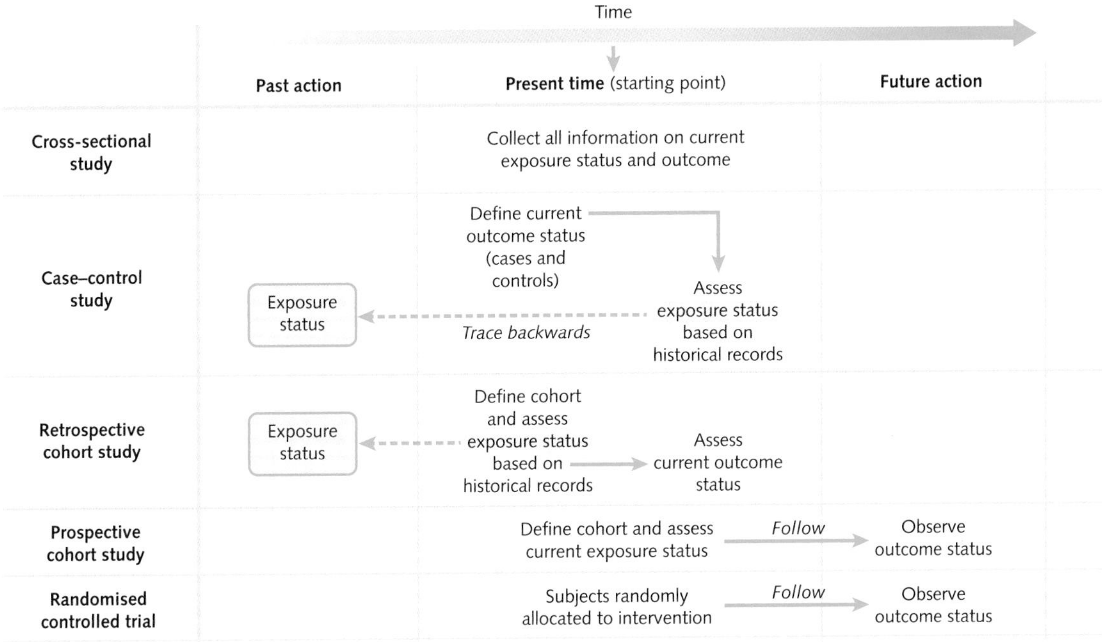

Fig. 5.2 Study design timeline.

- Despite this limitation, in some situations, observational studies are the only types of study that are practical.
- The different types of observational studies that will be reviewed in this book are:
  - Cohort studies
  - Case–control studies
  - Cross-sectional studies
  - Ecological studies
  - Case studies and case series.

COMMUNICATION

When would you choose an observational study design over an interventional study design?

You may consider using an observational study design to answer a specific research question if the equivalent interventional study design is:

- unethical, e.g. randomly allocating healthy people to radiation, to investigate whether exposure to radiation leads to a higher risk of cancer.
- inappropriate, e.g. are homosexual men at higher risk of acquiring HIV infection than heterosexual men?
- too expensive.
- unlikely to yield a significant result, e.g. for studying rare events such as a rare side effect of a drug.
- impracticable (unfeasible), e.g. is working on regular night shifts associated with a higher risk of ischaemic heart disease?

CLINICAL TRIALS

- Although there are many definitions of clinical trials, according to the National Institutes of Health ClinicalTrials.gov website (2012), they are 'generally considered to be biomedical or health-related research studies in human beings that follow a pre-defined protocol'. They include 'both interventional and observational types of studies'.

Types of clinical trials

- The National Institutes of Health defines five different types of clinical trials:
  1. *Treatment trials* – Involve testing new interventions (e.g. drugs, a new surgery procedure, a new radiological approach) or a combination of interventions
  2. *Prevention trials* – Involve investigating methods for the primary prevention (methods for preventing healthy people from developing a disease), secondary prevention (methods for slowing down the progression of a disease or for treating it in its early stage whilst the patient is still asymptomatic) and tertiary prevention (methods for preventing further physical deterioration in chronic symptomatic disease states) of a disease. These methods may include drugs, vaccines, lifestyle changes, etc.

3. *Diagnostic trials* – Involve investigating better procedures or tests for diagnosing a particular disease or condition.
4. *Screening trials* – Involve investigating ways for detecting a particular disease or health condition.
5. *Quality of life trials* – Involve exploring ways for improving the quality of life for individuals with a chronic disease.

Clinical trial phases

- Several clinical trial phases must be followed to ensure new drugs or treatments are safe and effective prior to incorporating them into clinical guidelines.
- The trials at each phase have a different purpose, helping scientists/clinicians answer different questions.
- We will go through the stages involved in turn, using the example of a new drug therapy to illustrate our points.

Pre-clinical trials

- Prior to starting clinic trials on a novel drug in humans, the first step is to show that it has some potential to be the next big thing! We demonstrate this by using in vitro (test tube experiments) and in vivo (animal studies) techniques at a laboratory to obtain preliminary toxicity, efficacy and pharmacokinetic information.

Phase I trials

- Once laboratory experiments show that a new drug has promise, the next step is to test its safety in humans.
- Phase I trials often involve only a small number of individuals (20–60), some of whom may be healthy volunteers.
- Phase I cancer trials often involve patients with advanced cancer who have already exhausted all current treatment options available to them, without much benefit.
- The protocol may involve giving very low doses of the new drug to the first group (or 'cohort') of patients and gradually increasing the doses for later groups.
- Using this dose escalation protocol allows researchers to identify:
  1. the safe dose range in humans
  2. the side-effect profile of the drug.
- These studies also involve investigating the most effective way of delivering the new drug, e.g. orally, intramuscularly, intravenously, subcutaneously, etc.
- If the new drug has been found to be reasonably safe, it can subsequently be tested in phase II clinical trials.

Phase II trials

- Phase II trials test the new drug in a larger group of people (100–300) to investigate whether it is effective (at least in the short term) and to further evaluate its safety profile.
- The methods used to assess how well the new treatment works depends on the disease type. For example, imaging techniques (e.g. X-rays, CT scans, MRI etc.) may be used to show whether a tumour is shrinking.
- The people chosen for phase II trials usually have the disease for which the drug is targeted.
- If the new drug shows an effect, and is shown to be safe enough, it can be then tested in phase III clinical trials.

Phase III trials

- Phase III trials usually involve comparing the new drug with the gold standard treatment (discussed in Chapter 14) currently in use, or with a placebo.
- Often these trials use a 'randomised controlled trial' study design whereby participants have an equal chance of being assigned to either the new drug or gold standard treatment (or placebo). Please refer to Chapter 6 for an in-depth discussion on RCTs.
- The main objective is to learn whether the new drug is better than, the same as or worse than the standard treatment.
- They also build on knowledge from the previous two trial phases regarding the safety and side-effect profile of the new drug.
- Phase III trials involve several thousand patients (1000–3000 or more), sometimes across different hospitals in different countries.
- The smaller the expected difference in effect size between the new drug and the standard treatment (or placebo), the greater the number of participants required for the trial to show this difference.
- Underpinned by ethical principle, an RCT will be stopped early if the side effects of the new treatment are too severe or if the outcome in one group (not necessarily the new treatment group) is better than the outcome in the other group(s).
- Phase III trials are needed before the new drug can be considered for use in routine clinical practice.

Phase IV trials

- Phase IV trials are carried out after the drug has been licensed, marketed and made available for all patients.
- The main objective of phase IV trials is to gather information on:
  - how well the drug works in various populations.
  - the long-term risks and benefits of taking the drug.

- the side effects and safety of the drug in larger populations.
- whether the drug can be used in combination with other treatments.
- These studies typically use an observational study design.

BRADFORD-HILL CRITERIA FOR CAUSATION

- Due to the nature of the study design, consistent evidence from RCTs will usually lead us to conclude that there is a causal relationship between the intervention (exposure) and the disease outcome.
- However, due to issues regarding the internal validity of observational studies, assessing for causation is less straightforward.
- Suppose we carry out an observational study to investigate whether smoking causes lung cancer. We use a cohort study design and collect the relevant data, comparing the incidence of lung cancer in smokers and in non-smokers. To exclude the role of chance we carry out a statistical test, which yields a P-value < 0.05, thus providing evidence that the study is externally valid. Can we therefore conclude that smoking causes lung cancer? NOOOOOOOO!!! Well, not yet!
- As discussed in Chapter 1, we must first determine the internal validity of the study. This involves ensuring that the study was run carefully (research design, how variables were measured, etc.) and that the observed effect(s) are likely to be produced solely by the intervention being assessed (and not by another factor).
- The three main threats to internal validity are:
  - confounding
  - bias
  - causality.
- We exclude bias (discussed in Chapter 7) and confounding (discussed in Chapter 13) as the likely explanation for our findings. At this stage, we can safely conclude that there is a true *association* between smoking and lung cancer.
- Association, however, does not mean causation.
- In 1965, Austin Bradford-Hill proposed a series of considerations to help assess evidence of causation, which are known as the 'Bradford-Hill criteria'.
- These criteria serve as a guide and do not all need to be fulfilled before concluding that the relationship between two variables is causal.
- Observational studies can never establish that the relationship between two variables is causal. To demonstrate this point, let's return to the cohort study example discussed in Chapter 7 under the 'Confounding' subsection. A well-conducted cohort study showed that taking hormone replacement therapy (HRT) was associated with a reduced risk of coronary heart disease (CHD). However, a subsequent RCT showed that HRT does not reduce the risk of CHD. It turned out that women who took HRT were also more likely to be living a healthy lifestyle, and it was this that led to a reduction in CHD. Therefore, due to issues regarding the internal validity of observational studies, we must rely on well-conducted RCTs to establish a causal relationship between two variables.
- Figure 5.3 summarises the steps involved in assessing whether there is an association or causation

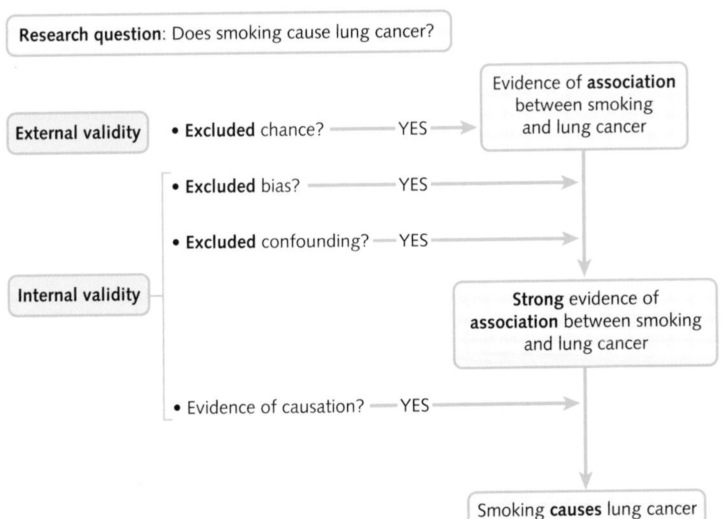

Fig. 5.3 Association versus causation.

between two variables. You must rely on evidence from multiple studies when assessing for evidence of causation. Let's go through the checklist of criteria in turn.

Strength of association

- The strength of the association is defined by the actual size of the association between two variables, as measured using the appropriate statistical test.
- The stronger the association:
  - the more likely that the relationship between the two variables is causal.
  - the less likely the relationship is due to confounding or bias.
- A small association does not rule out a casual effect. There is still an association!
- Regarding risk ratios (discussed in Chapter 7), those under 1.5 are generally regarded as pretty weak whilst those greater than 4.0 are strong.

Consistency

- The association is consistent when the results are replicated:
  - by different people
  - in different places
  - using different populations
  - using different study designs.
- Numerous studies must be carried out before a statement can be made about the causal relationship between two variables. However, because different exposure levels and other parameters may reduce the effect of the causal factor, a lack of consistency doesn't automatically rule out a causal association.

Specificity

- An association is specific if there is a one-to-one relationship between the cause and outcome. In other words, in the ideal situation, a single putative cause produces a specific effect. However, this is not always the case in medicine, where most exposures (e.g. smoking, diet) lead to numerous outcomes (e.g. lung cancer, heart disease).
- Absence of specificity in no way negates a causal relationship.

Temporal sequence

- The exposure *must* always precede the outcome. If there is an expected delay between the exposure and effect, then the effect must occur after that delay. This is the only absolutely essential criterion.
- The study design sometimes dictates whether it is easy to establish temporality. For example, as the exposure is measured at the start of the study, the temporal relationship between exposure and outcome is clear in prospective cohort studies.
- When measurements of the putative cause and the effect are made at the same time, as is the case in cross-sectional and case–control studies, it is difficult to establish a temporal sequence between the exposure and outcome; therefore, 'reverse causality' may be an issue. For example, case–control studies have shown that the inflammatory marker C-reactive protein (CRP) is higher in patients who have had a myocardial infarction. For a while, there was a feasible hypothesis that CRP levels could be used as a biomarker of myocardial infarction risk. However, clever Mendelian randomisation studies refuted this hypothesis. Instead, the inflammatory process associated with myocardial infarction was causing an increase in the levels of CRP (not the other way around).

Biological gradient (dose–response)

- There should be a direct relationship between the level of exposure and the risk of disease (or incidence of effect). This relationship may not be a simple linear relationship.
- In some cases, greater exposure leads to a lower incidence of effect. The presence of a dose–response relationship provides strong evidence that a causal relationship exists.
- However, as with specificity (discussed above), the absence of a dose–response relationship does not rule out a causal relationship. This is because in some cases, the mere presence of the exposure can trigger the effect.
- Conversely, a relationship may only exist above a certain exposure threshold.

Biological plausibility

- The apparent cause and effect must be plausible in the light of current knowledge. For example, is there a biological mechanism by which the exposure alters the risk of a disease?
- If a biological explanation appears to be outside the scope of current scientific knowledge, additional studies may be required before a true mechanism can be postulated. Consequently, the lack of a known mechanism should not rule out causality.

Coherence

- The association must be coherent with our existing knowledge within the relevant field.
- There should be no competing or conflicting information.

Reversibility (experimental evidence)

- Removing the exposure should reduce or prevent the disease outcome.
- Ideally, such evidence should come from RCTs.

Analogy

- It is necessary to determine whether other factors similar (or analogous) to the putative cause may also be causing the effect. For example, does a similar drug have the same effect on the disease outcome?
- Bradford-Hill suggests that existing similar associations would support causation.

CHOOSING THE RIGHT STUDY DESIGN

- There are a number of factors that must be taken into account when choosing the best study design to investigate your research question.
- In reality, the following four key issues are usually taken into account:
  1. The aim of the study
  2. The advantages and disadvantages of different study designs
  3. The resources available
  4. Ethical considerations.
- The advantages and disadvantages of the various types of studies covered above will be discussed in their respective chapters.
- Earlier in this chapter we introduced the idea that both interventional and observational studies play a role in clinical research. Once you've decided on your broad study design, the next step is to determine which type of study (e.g. cohort, case–control) best answers the research question.
- The flowchart shown in Fig. 5.4 may assist you in choosing among the different types of study designs.
- As shown in Fig. 5.4, it would be sensible to use a case–control or retrospective cohort study rather than a prospective cohort study:
  - if the outcome is rare.
  - if there is a relatively long time lag between the exposure and the outcome. This is also known as a long induction and latent period.
  - if there is a dynamic population due, for instance, to people moving in or out of the area. This is because it would be difficult to keep track of study participants who live in a population that is constantly changing; a fixed source population is preferred for cohort studies.

Using the hierarchy of evidence

- If a lot of research has already been carried out on the research question but there is no obvious answer, it may be appropriate to carry out a systematic review and meta-analysis.
- If observational studies show there is an association between two variables, but you are unsure whether there is a causal link between them, it may be appropriate to carry out an interventional study.
- If ecological or case–control studies have shown that there may be an association between two variables, moving up the hierarchy of evidence (discussed in Chapter 1), the next step may be to carry out a cohort study. However, if a number of case reports suggest that there may be an association between two variables, jumping straight to a cohort study would not be rational. It would be sensible to first gather additional evidence of association using a cheaper and less resource intensive study, such as using an ecological or cross-sectional study design. The graph shown in Fig. 5.5, which is based on the hierarchy of evidence, illustrates this point.
- Referring to Fig. 5.5, it is important to understand the following key points:
  - You are able to obtain more reliable evidence of causality from studies which are higher up in the hierarchy of evidence.
  - The initial discovery of a possible association between two variables doesn't always come from a case report. In other words, the starting point on the time axis (horizontal axis) isn't fixed.
  - If a study shows there may be an association between two variables, studies higher up in the hierarchy of evidence don't always agree with this finding. Therefore, time doesn't always equate to gathering more evidence of causality (despite the graph showing otherwise).

WRITING UP A RESEARCH STUDY

- The following guideline can be used for writing most types of research studies (e.g. cohort, case–control, cross-sectional).
- There are separate specific guidelines on how to report systematic reviews (Chapter 4), RCTs (Chapter 6) and case reports (Chapter 11).
- The following guideline will cover the following sections:
  - Title
  - Abstract
  - Introduction
  - Methods

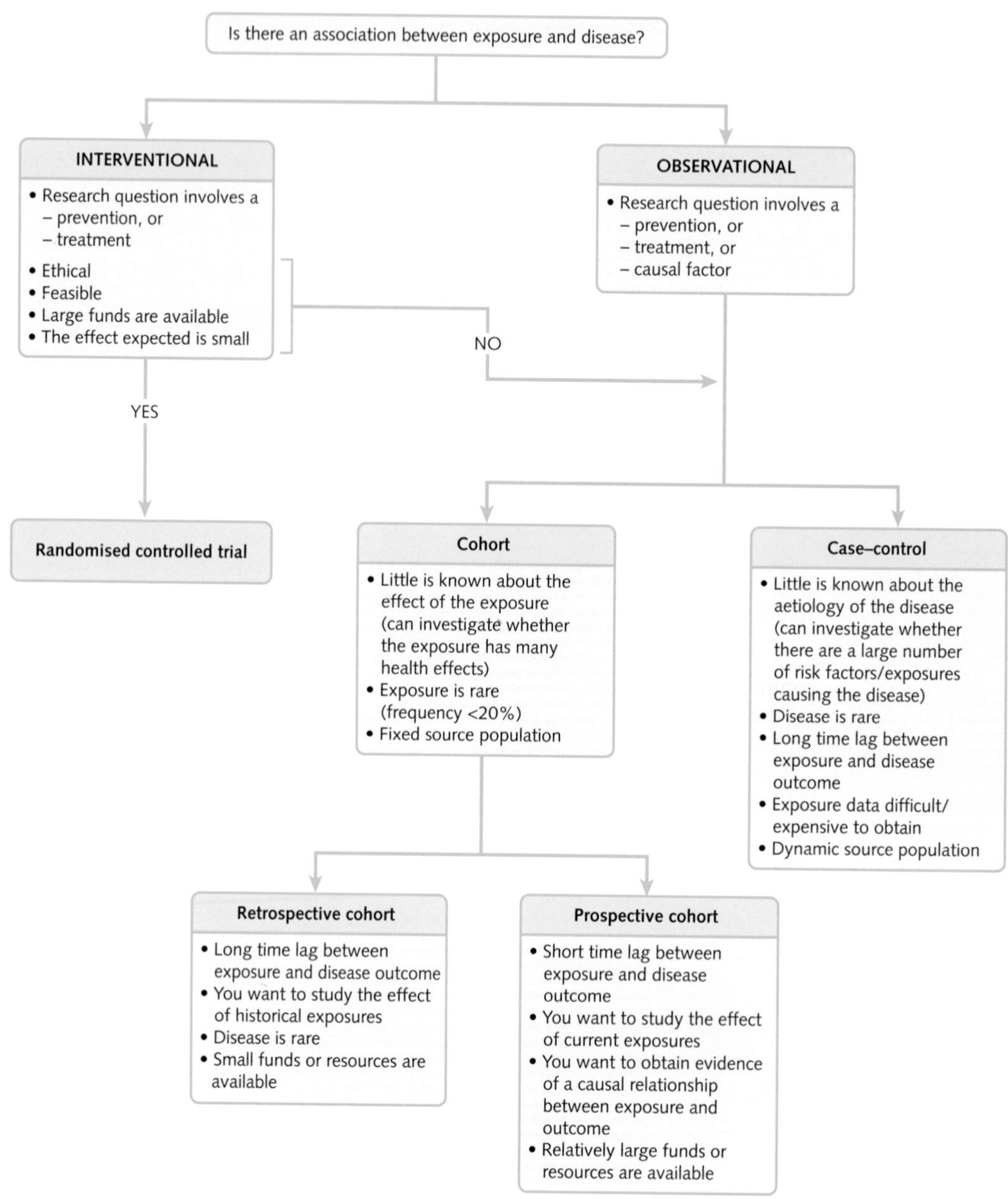

Fig. 5.4 Flowchart for choosing the right type of study.

- Results
- Discussion
- References.

Title

- The title is essentially a highly condensed version of the abstract.
- Your objective is to use the fewest number of words to accurately describe the content of the paper.

Abstract

- There is usually a strict word limit for the abstract, so carefully read the journal guidelines before you begin!

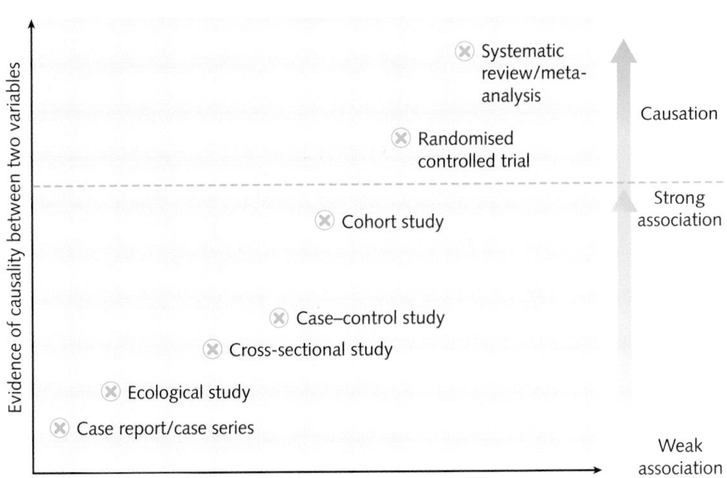

Fig. 5.5 Evidence of causality: choosing the right type of study.

- The abstract will help readers discern whether they are interested (or not) in reading the research report.
- For obvious reasons, the abstract is written after the rest of the paper is completed.
- As it is a summary of the work done, it should be written in the past tense.
- Complete sentences should be used to summarise the following elements of the study:
  - Purpose of the study – Background to the study, research question and objectives.
  - Methods – Brief description of the study protocol.
  - Results – Specific summarised data should be included; the results of any important statistical tests should be stated, including the confidence interval and *P*-value.
  - Discussion – Important reflective points.
  - Conclusion – Key finding/s from the study; any questions that follow from the study.
- The abstract should be engaging and to the point, highlighting only the key details from the main text.

Introduction

- You should grab the readers' attention at the start of the introduction, highlighting the important issues that your paper addresses.
- The purpose of the Introduction is to discuss the rationale behind the study.
- The opening sentence should take the reader straight to the issue.
- It is important to refrain from describing everything that is known about the topic. Instead, you should set the scene, citing the best evidence available, ideally from systematic reviews.
- By the end of the introduction, the reader should understand:
  - why your research was needed.
  - what was innovative about your work.
  - whether any controversies were addressed.
  - who will potentially benefit from the research.
- The Introduction should end with a clear research question, i.e. a specific hypothesis/objective.
- You should write the various sections of the paper using the active voice rather than the passive voice. For example, 'We compared the effect of drug A with . . .' rather than 'The effect of drug A was compared to . . .'.

Methods

- The objective of this section is to document all the methods used in your study, so that a reader would know exactly how to repeat the study.
- If necessary, you should include a clear statement of ethics committee approval and that subjects gave their informed consent for participating in the study.
- For studies handling quantitative data, you should:
  - specify the study design (e.g. observational or interventional, prospective or retrospective, controlled or uncontrolled).
  - describe how and why you chose the study sample, including details on:
    - how the sample size was determined. Was a sample size calculation performed prior to starting the study?
    - how participants were recruited for the study.
    - the sampling strategy, i.e. how you ensured the sample was representative of the population you chose to study.

    - your inclusion and exclusion criteria.
    - any steps taken to ensure selection bias was avoided.
  - describe the intervention and the comparison group.
  - identify the main study outcome variables, including specific details on:
    - what outcome was measured. Were there primary and secondary outcomes?
    - when the outcome was measured.
    - any steps taken to ensure measurement bias was avoided.
  - state which statistical methods were used to analyse your data.
- For studies handling qualitative data, you should:
  - explain why a qualitative approach was appropriate for answering your research question (as opposed to a quantitative approach).
  - explain how you selected the study participants and in which setting.
  - describe what methods were used for collecting data.
  - describe what methods were used for analysing the data, and whether any quality control measures were implemented.
  - include specific details on any steps taken to avoid bias when collecting or analysing the data.

HINTS AND TIPS

The primary outcome variable is the outcome of greatest importance. Data on secondary outcomes are used to evaluate any additional effects caused by the intervention/exposure. It is usually the primary outcome on which sample size calculations are based.

Results

- The purpose of the Results section is to present and illustrate your findings.
- This section should be a completely *objective* report of the results.
- In summary, you should:
  - summarise your data in the main text and illustrate them, if appropriate, with tables and figures.
  - provide some context to a statistical test before describing the result, i.e. describe the question that is going to be addressed by a particular statistical test.
  - analyse the data using appropriate statistical tests, stating:
    - the P-value
    - the 95% confidence interval of the mean (or proportion).
- You should avoid:
  - presenting the data more than once.
  - interpreting the results (save this for the Discussion section).
- The text should complement any tables or figures, not repeat the same information.
- As always, you should use the past tense when referring to your results.

HINTS AND TIPS

For each figure or table, you should remember to include a legend which:
- is numbered consecutively.
- consists of a title.
- conveys information about what the table or figure tells the reader.

Each table or figure must be sufficiently complete so that it stands on its own, separate from the text.

Discussion

- The objective of the Discussion is to provide an interpretation of your results, using evidence from the literature to make your conclusions.
- The Discussion should start with a sentence that describes your principal finding.
- The strengths and weaknesses of the study design should both be discussed to help you interpret the validity of the findings.
- The results should be discussed with reference to previous research. Do your results:
  - fit in with what is already known about the topic?
  - reach different conclusions to those stated in the literature? If so, why?
- It is important to explain all your observations as much as possible. For example:
  - what are the possible mechanisms linking one variable to another?
  - what are the policy and practice implications of your results?
- You should end the Discussion with a paragraph highlighting any questions left unanswered and ideas for future research.
- Again, refer to work done by specific individuals (including yourself) in the past tense.

References

- All sources of information referred to in the research paper should be acknowledged in the references section at the end of the paper.
- The Harvard Referencing System is a collection of rules that standardises the format in which common types of material (e.g. books, journal articles, websites) are referenced.

Journal articles

Journal articles are usually laid out like this:

Authors(s). (Year) Title of article. *Title of journal*. Volume number (part/issue): Page number.

The title of the journal is usually abbreviated. For example,

Doll R and Hill AB. (1954) The mortality of doctors in relation to their smoking habits. *Br Med J*. 1(4877): 1451–1455.

Books

Books are usually laid out like this:

Authors(s). (Year) *Title of book*. Edition. Place of publication: Publisher.

For books with one or more editors, you include the abbreviation (ed.) or (eds) after their surname. You only include the edition if the book is not in its first edition. For example,

Khot A and Polmear A. (eds) (2010) *Practical General Practice: Guidelines for Effective Clinical Management*. 6th edn. Edinburgh: Elsevier, Churchill Livingstone.

Chapters in books

Chapters in books are usually laid out like this:

Authors(s). (Year) Title of chapter. In: Author(s)/Editor(s). *Title of book*. Edition. Place of publication: Publisher.

For example,

Jeremy JY, Kaura A, Sablayrolles JL and Angelini GD. (2010) Saphenous vein graft attrition. In: Escaned J and Serruys PW (eds) *Coronary Stenosis. Imaging, Structure and Physiology*. Toulouse, France: PCR Publishing.

Websites

A website should be treated similarly to a print work; i.e. it should have an author or editor and a title. You should include the *full* address of the website and also the date on which the page was accessed. Websites are usually laid out like this:

Authors(s). (Year) Website title. Web address [accessed day month year].

For example,

The foundation programme. (2012) Academic Programmes. http://www.foundationprogramme.nhs.uk/pages/academic-programmes [accessed 14 May 2012].

Dissertations and theses

These are usually laid out like this:

Authors(s). (Year) *Title*. Designation (Level, e.g. MSc, PhD), Institution.

If the piece of work has not been published, you include this after the title. For example,

Wayne B. (2012) *How I Became Batman!* Unpublished dissertation (MSc), DC University.

Verbal materials: interviews

Interviews are usually laid out like this:

Named Person(s). (Year) *Title for interview*. Conducted by (name) on (date) at (location).

For example,

Simpson H. (2012) *Interview on the World's Best Doughnut*. Conducted by Kaura A, on 21 November 2010 at Springfield nuclear power plant, USA.

Unpublished material: lecture notes

Lecture notes are usually laid out like this:

Lecturer(s). (Year) *Title of lecture*. Course/module name, Institution where delivered, Date delivered [Lecture notes taken by (name)].

For example,

Parker P. (1984) *How to Become a Spiderman (or Spiderwoman)!* BSc Genetics, Marvel University, 14 June 1984 [Lecture notes taken by Kaura A].

Randomised controlled trials

Objectives

By the end of this chapter you should:

- Be able to identify and critically appraise randomised controlled trials.
- Know the steps involved in carrying out a randomised controlled trial.
- Understand the key differences between the various types of randomised controlled trial study designs used in clinical practice.
- Be able to interpret the results of a randomised controlled trial.
- Know how to interpret and calculate the 'numbers needed to treat' for benefit or harm.
- Understand the common sources of bias implicated in randomised controlled trials.
- Understand the terms confounding and causality in relation to randomised controlled trials.
- Be able to list the advantages and disadvantages of randomised controlled trials.
- Know how a randomised controlled trial is reported.

A methodological checklist on how to critically appraise randomised controlled trials is provided in Chapter 19.

WHY CHOOSE AN INTERVENTIONAL STUDY DESIGN?

- As introduced in Chapter 5, interventional studies test whether intervening in some way leads to a measurable variation in the outcome.
- The intervention usually involves a particular treatment or practice.
- As highlighted by Hennekens (1987), interventional studies test either preventative or therapeutic interventions, including:
    - prophylactic agents
    - therapeutic agents
    - surgical procedures
    - diagnostic agents
    - health service strategies.
- Therapeutic trials are conducted on individuals with a particular disease to evaluate whether a certain procedure or agent has an effect on a specific outcome, such as symptomatic relief or reduced mortality.
- Preventative trials are conducted to investigate whether a certain procedure or agent reduces the risk of developing a particular disease. The individuals (or entire communities) enrolled at the beginning of the trial should be free from that disease, but deemed to be at risk.
- Regardless of whether the trial is based on therapeutic or preventative research:
    - the intervention being tested is allocated (not always randomly) by the investigator to a group of participants (the test group).
    - the study participants are followed up, prospectively, to compare the test group to the control group (gold standard treatment, placebo or no treatment).
- Let's start by discussing one of the most commonly used interventional study designs, the parallel randomised controlled trial (RCT).

PARALLEL RANDOMISED CONTROLLED TRIAL

Study design

- An RCT is an interventional study during which study participants are randomised to different treatment options.
- It is this process of randomisation that makes RCTs the most rigorous method for determining a cause–effect relationship between an intervention and an outcome, thus placing RCTs at the top of the hierarchy of evidence (Fig. 1.5).
- They are only bettered when the results of several RCTs are pooled together in a meta-analysis, as part of a systematic review (discussed in Chapter 4).
- A 'parallel' RCT involves randomly assigning individuals from the sample population to different

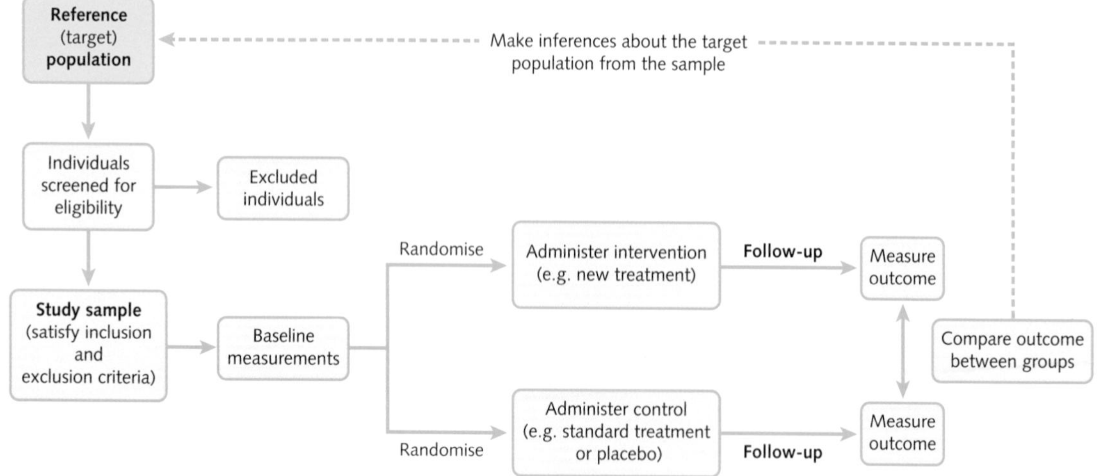

Fig. 6.1 Parallel RCT study design.

interventions (usually two, the intervention and control 'arm' (e.g. gold standard treatment or placebo), but there may be more than two arms). These groups are then followed up prospectively to assess the effectiveness of the intervention compared with the control. This parallel study design is illustrated in Fig. 6.1.

- The essential steps involved in a parallel RCT are:
    1. Formulate the *hypothesis* (discussed in Chapter 1). For example,

       We hypothesise that the 2-year mortality risk in patients receiving treatment A is 30% lower than the mortality risk in patients receiving standard treatment.
    2. Define the methods of recruitment, including the *inclusion* and *exclusion criteria.*
    3. Define the *intervention* (discussed above).
    4. Define the comparison group.
    5. Determine the *sample size.*
    6. Specify the *outcome measures* that will be used to assess the effectiveness of the intervention.
    7. Obtain ethical approval.
    8. Obtain *informed consent* before the study participants are randomised to either the intervention or control.
    9. Generate and conceal an allocation sequence to ensure *randomisation.*
    10. Indicate whether the assessors and/or study participants have any knowledge of the treatment allocation (*blinding*).
    11. Perform an *intention to treat* analysis.

Inclusion/exclusion criteria

- There should be a clear statement highlighting which individuals are eligible to participate in the RCT.
- Some individuals are excluded if it is too risky (contraindicated) to give them the new intervention or to deny them the conventional (gold standard) treatment.
- Some investigators restrict eligibility:
    - if they feel the intervention will have a different effect in different groups of people. Therefore, to ensure the internal validity of the findings, patients with multiple co-morbid conditions are often excluded.
    - By focusing on patients with a higher event rate, which:
        - lowers the required sample size (by increasing the power of the study).
        - shortens the required follow-up period.
- Having strict inclusion or exclusion criteria limits the generalisability and thus the external validity of the RCT. If the inclusion or exclusion criteria are too restrictive, the results of the study can only be applied to a select group of patients. However, these trials provide data that are often used to inform the justification of the intervention for all patients. The resulting guidelines may therefore offer a simplistic, potentially inadequate approach to using the intervention in clinical practice.
- Members of the population may be excluded if they have certain co-morbid conditions or have particular demographic features (race, age, gender etc.). For example, trials on the treatment of hypertension were, for decades, limited to patients under 80 years old. There was therefore no evidence on which to base a decision on treating hypertension in the older patient. As a result, the myth that hypertension in the elderly did not require treatment was allowed to persist, at the expense of the lives of many older patients!

Excluding patients with co-morbid conditions

The question of excluding patients with co-morbidities, such as those with cardiac, pulmonary or renal disease, is complex. These patients are more likely to die from, or to become ill with, conditions unrelated to the intervention being tested, therefore weakening the power of the trial to detect a real benefit from the intervention. Having never been tested in those with co-morbidities (often elderly patients), the intervention may perform unpredictably in these patients when used in clinical practice.

HINTS AND TIPS

The patient groups commonly under-represented in trials include:

- pregnant women
- children
- individuals with co-morbidities
- the elderly
- individuals with mental illness, including dementia.

Choice of comparator

- An important feature of an RCT is that it should be comparative.
- Once you've defined the intervention, the next step is to choose the comparator.
- The intervention and comparison groups are known as the 'arms' of the trial.
- There may be more than one comparison group, e.g. comparing the intervention to the gold standard treatment (best available treatment) and a placebo.
- The comparator chosen (known as the control) will influence how we interpret the evidence about the intervention from the trial.
- If the control chosen is an inert treatment (placebo), the intervention may show a more favourable outcome (i.e. the importance of the new intervention may be overstated) than if the control was another active treatment, such as the gold standard. Placebos or using no treatment at all are known as negative controls. Using the gold standard treatment is known as a positive control.
- As highlighted by the Declaration of Helsinki, item 32, comparing the active intervention against a placebo when an active treatment exists would be unethical:

The benefits, risks, burdens and effectiveness of a new intervention must be tested against those of the best current proven intervention, except in the following circumstances:

- *The use of placebo, or no treatment, is acceptable in studies where no current proven intervention exists; or*
- *Where for compelling and scientifically sound methodological reasons the use of placebo is necessary to determine the efficacy or safety of an intervention and the patients who receive placebo or no treatment will not be subject to any risk of serious or irreversible harm.*

HINTS AND TIPS

A placebo is a treatment which looks, feels and even tastes like the new interventional drug being tested but contains no active ingredients whatsoever.

Sample size

- The RCT should have enough subjects to detect the smallest difference in effect size between the two study arms that is clinically important. This effect size should be informed by clinical judgement, not by the effect sizes observed in previous studies.
- A larger sample size is required if the *clinically* significant difference in effect size is small. In other words, more data are required to distinguish a small treatment effect from a random sampling error.
- In addition to the effect size, the size of the sample is dependent on:
  - the power of the study (often set at 80 or 90%)
  - the stated level of statistical significance (often $P = 0.05$)
  - the standard deviation of the data for each group.
- Please refer to the section 'Statistical power' in Chapter 3 for a discussion on how to calculate the sample size for a comparative study.
- If the sample size has not been given in a research paper or if the calculated sample size was not achieved, the study may have been too small to detect a clinically significant difference in effect size between the two groups.

The outcome measure

- The outcome is what is measured in all subjects after they have been treated with the intervention or control.

- The outcome measured as part of the trial should give the investigator an indication of the effectiveness of the intervention (and the control).
- Various aspects of the outcome need to be considered to properly assess the effectiveness of the treatment:
  - *Disease aspect*: Mortality or survival rate, lab tests, complications, major events, side effects, etc.
  - *Patient aspect*: Health-related quality of life, symptoms, activities of daily living, etc.
  - *Economic aspect*: Service utilisation (e.g. length of stay or number of GP visits) or social disruption (e.g. returning to work).
- The outcome measured should be:
  - precisely defined; this reduces or prevents misclassification
  - measureable
  - repeatable
  - reliable
  - relevant from both a healthcare professional and patient point of view.
- It is important to specify how and at what time points these outcomes should be measured.
- While many outcome measures may be assessed in a single trial, it is important to define a primary outcome variable, which:
  - is the outcome of greatest importance.
  - has the strongest influence on the conclusions of the trial.
  - will inform the sample size calculations.
- Data on secondary outcomes are used to evaluate any additional effects caused by the intervention.
- While the sample size may be large enough to determine a treatment effect based on the primary outcome, it may be too small to detect a clinically important difference on secondary outcomes.

Ethical issues

- All research studies must receive research ethics committee approval before being undertaken.
- Considering that the investigators are 'intervening' in peoples' lives, RCTs raise a number of important ethical issues, including:
  - Clinical equipoise
  - Informed consent.

Clinical equipoise

- Healthcare professionals treating the patients must have sufficient doubt about the relative effectiveness of the treatments being compared.
- There must be no evidence that the new intervention is better, worse or the same as:
  - any of the treatments currently being used in clinical practice, or
  - the placebo.
- As highlighted earlier in this chapter, if an effective treatment is available, the new intervention should be compared against this, not a placebo.
- If these criteria are satisfied, the trial has 'clinical equipoise'.

HINTS AND TIPS

There is clinical equipoise if there is an equal chance of benefit, harm or no effect, regardless of which treatment arm of the trial a study participant is randomised to.

Informed consent

- *Informed* consent must be obtained from all patients recruited to an RCT.
- Two key steps must be addressed to ensure that an individual gives valid informed consent to participate in a trial:
  - Disclosure of information
  - Capacity of the subject.
- *Disclosure* requires the investigator to supply the subject with an adequate amount of information so that he or she can make an autonomous decision about whether to participate in the trial.
- The investigator should use lay language to communicate the details of the study to the eligible subjects.
- According to the Declaration of Helsinki, item 24:

> *Each potential subject must be adequately informed of the aims, methods, sources of funding, any possible conflicts of interest, institutional affiliations of the researcher, the anticipated benefits and potential risks of the study and the discomfort it may entail, and any other relevant aspects of the study.*

- The next step is to ensure that the patient has the *capacity* to make a decision about participating in the trial.
- The potential subject must understand the information provided, weigh up the risks and benefits of taking part in the trial and then communicate his or her decision to the investigator.
- The consent must be voluntary; i.e. the decision made is not subject to external pressure such as coercion or manipulation.
- Ideally, the consent should be confirmed in writing; however, if this is not possible, it is important to ensure that non-written consent is formally documented and witnessed.
- There is usually a 'cooling-off period' to allow subjects sufficient time to change their minds if they wish to do so.

- Whether or not the individual decides to participate in the trial, his or her future access to health services or treatment should not be affected.

What if the intervention is perceived by the study participants to be better and more desirable than the control?

- This may happen if the intervention is a full programme of care, while the control is usual care. For example, in 2009, an RCT assessed the effectiveness of supervised exercise therapy compared with usual care, in patients with patellofemoral pain syndrome. Outcome measures included assessing pain scores, functional status and patient recovery. The intervention group received a standardised exercise programme for 6 weeks and the control group were assigned usual care, which compromised a 'wait and see' approach of rest during periods of pain. In trials similar to this, it is not possible to mask the intervention; i.e. the study participants are able to tell which study arm they have been randomly allocated to.
- In an attempt to prevent subjects from dropping out of the trial if they are allocated to the control group, some investigators decide in advance to offer the new intervention to all subjects randomly allocated to the control group after the end of the trial, assuming the intervention proves to have a beneficial effect. This will have to be taken into account when the trial finances are being considered.

Randomisation

- Each study participant has the same probability of being allocated to a particular treatment arm. This process is known as random allocation, which forms the essence of RCTs.
- Randomisation ensures that those patient characteristics which may affect the outcome measure are distributed evenly between the groups. With this in mind, provided that the trial is reasonably large, any observed differences between the study arms are due to differences in the treatment alone and not due to the effects of confounding factors (known or unknown) or selection bias (discussed below). In other words, large, well-conducted RCTs have internal validity.

Methods of randomisation

- There are four main methods used to randomise patients to the different study arms:
  1. Simple randomisation.
  2. Block randomisation.
  3. Stratified randomisation.
  4. Minimisation.

Simple randomisation

- Random numbers can be generated using a computer program:
  - As a patient enters the trial, the computer program provides an allocation *code* which refers to a particular treatment.
  - An alternative approach is to produce a computer-generated list of sequential random allocations to the different treatment arms.

Block randomisation

- Considering it can take many months before a sufficient number of subjects have been entered into a trial, block randomisation is used to ensure that the number of participants assigned to each treatment arm are very similar at any stage during the recruitment process. A computer randomisation software can be programmed to ensure that every 'block' of patients (e.g. every hundred) contains an equal number allocated to each arm of the trial. This method is commonly used in smaller trials.

Stratified randomisation

- Stratified randomisation is used to ensure that important baseline confounding factors are more evenly distributed between the treatment arms rather than leaving it to chance.
- The confounding factors balanced by stratification are usually those that are important prognostic factors for the particular disease you are investigating. For example, in a trial of women with breast cancer, it may be important to have similar numbers of pre- and post-menopausal women in each treatment group. Prior to randomisation, participants would be separated into two different groups (strata) according to their menopausal status. Equal numbers of participants would then be randomly allocated to each treatment arm within the strata. To ensure that there are an equal number of participants in each treatment arm, this method of treatment allocation, within each stratum, may be based on the block randomisation method (discussed above).

Minimisation

- Similar to stratified randomisation, minimisation may be used to balance the numbers of prognostic factors in each treatment arm.
- In minimisation, the first participant is allocated a treatment at random. Each subsequent participant is allocated to the intervention arm that would lead to a better balance between the groups in the variable (prognostic factor) of interest.

HINTS AND TIPS

Patients are not always randomly allocated in equal proportions to the different treatment arms. For example, an investigator may choose a randomisation method to ensure that 60% of the study participants receive the intervention while 40% receive the usual treatment. This is still random allocation, as each study participant will have the same 60% probability of being allocated to the intervention. The investigators may wish to obtain extra information about the novel intervention if sufficient information is already known about the effectiveness of the usual treatment.

Allocation sequence concealment

- The second part of randomisation is to ensure that the random allocation sequence is concealed. This involves making sure that the patients and the investigators enrolling the patients cannot foresee treatment group assignment. If this allocation process is not adequately concealed, there is potential for selection bias and confounding (discussed below).
- Examples of adequate concealment include:
  - central randomisation at a site remote from the trial location (usually the gold standard).
  - using sequentially numbered, opaque, sealed envelopes (however, this approach is open to tampering).
  - coding and packaging drugs at an independent pharmacy in a drug trial.

HINTS AND TIPS

Concealment is different to blinding; while the allocation sequence can *always* be concealed *at the time of recruitment* in an RCT, the feasibility of blinding depends on the particular interventions being investigated. Therefore, while all interventions are technically concealable, they are not all blindable!

HINTS AND TIPS

If randomisation has been successful, the two treatment arm groups should be similar. The investigators can assess this by measuring and comparing various baseline characteristics, such as age, gender and disease severity, between the two groups. Large differences in the baseline characteristics may be due to:

- random allocation not being random, due to issues with generating or concealing the allocation sequence.
- chance variation, especially if the sample size is small.

Blinding

- Blinding refers to patients and investigators (including those involved in recruitment and assessing the outcome) having no knowledge of treatment allocation.
- Traditionally, blinded RCTs have been classified as 'single-blind', 'double-blind' or 'triple-blind'. However, due to inconsistency in definitions of these terms and lack of clarity in journals, it is better to specify who exactly was blinded and how.
- If the intervention is an active drug, it is possible for both the subject and investigator to be blind to treatment allocation if the comparison group takes an inactive placebo, which looks, tastes and feels exactly like the active drug.
- RCTs may also use an active placebo that mimics the common side effects of the drug under study. For example, in a study assessing the effects of morphine and gabapentin (painkillers) on neuropathic pain, lorazepam was chosen as an active placebo as it mimicked the side effects of the painkillers (dizziness and sleepiness).
- It is important to note that blinding may not be possible if the RCT involves:
  - a technology, e.g. surgery versus chemotherapy.
  - a programme of care, e.g. exercise therapy versus medication.
- In these studies, known as open-label trials, randomisation should still be used and the outcome assessor should still be blind (if possible) to which treatment the participant received.

CONFOUNDING, CAUSALITY AND BIAS

Confounding

- Confounding occurs when the exposure of interest is not only associated with the risk of disease but also associated with a third variable that provides an alternative explanation for any association measured between the exposure and disease (please refer to Chapter 13 for an in-depth discussion on confounding).
- As discussed above, the aim of random allocation is to ensure that the treatment groups are similar in composition with respect to prognostic factors, demographics or any other factor. In other words, randomising trial

participants reduces confounding between treatment groups. Therefore, any differences in outcome are due to actual differences in the treatment.

- Confounding would be an issue if, for example, being male was a poor prognostic factor for a given disease, and the distribution of sexes was not equal between the treatment groups investigating that disease.

Causality

- RCTs are considered as the most rigorous of all methods of determining whether a cause–effect relationship exists between an intervention and outcome.
- As the exposure is assigned at the start of the study, the temporal relationship between exposure and outcome is clear.
- For a more in-depth discussion on causality, please refer to the Bradford-Hill criteria, which are discussed in Chapter 5.

Bias

- The reliability of the results of an RCT also depends on the extent to which potential sources of bias have been avoided. For an introduction to systematic error and bias, please refer to the 'Bias' section in Chapter 7. Systematic error can be divided into selection bias and measurement bias (Fig. 6.2).
- As there is usually more interest in showing that an intervention works than in showing that it has no beneficial effect, bias in RCTs tends to lead to an exaggeration in the importance or effectiveness of a new intervention.

Selection bias

- Selection bias occurs when the association between an intervention and outcome is different for those who complete the study, compared with those who are in the target population. Selection bias may exist when procedures for subject selection or factors that influence subject participation affect the outcome of the study. The main types of selection bias that may occur in RCTs include:
  - Bias associated with randomisation
    - Random sequence generation bias
    - Allocation of intervention bias.
  - Bias during study implementation
    - Contamination bias
    - Loss-to-follow-up bias.

Bias associated with randomisation: random sequence generation bias and allocation of intervention bias

- If the randomisation sequence is not truly random (random sequence generation bias), there is potential for selection bias.

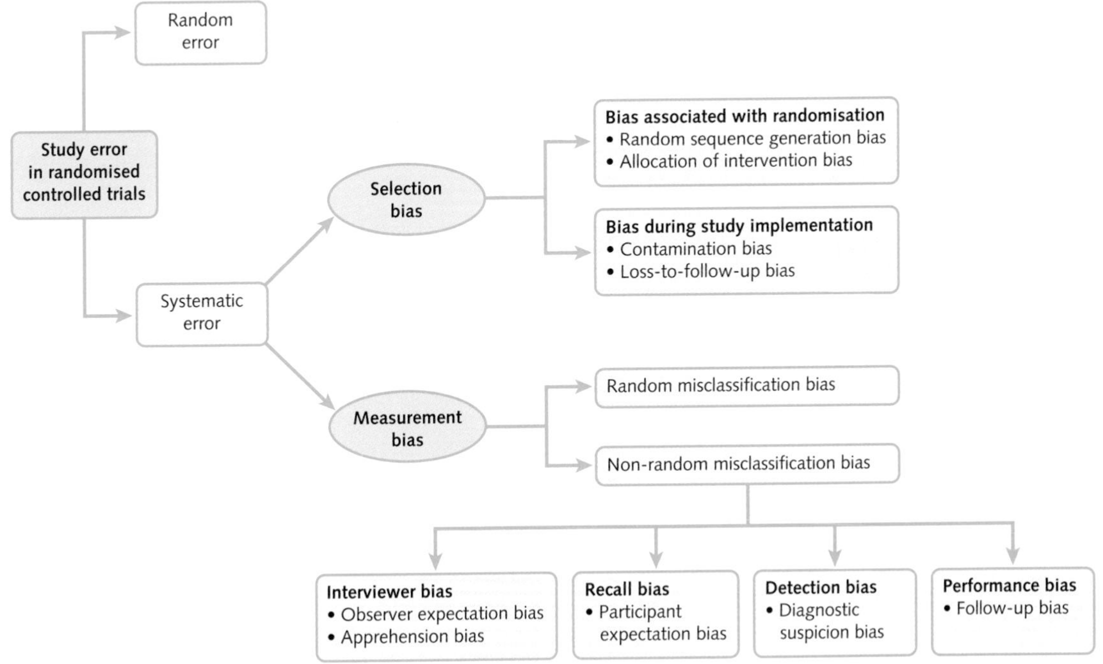

Fig. 6.2 Study error in randomised controlled trials.

- Even if the randomisation sequence is truly random, selection bias may still be an issue if allocation is not concealed at the time of recruitment (allocation of intervention bias):
  - The investigator may recruit patients for the intervention based on their prognosis.
  - A patient may decide to take part in the trial only if they are allocated to one treatment arm and not the other.
- This will lead to systematic differences between the participants in the different treatment groups. Therefore, differences in the outcome may be explained by pre-existing differences between the groups rather than due to differences that exist between the treatments.
- There is empirical evidence confirming that the effects of new interventions can be exaggerated if an RCT has poor allocation concealment. One study has shown that the intervention effect size may, on average, be exaggerated by as much as 40%.

Bias during study implementation: contamination bias

- Contamination may be an issue if there is unintentional (or intentional) application of the intervention in the control group. Alternatively, there may be unintentional (or intentional) failure to give the intervention to those study participants randomly assigned to it.
- The intervention effect is biased towards the null.
- Contamination bias occurs more frequently in community RCTs because of the relationships that exist between members who reside in different communities and due to interference from the media or other health professionals.
- Group randomisation (i.e. in cluster randomised trials) reduces the likelihood of contamination bias.

Bias during study implementation: loss-to-follow-up bias

- Attrition refers to the loss of subjects during the course of a trial; i.e. these subjects are lost to follow-up.
- Loss-to-follow-up bias (or attrition bias) refers to systematic differences between the treatment groups in terms of the number of subjects lost, or differences in characteristics between those not adhering to the study protocol and those who remain in the study.
- Attrition applies to those subjects:
  - excluded after the allocation process, e.g. if they don't actually satisfy the eligibility criteria.
  - who don't adhere to the treatment course (regardless of whether outcome measurements are still taken). If the subject knows which treatment he has been allocated to, this may affect his decision regarding treatment withdrawal or compliance.
  - who won't comply with having outcome measurements taken (regardless of whether they adhered to the treatment course).
  - who are lost to follow-up for any reason, e.g. they move out of the area, or they die when out of the area and their death is not reported to the investigators.
- It is important to consider not only why subjects were lost to follow-up but also how many.
- As mentioned above, it is possible that those subjects lost to follow-up have different characteristics to those who adhere to the trial protocol.
- The reliability of the results are therefore in question if these two parameters (reason for loss to follow-up and the number of subjects affected) are not comparable between the two treatment groups. For example, participants may drop out due to the side effects caused by the new intervention. Excluding these participants from the analysis could result in an overestimation of the effectiveness of the intervention, especially when the proportion of people dropping out varies between the treatment groups (thus causing attrition bias). In an attempt to try and minimise the degree of attrition bias, an intention to treat analysis (ITT) is usually performed (discussed below).

HINTS AND TIPS

One technique commonly used to assess the likely impact of attrition (loss-to-follow-up) is to calculate the percentage of participants affected. If attrition affects:

- <5% of the study participants, bias will be minimal.
- >20%, then bias is likely to be considerable.

The potential impact of loss to follow-up can be assessed by carrying out a 'best case worst case' sensitivity analysis (discussed below).

Measurement bias

Measurement bias occurs when the information collected for the exposure and/or outcome variables is inaccurate. This type of bias can be divided into random or non-random misclassification bias.

Random misclassification bias

Random misclassification bias (also known as non-differential misclassification bias) can occur when misclassification is the same across the groups being compared. For example, the outcome is equally misclassified in both treatment arms. The treatment groups therefore seem more similar than they actually are, leading to an underestimation (dilution) of the true effect of the intervention on the disease outcome. Random misclassification bias is discussed in further detail in Chapter 7.

Non-random misclassification bias

Non-random misclassification bias (also known as differential misclassification bias) occurs only when misclassification is different in the treatment groups being compared. It can lead to the intervention effect on the disease outcome being biased in either direction. The main types of non-random misclassification bias that may occur in RCTs include:

- Performance bias
  - Follow-up bias
- Detection bias
  - Diagnostic suspicion bias
- Recall bias
  - Participant expectation bias
- Interviewer bias
  - Observer expectation bias
  - Apprehension bias.

Performance bias

- Performance bias may exist if the investigators were not kept blind to the treatment allocation.
- Performance bias is a type of non-random misclassification measurement bias.
- It refers to systematic differences between the two treatment groups in the care that is provided, other than having different treatments.
- If the investigator knows which treatment arm the patient was allocated to, this may bias the results, either intentionally or unintentionally. Depending on treatment allocation, the investigator may:
  - administer other effective interventions (co-interventions)
  - perform different investigations
  - provide additional advice.

  This type of bias is known as follow-up bias.
- However, as alluded to previously, blinding is not always possible!
- It is important to think about the likely size and direction of the bias caused by lack of sufficient blinding. Studies have shown that the intervention effect size may be exaggerated by as much as 17%.

Detection bias

- Detection bias refers to systematic differences between the groups in how the outcomes are measured.
- It is a type of non-random misclassification measurement bias.
- Similar to the concept behind performance bias, failure to blind the investigators assessing the outcome can lead to variation in how the outcome is measured between the groups. This is especially the case if the outcomes measured are subjective. In other words, knowledge of the subject's prior exposure status to a putative cause may have an influence on the intensity (and possibly the outcome) of the diagnostic process. This type of detection bias is known as diagnostic suspicion bias.
- In addition to ensuring that the outcome assessors are kept blind to treatment allocation (and other important confounding factors), valid and reliable methods should be used to determine precisely defined outcomes in all subjects.
- It is important that an RCT has an appropriate length of follow-up to identify the outcome of interest. For example, for outcomes that occur late following an exposure, an RCT with a relatively short follow-up period will give an imprecise estimate of the effect, which may lead to detection bias.

Recall bias

- If the subject knows which treatment he has been allocated to, this may affect his decision regarding his beliefs about the effectiveness of the treatment. For example, subjects who *knowingly* receive a new treatment for chronic pain may expect that it is having a positive effect on their pain levels. They are therefore more likely to perceive having less pain compared to if they were knowingly allocated to the usual treatment. This type of bias, known as participant expectation bias (a type of recall bias), can be prevented if the subjects are kept blind to their treatment allocation.

Interviewer bias

- Please refer to Chapter 7 on cohort studies for a discussion on interviewer bias, which may be an issue when questioning subjects about their disease status.

INTERPRETING THE RESULTS

- After randomisation, individuals are followed up to ascertain whether there is an association between the intervention and outcome.
- As RCTs are prospective, it is possible to estimate a number of outcome measures, including:
  - *Risk ratio (or odds ratio)*: The ratio of the event rate in the intervention group and in the control group (discussed in Chapter 7 (risk ratio) and 8 (odds ratio)).
  - *Risk difference*: The difference between the intervention and control groups, as a rate (discussed in Chapter 7).
  - *Intervention event rate*: The incidence of the event in the intervention arm. The event may be cure, death, side effect, etc.

- *Control event rate*: The incidence of the event in the control arm.
- *Number needed to treat* (*NNT*): Discussed below.
- The types of statistical methods used in RCTs depend on the characteristics of the data (discussed in Chapter 15).
- Regardless of the statistical method used, the following should be considered when analysing an RCT:
    - Interim analysis
    - Adjusting for confounders
    - Intention to treat analysis
    - Sensitivity analysis
    - Subgroup analysis
    - Numbers needed to treat for benefit and harm.

Interim analysis

- The investigators may wish to carry out some preplanned interim analyses to assess whether the RCT should be stopped early. For example, an RCT may be stopped early if the intervention produces an effect that is larger than the expected benefit or harm.

Adjusting for confounders

- If a simple randomisation approach is used in a small RCT, key prognostic factors (which are measured at baseline, at the start of the trial) may be distributed unevenly in the intervention and control groups. If this is the case, it is possible to mathematically adjust the study results by taking into account those confounders that are strongly related to the outcome and are distributed unevenly between the treatment arms.
- Please refer to Chapter 15 for a discussion on the statistical methods used to adjust the exposure–outcome relationship for the effects of one or more confounders.

Intention to treat analysis

- ITT analysis refers to the analysis that compares outcomes based on the original treatment arm that each individual participant was randomised to, regardless of violations to the protocol. In other words, patients are analysed in the treatment groups to which they were randomised to and not on the basis of whether their allocated treatment course was actually completed.
- As highlighted above, reasons for these protocol violations may include:
    - subjects being lost to follow-up.
    - ineligibility, i.e. subjects who should not have been enrolled in the study in the first place!
    - non-compliance to the allocated treatment; e.g. an individual stops taking the intervention after 5 days of starting the treatment course.
- An ITT analysis is usually performed, as the treatment groups are only comparable at the time of randomisation. People who violate the protocol tend to be systematically different from those who comply.
- ITT therefore provides an unbiased comparison of the treatments.
- An analysis including only those who adhered to their allocated treatment is known as a 'per-protocol' or 'on-treatment' analysis. Figure 6.3 illustrates the difference between the ITT and per-protocol analyses.

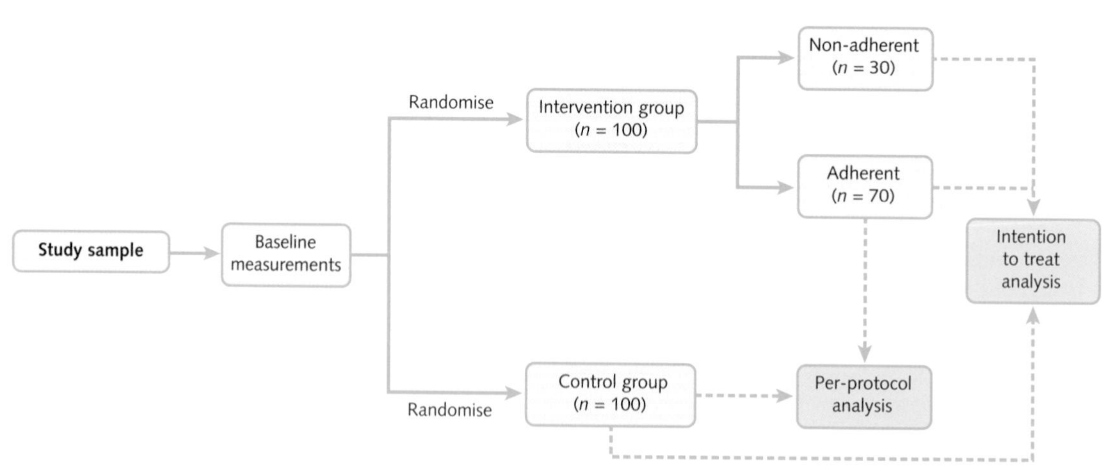

Fig. 6.3 Intention to treat versus per-protocol analysis.

Efficacy versus effectiveness

- If the aim of the trial is to assess:
  - the effectiveness of the intervention, you are wondering how well it works in clinical practice (i.e. in those *offered it*). The ITT is the most appropriate analysis to assess effectiveness.
  - the efficacy of the intervention, you are wondering whether the intervention works in the people who *actually receive it*. The per-protocol analysis is the most appropriate analysis to assess efficacy.

Sensitivity analysis

- It is important to keep track of the study participants and measure outcome data from as many of those who remain in the study as possible.
- When interpreting the findings, a detailed account of what happened to all the subjects should be included.
- It may be impossible to include a particular individual in the analysis if there is missing data, unless you use:
  - interim data, if available
  - statistical modelling.
- A 'best case worst case' sensitivity analysis can be used to assess the impact that loss to follow-up had on the data.
  - In the best case scenario, all the subjects lost to follow-up are assigned the best possible outcome, e.g. no adverse event, if this was the primary outcome.
  - In the worst case scenario, all the subjects lost to follow-up are assigned the worst possible outcome.
- The study findings are questionable if:
  - there is a high loss to follow-up.
  - there is a wide range for the best and worst case sensitivity results.
- For example, in a hypothetical RCT, only 80 of the 140 participants assigned to the intervention arm adhered to the treatment and were available for follow-up.
  - The rate of loss to follow-up was therefore (140 − 80)/140 = 42.9%, which is very high!
  - Suppose the primary disease outcome occurred in 25% (20 of 80) of the participants who were successfully followed up in the intervention arm. The results of the 'best case worst case' sensitivity analysis would be:
    - Best case: 20/140 = 14.3%.
    - Worst case: (20 + 60)/140 = 57.1%.
  - You would be cautious when interpreting the findings as:
    - there is a high loss to follow-up rate (42.9%).
    - there is a wide range for the best and worst case sensitivity results (14.3 to 57.1%).
- Conversely, if the best case and worse case scenarios have no significant impact on the study results, then loss to follow-up is not an issue.

Subgroup analysis

- If the investigators identify clinical characteristics or prognostic factors that affect the primary outcome, these can be evaluated in pre-specified subgroup analyses. For example, if you thought that the treatment effect would be different in Caucasians compared to non-Caucasians, you would collect information on ethnicity, so that the outcome could be evaluated within the ethnicity subgroups.
- Note that these subgroups must be predefined. At the end of a trial, if the investigators find that the results are negative, they may be tempted to search for subgroups in whom the outcome result is significant. They may then announce that the treatment is effective in, say, men aged under 40 years. This is unlikely to be a real result. The nature of statistical significance dictates that, if you look at 20 subgroups (when $P = < 0.05$), one will appear to show a significant result purely by chance.

Numbers needed to treat for benefit and harm

- As healthcare professionals, it is useful to know how many patients need to receive a particular treatment in order to prevent one case of disease. This is determined by calculating the number needed to treat to benefit (NNTB):

$$\text{NNTB} = \frac{1}{|\text{Risk difference between two treatment groups}|}$$

The vertical bars in the formula indicate that we use the absolute (positive) value of the risk difference.

- However, in medicine, an intervention may also have the potential to do harm. This is expressed as the number needed to treat to harm (NNTH).
- The formula for the NNTH is the same as that used for the NNTB.
- *The nature of the outcome measure determines whether the NNTB or the NNTH should be used.*

NNTB example

- Suppose we carry out an RCT investigating whether a new drug, AK87, reduces the risk of disease compared to the regular drug. All study participants were disease-free at the start of the trial. Two sets of hypothetical results, from 'Trial 1' and 'Trial 2' are

Fig. 6.4 Calculating the number needed to treat to benefit.

	Risk of disease per 1000		Risk ratio (R_1/R_0)	Risk difference per 1000 ($R_1 - R_0$)	NNTB
	Regular drug (R_0)	New drug (AK87) (R_1)			$\frac{1 \times 1000}{\lvert R_1 - R_0 \rvert}$
Trial 1	109	47	0.43	−62	16.1
Trial 2	10.9	4.7	0.43	−6.2	161.3

summarised in Fig. 6.4. In both sets of data, patients randomised to AK87 were less likely to develop the disease.

- The risk ratio, which indicates the increased (or decreased) risk of disease associated with the exposure of interest, is the same in both trials. With a risk ratio of 0.43, AK87, reduces the risk of disease by 57%.
- The risk difference gives an indication of whether the risk of the disease is common. Referring to Trial 1, for every 1000 people treated with AK87, we would expect to prevent 62 of the 109 cases of newly diagnosed disease that would have occurred amongst those patients on the regular drug.
- The NNTB of 16 means that for every 16 patients treated AK87, we would prevent 1 case of disease.
- Moving on to the data set from Trial 2:
  - the rate of disease is only 10% of that observed in Trial 1.
  - the NNTB is 161.3.
  - you would need to treat 161 patients with AK87 to prevent 1 case of disease.
- Despite both trials showing that AK87 reduced the risk of disease by 57%, the rate of disease was relatively low in Trial 2, therefore it may not be worthwhile financing the new drug for use in clinical practice based on the results of Trial 2 alone. Furthermore, it is also important to consider whether there are any adverse side effects before any drug licensing decisions are made.

NNTH example

- Sticking with our example above, the new drug, AK87, was found to be associated with an adverse, potentially fatal, side effect.
- Suppose the rates of this adverse effect in Trial 2 are 180 per 1000 patients in the new drug group and 43 per 1000 patients in the regular drug group.
- The NNTH is therefore:

$$\frac{1}{|180 - 43|} \times 1000 = 7.3 \text{ patients}$$

- Therefore, putting all our findings for Trial 2 together, we need to treat 161 patients with AK87 to prevent 1 case of disease but only 7 patients to cause 1 case with an adverse effect.
- Assessing this benefit-to-harm ratio, we can safely conclude that this new drug is more harmful than beneficial.

TYPES OF RANDOMISED CONTROLLED TRIALS

Two or more parallel groups

- Our discussion on RCTs, so far, has focused on comparing two groups, an intervention and a control group. However, it is possible to compare more than two treatments provided the groups are independent of each other.

Cross-over trial

- In a cross-over trial, each subject acts as his or her own control, receiving all the treatments in a particular sequence.
- Random allocation determines the sequence in which each subject receives the treatments (Fig. 6.5).
- Understandably, it is important to avoid the carry-over effect of the first treatment into the period during which the second treatment is allocated. This is achieved by having a washout period between the treatments, i.e. a gap, during which no treatment is given.
- The different treatments are compared within the same group of patients, therefore:
  - fewer subjects are needed in a crossover trial compared with an equivalent parallel group trial. As previously discussed, the treatments are compared between different groups of patients in a parallel group trial.
  - the differences between the patients are accounted for explicitly.
- This study design is usually used to test treatments for chronic conditions such as hypertension or for long-term illnesses. Conversely, testing treatments for acute conditions (e.g. antibiotics for a urinary tract infection) may not be feasible with this type of study design as the patient may be cured after the first treatment.
- Cross-over trials are likely to take less time than the equivalent parallel group design.

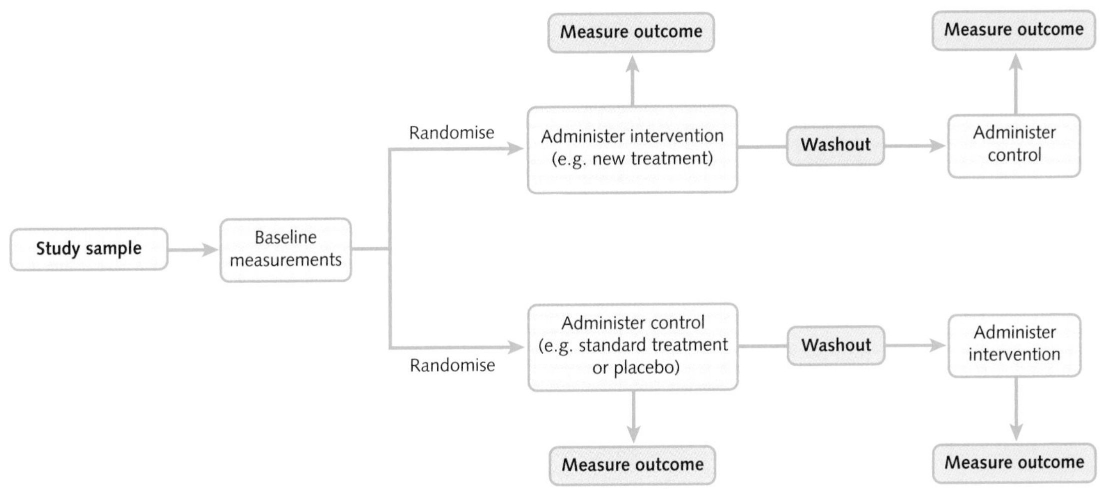

Fig. 6.5 Cross-over RCT study design.

Factorial trial

- A factorial trial is where two or more interventions are evaluated *simultaneously* and compared with a control group in the same trial.
- This type of RCT is commonly used to evaluate interactions between different treatments.
- A factorial design can be displayed as a 2×2 table (Fig. 6.6). As shown, there are four groups in a trial comparing two interventions.

Cluster trial

- Cluster randomised trials involve groups of patients, clinics or communities, as opposed to individuals.
- These clusters are randomised to receive the intervention or a control.
- Comparisons are made between these clusters rather than between individuals.
- A cluster trial is appropriate when evaluating interventions that are likely to have a group effect. Such interventions include preventative health services (e.g. smoking cessation programmes or vaccines).

		Randomisation of B	
		Drug B	Control B
Randomisation of A	Drug A	Drug A & Drug B	Drug A & Control B
	Control A	Control A & Drug B	Control A & Control B

Fig. 6.6 Factorial RCT study groups.

Superiority versus equivalence trials

- It is important to distinguish between superiority and equivalence trials. They differ in terms of the primary objective of each trial.
- Both types of trials are discussed in further detail in the 'Cost minimisation analysis' section in Chapter 18.

Superiority trial

- The objective of a superiority trial is to determine whether a new intervention is *better than* the control (e.g. placebo or usual treatment).
- The null hypothesis is that there is no difference between the two groups.
- The alternative hypothesis is that the new intervention is better than the control.

Equivalence trial

- The objective of an equivalence trial is to determine whether a new intervention is *similar* in effectiveness to the usual treatment.
- This type of trial is used if the new intervention has certain advantages such as:
  - being cheaper to manufacture.
  - being cheaper to monitor.
  - having fewer side effects.
- The null hypothesis is that the difference in outcome between the two intervention groups is greater than x (a pre-set value).

- The alternative hypothesis is that the difference in outcome between the two intervention groups is less than x.

ADVANTAGES AND DISADVANTAGES

What are the advantages and disadvantages of randomised controlled trials (Fig. 6.7)?

HINTS AND TIPS

It is sometimes necessary to use the results of observational studies to examine the effectiveness of an intervention in patient groups excluded from a trial.

KEY EXAMPLE OF A RANDOMISED CONTROLLED TRIAL

- The 4S secondary prevention trial was the first RCT that demonstrated that long-term simvastatin treatment lowered the 10-year mortality of coronary heart disease (CHD) in those who had a previous myocardial infarction or angina.
- While it would be possible to discuss all aspects of the study design in a lengthy essay, we will only focus on some of the key methodological issues (Fig. 6.8).

REPORTING A RANDOMISED CONTROLLED TRIAL

- Clinical trials should be reported according to the CONSORT (Consolidated Standards of Reporting Trials) guidelines.
- It is for *reporting* RCTs only. It should not be used as a checklist for conducting or critically appraising an RCT.
- Many journals, including the *Lancet* and the *BMJ*, request for authors to comply with the CONSORT guidelines.
- Systematic reporting of the results should make critical appraisal easier as the relevant information is more likely to be included in the report.
- The CONSORT statement has been included in Fig. 6.9. It is strongly recommended that this statement is read in conjunction with the CONSORT 2010 Explanation and Elaboration document (see 'Further Reading') to assist you in understanding all the items on the guideline.
- The CONSORT statement 2010 flow diagram is shown in Fig. 6.10. The flow diagram depicts a passage of participants through an RCT. Inclusion of numbers of participants at various stages of a trial (enrolment, intervention, allocation, follow-up and analysis) allows you to assess whether the investigators have done an accurate ITT analysis.

Fig. 6.7 Advantages and disadvantages of randomised controlled trials.

Advantages	Disadvantages
Provides the strongest evidence of any study design to determine the effectiveness or safety of a given intervention.	Limitations to external validity due to: • Strict eligibility criteria regarding patient characteristics • Recording unrepresentative outcome measures • Using difficult study procedures.
Has the most rigorous study design to determine whether a cause–effect relationship exists between an intervention and outcome (there is a clear temporal sequence – exposure precedes outcome).	Difficult to detect small effects as this would require a very large sample size. This may be an issue when investigating: • Rare outcomes (e.g. sudden infant death syndrome) • Uncommon adverse outcomes (e.g. a rare side effect of a drug).
Prospective study design, therefore able to measure disease risk.	Costly to study late outcomes which require long periods of follow-up
Enables blinding; therefore, bias is minimised	Relatively expensive.
Randomisation can control for known or unknown confounders.	The efficacy of the intervention may be different under trial conditions, where protocols are strictly followed, compared to normal practice.

Fig. 6.8 4S secondary prevention trial study design.

Study design	4S secondary prevention trial	Comments
Recruitment	*Inclusion criteria*: • Men and women aged 35–70 years • History of angina pectoris or acute myocardial infarction *Exclusion criteria*: • A long list of conditions, including patients on antiarrhythmic therapy and patients with congestive heart failure requiring treatment with digoxin, diuretics or vasodilators.	There is a clear statement highlighting which individuals are eligible to participate in the RCT. To ensure internal validity of the findings, patients with multiple co-morbid conditions were excluded. However, this limits the generalisability and thus the external validity of the RCT.
Intervention and control	Eligible patients were randomised to receive either simvastatin or similar placebo tablets.	To minimise performance bias, placebo tablets were used as a control.
Outcome	Primary outcome: total mortality. Secondary outcome: major coronary events.	Suitable outcome measures were recorded.
Power	The study was planned to have 95% power to detect a 30% reduction in total mortality at $\alpha = 0.05$. To achieve this power, the statistical analysis specified that 4400 patients needed to be recruited and followed up until the occurrence of 440 deaths, unless the trial was stopped early on the basis of an interim analysis.	Sample size calculations were based on the study having a relatively high amount of power, which is commendable. However, a very large sample size was required to achieve this power.
Randomisation	• Randomisation was stratified for clinical site and number of previous myocardial infarctions • 2223 patients were randomly assigned the placebo • 2221 patients were randomly assigned simvastatin treatment	Consideration was given to potential confounding factors when randomising patients. Stratified randomisation was used to ensure that there were an equal number of patients with these confounding factors in both treatment arms.
Ethics	• The study protocol was approved by regional and national ethics committees • Informed consent was obtained • There was no prior strong evidence of the effectiveness of simvastatin; therefore there is clinical equipoise	Ethical issues were all addressed prior to starting the RCT

Results	• The study was stopped after the 3rd interim analysis due to the simvastatin group having a beneficial effect (therefore not maintaining clinical equipoise)
	• The total mortality risk was:
	  • 11.5% in the placebo group
	  • 8.2% in the simvastatin group
	• The relative risk was 0.70
		Despite stopping the trial early, 438 patients died; thus the power calculations were satisfied. The NNTB is:
		$\frac{1}{\lvert 11.5 - 8.2 \rvert} \times 100 = 30.3$ patients
		Therefore, you would need to treat 30 patients with simvastatin to prevent one case of all-cause mortality.

Fig. 6.9 The CONSORT 2010 statement.

Section/topic	Item no.	Checklist item
Title and abstract		
	1a	Identification as a randomised trial in the title
	1b	Structured summary of trial design, methods, results, and conclusions (for specific guidance see CONSORT for abstracts)
Introduction		
Background and objectives	2a	Scientific background and explanation of rationale
	2b	Specific objectives or hypotheses
Methods		
Trial design	3a	Description of trial design (such as parallel, factorial) including allocation ratio
	3b	Important changes to methods after trial commencement (such as eligibility criteria), with reasons
Participants	4a	Eligibility criteria for participants
	4b	Settings and locations where the data were collected
Interventions	5	The interventions for each group with sufficient details to allow replication, including how and when they were actually administered
Outcomes	6a	Completely defined pre-specified primary and secondary outcome measures, including how and when they were assessed
	6b	Any changes to trial outcomes after the trial commenced, with reasons
Sample size	7a	How sample size was determined
	7b	When applicable, explanation of any interim analyses and stopping guidelines
Randomisation		
Sequence generation	8a	Method used to generate the random allocation sequence
	8b	Type of randomisation; details of any restriction (such as blocking and block size)
Allocation concealment mechanism	9	Mechanism used to implement the random allocation sequence (such as sequentially numbered containers), describing any steps taken to conceal the sequence until interventions were assigned
Implementation	10	Who generated the random allocation sequence, who enrolled participants and who assigned participants to interventions
Blinding	11a	If done, who was blinded after assignment to interventions (for example, participants, care providers, those assessing outcomes) and how
	11b	If relevant, description of the similarity of interventions
Statistical methods	12a	Statistical methods used to compare groups for primary and secondary outcomes
	12b	Methods for additional analyses, such as subgroup analyses and adjusted analyses
Results		
Participant flow (a diagram is strongly recommended)	13a	For each group, the numbers of participants who were randomly assigned, received intended treatment and were analysed for the primary outcome
	13b	For each group, losses and exclusions after randomisation, together with reasons
Recruitment	14a	Dates defining the periods of recruitment and follow-up
	14b	Why the trial ended or was stopped
Baseline data	15	A table showing baseline demographic and clinical characteristics for each group
Numbers analysed	16	For each group, number of participants (denominator) included in each analysis and whether the analysis was by original assigned groups
Outcomes and estimation	17a	For each primary and secondary outcome, results for each group, and the estimated effect size and its precision (such as 95% confidence interval)
	17b	For binary outcomes, presentation of both absolute and relative effect sizes is recommended

Fig. 6.9 The CONSORT 2010 statement—cont'd.

Section/topic	Item no.	Checklist item
Ancillary analyses	18	Results of any other analyses performed, including subgroup analyses and adjusted analyses, distinguishing pre-specified from exploratory
Harms	19	All important harms or unintended effects in each group (for specific guidance see CONSORT for harms)
Discussion		
Limitations	20	Trial limitations, addressing sources of potential bias, imprecision and, if relevant, multiplicity of analyses
Generalisability	21	Generalisability (external validity, applicability) of the trial findings
Interpretation	22	Interpretation consistent with results, balancing benefits and harms, and considering other relevant evidence
Other information		
Registration	23	Registration number and name of trial registry
Protocol	24	Where the full trial protocol can be accessed, if available
Funding	25	Sources of funding and other support (such as supply of drugs), role of funders

We strongly recommend reading this statement in conjunction with the CONSORT 2010 Explanation and Elaboration for important clarifications on all the items. If relevant, we also recommend reading CONSORT extensions for cluster randomised trials, non-inferiority and equivalence trials, non-pharmacological treatments, herbal interventions, and pragmatic trials. Additional extensions are forthcoming: for those and for up-to-date references relevant to this checklist, see http://www.consort-statement.org.

Schulz KF et al., 2010. Ann. Int. Med. 152. Reproduced with permission.

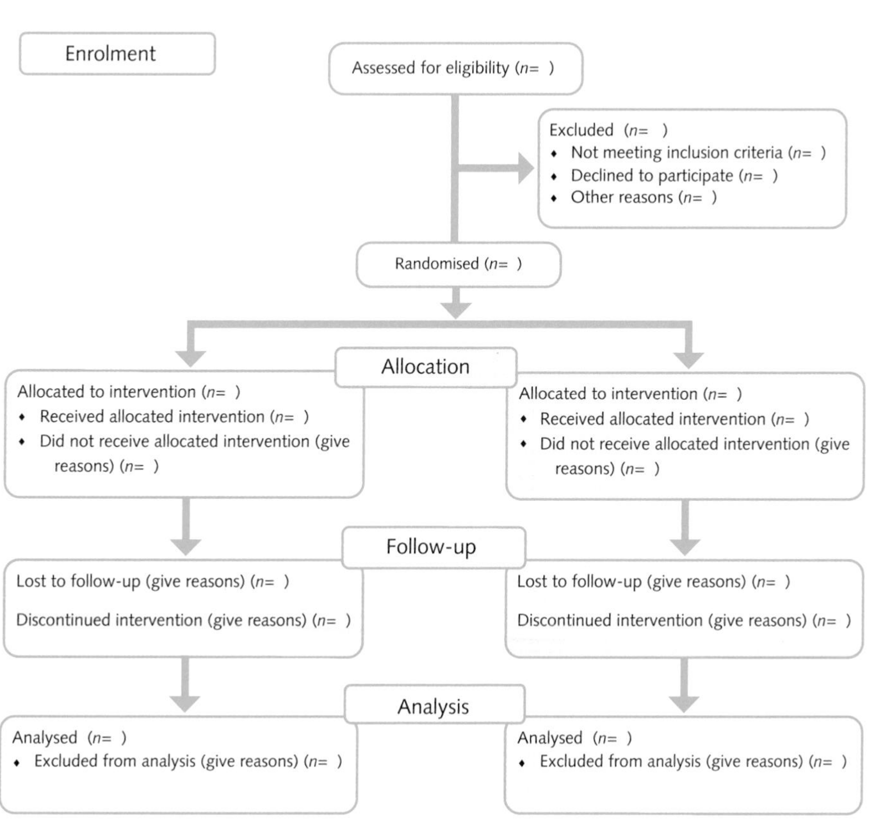

Fig. 6.10 The CONSORT 2010 statement flow diagram. (Schulz KF et al. (2010) Ann. Int. Med. 152. Reproduced with permission.)

Cohort studies

Objectives

By the end of this chapter you should:

- Be able to identify and critically appraise cohort studies.
- Know the steps involved in carrying out a cohort study.
- Understand the differences between prospective and retrospective cohort studies.
- Be able to calculate and interpret the risk ratio and its 95% confidence interval.
- Know the difference between the risk ratio and the risk difference.
- Understand the terms confounding and causality in relation to cohort studies.
- Be able to define the term bias and understand the different types of bias implicated in cohort studies.
- Be able to list the advantages and disadvantages of both prospective and retrospective cohort studies.

A methodological checklist on how to critically appraise cohort studies is provided in Chapter 19.

STUDY DESIGN

A cohort study is a form of observational study that aims to investigate whether exposure of subjects to a certain aetiological factor will affect the incidence of a disease in the future (Fig. 7.1). Cohort studies have the following design properties:

- The subjects (cohort) chosen for the study should represent the population to which the results will be generalised.
- For ease of data collection, the cohorts are usually chosen from a similar source: for example, people who are enrolled at the same university, work in a particular occupation or live in the same area.
- As we are assessing the aetiological effect of a risk factor, it is imperative that the cohorts are disease-free at the start of the study.
- The exposures of interest are then measured at baseline in these subjects.
- The subjects are followed up over time to see whether those who were exposed develop the disease at a different rate than those not exposed.
- The length of follow-up chosen should allow enough time for a sufficient number of subjects to develop the disease of interest.
- As subjects are followed up over time, there is the possibility of individuals being lost to follow-up.
- It is important to maintain regular contact with subjects to minimise dropout rates.
- In 'prospective' cohort studies, the data on exposure are recorded from the (disease-free) study subjects in the present time. The disease outcome is subsequently measured in these same subjects in the future.
- In 'retrospective' cohort studies (also referred to as 'historical' cohort studies), data on exposure are obtained from pre-existing records and we measure disease outcome in these subjects in the present time (Fig. 7.2).
- As explained above, when carrying out an aetiological study, you start by identifying your disease-free cohort. You then question whether the incidence of disease is greater in people exposed to a suspected cause than those not exposed.
- Non-aetiological cohort studies can also be used in clinical medicine. For example, people with a particular condition or disease can be followed up over time to evaluate different outcomes, such as survival rates.

HINTS AND TIPS

While case–control studies start by identifying your subjects based on whether they have the outcome of interest (cases), cohort studies start by identifying a group of subjects (cohort) who are followed up for a set period of time to assess whether they develop the outcome.

COMMUNICATION

What research questions are best answered with a cohort study design?

Most cohort studies assess the harm or benefit of a risk factor, especially if little is known about the effect of this exposure. Specifically, the cohort study design is best suited to answering research questions:

- where the exposure is rare.
- where it would be impossible, or unethical, to expose subjects deliberately to the risk factor (e.g. if investigating the effects of smoking or alcohol).
- where the number of subjects needed to detect an effect are too great for a randomised controlled trial to be feasible. However, note that when a disease is very rare, the numbers needed may be too large for a prospective cohort study, and a retrospective cohort study design or a case–control study is preferred.
- in a retrospective study design:
  - if the exposure to risk has already occurred
  - if there is a long time lag between exposure and disease outcome.
  - if the disease outcome is rare.
- in a prospective study design:
  - if there is a short time lag between exposure and disease outcome

INTERPRETING THE RESULTS

We can use a 2×2 table to summarise the number of exposed and unexposed subjects who do and do not go on to develop the disease of interest (Fig. 7.3).

Risk

In cohort studies, as subjects are followed up longitudinally over time, we can estimate the proportion of new cases of disease that occur by calculating the *risk* in the study sample. It is a measure of the probability (between 0 and 1) of developing the disease in the stated time period:

$$\text{Risk of disease} = \frac{\text{Number of new cases of disease over study period}}{\text{Total number of subjects initially disease-free}} = \frac{d_1 + d_0}{n}$$

Sometimes it may be useful to present values for 100 times the risk, which describes the risk of disease for every 100 people in the exposed or unexposed group.

Risk ratios

The risk of developing the disease in the population can be compared between the exposed and unexposed groups by calculating the *risk ratio* (also referred to as the *relative risk*). The risk of disease in the exposed group is divided by the risk of disease in the unexposed group:

$$\text{Risk ratio} = \frac{\text{Risk in exposed group}}{\text{Risk in unexposed group}} = \frac{d_1/(d_1 + h_1)}{d_0/(d_0 + h_0)}$$

The risk ratio indicates the increased (or decreased) risk of disease associated with the exposure of interest. The risk ratio can take any value between 0 and infinity, for example:

- If the risk ratio is 1, the risk of disease is the same in the exposed and unexposed groups.
- If the risk ratio is 2, the exposure of interest doubles the risk of disease.
- If the risk ratio is 0.5, the exposure of interest halves the risk of disease.
- If the risk ratio is 0.25, the exposure of interest reduces the risk of disease by 75%.

The example at the end of this chapter demonstrates the application of these formulae in a real cohort study investigating the connection between smoking and mortality.

HINTS AND TIPS

It is important to interpret the risk ratio alongside the underlying risk of disease in the population. A large risk ratio may have a limited clinical implication if the underlying risk of disease is very small.

Confidence interval for a risk ratio

In Chapter 3 we introduced the concept of confidence intervals for differences between means or proportions. By adding or subtracting $1.96 \times$ the standard error of the difference, we learned how to calculate the 95% confidence interval. However, an alternative approach must be used when calculating the 95% confidence interval for a risk ratio as the interval cannot take values less than 0.

For example, if the risk ratio was 0.41 and the standard error of the risk ratio was 0.30, then the 95% confidence interval would be −0.18 to 1.0. However, the lower limit of −0.18 is an unfeasible value for a risk ratio.

To get around this problem, the 95% confidence interval for a risk ratio is calculated using an error factor with the following two formulae:

$$\text{Error factor} = \text{exponential}\,(1.96 \times \text{standard error (log risk ratio)})$$

Total population

Disease-free – 'healthy'

Disease

'Healthy' sample

Unexposed to factor

Exposed to factor

Follow-up

Remains 'healthy'

Develops disease

Remains 'healthy'

Develops disease

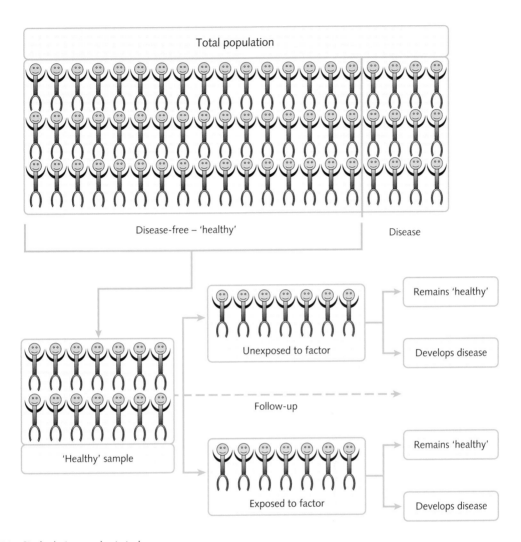

Fig. 7.1 Study design – cohort study.

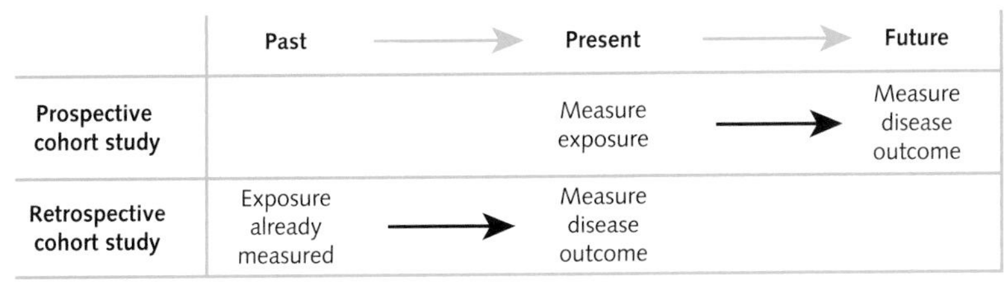

	Past →	Present →	Future
Prospective cohort study		Measure exposure →	Measure disease outcome
Retrospective cohort study	Exposure already measured →	Measure disease outcome	

Fig. 7.2 Prospective versus retrospective cohort studies.

where

$$\text{the SE of log RR} = \sqrt{\frac{1}{d_1} + \frac{1}{h_1} + \frac{1}{d_0} + \frac{1}{h_0}}$$

95% confidence interval for a risk ratio

$$= \frac{\text{Risk ratio}}{\text{Error factor}} \text{ to Risk ratio} \times \text{Error factor}$$

The error factor is defined as the 95th percentile divided by the median. It is a measure of the spread of the distribution, and is usually denoted by 'EF'. For the purposes of your undergraduate training, you do not need to understand the formula for the confidence interval for a risk ratio.

		Exposure		
		Yes	*No*	*Total*
Disease	*Yes*	d_1	d_0	$d_1 + d_0$
	No	h_1	h_0	$h_1 + h_0$
	Total	$d_1 + h_1$	$d_0 + h_0$	$n = d_1 + d_0 + h_1 + h_0$

d = disease *h* = healthy 1 = exposed 0 = unexposed

Fig. 7.3 Observed frequencies.

HINTS AND TIPS

If you're still not sure how to calculate the risk ratio or the confidence interval for a risk ratio, try using an online calculator that walks you through the basic steps. One example, accessible online, is http://www.hutchon.net/confidRR.htm

Risk difference

In addition to calculating the risk ratio, the association between an exposure and disease can also be determined in cohort studies by interpreting the *absolute risk difference*. As the name suggests, this measure is calculated by working out the difference in risk between exposed subjects and unexposed subjects:

$$\text{Risk difference} = \text{Risk in exposed group} - \text{Risk in unexposed group} = \frac{d_1}{(d_1 + h_1)} - \frac{d_0}{(d_0 + h_0)}$$

Calculating the 95% confidence interval for a risk difference is described in the Chapter 3 section 'Confidence interval for the difference between two independent proportions'.

The risk difference describes the absolute change in risk that is attributable to the exposure of interest and can take any value between −1 and +1:

- If the exposure has no effect on the risk of disease, the risk difference will be equal to 0.
- If the exposure reduces risk of disease, the risk difference will be less than 0.
- If the exposure increases the risk of disease, the risk difference will be greater than 0.

However, the clinical importance of a risk difference usually depends on the underlying risk of disease. For example, a risk difference of 0.03 (or 3%) may represent a small, clinically insignificant change from a risk of 37 to 40%. On the other hand the exposure may be clinically significant if the change in risk is from 1 to 4%.

HINTS AND TIPS

It is easier to interpret the risk difference if we multiply the value by 100, which describes how many people have avoided (or incurred) the disease for every 100 exposed to the risk factor of interest.

Risk ratio versus risk difference

What is the difference between the risk ratio and the risk difference? Figure 7.4 highlights the key differences.

CONFOUNDING, CAUSALITY AND BIAS

Due to the methodology involved, there are three general issues that must be addressed when appraising observational studies:

1. Confounding
2. Causality
3. Bias.

Confounding

- Confounding occurs when the exposure of interest is not only associated with the risk of disease but also with a third variable that provides an alternative explanation for any association measured between the exposure and disease (please refer to Chapter 13 for an in-depth discussion on confounding).

Fig. 7.4 Risk ratio versus risk difference.

Risk ratio	Risk difference
A measure of the *strength* of the association between exposure and disease.	A measure of the *impact* of exposure In clinical trials, the number needed to treat is derived from the risk difference (please refer to Chapter 6).
Useful if the relative difference in risk of disease between the exposed and unexposed groups is of interest. Useful when comparing the size of the effect for several exposure factors.	Useful if the actual size of the difference between the risk of disease in the exposed and unexposed groups is of interest.
Values range from 0 to 1.	Values range from −1 to +1.
Risk ratios are unitless.	Risk differences have units.

- Provided the confounding factors are recognised and measured at the start of the study, they may be controlled for at the study design level or when analysing the results of the cohort study (discussed in Chapter 13).
- A famous example of confounding in cohort studies is the apparent association of hormone replacement therapy (HRT) with a reduction in the risk of coronary heart disease (CHD). However, a subsequent randomised controlled trial showed that HRT does not reduce the risk of CHD. It was found that women who took HRT were more likely to be living a healthy lifestyle, and it was this that led to a reduction in CHD (the 'healthy user' effect).

Causality

- Among observational studies, a prospective cohort study provides the best evidence of causality between an exposure and outcome.
- As the exposure is measured at the start of the study, the temporal relationship between the exposure and outcome is clear.
- However, in retrospective cohort studies, reverse causality may be an issue, as the temporal sequence between the exposure and outcome was not observed.
- For a more in-depth discussion on causality, please refer to the Bradford-Hill criteria, which are discussed in Chapter 5.

Bias

- Study error can broadly be categorised into two main groups: random error and systematic error (Fig. 7.5).
- Random error occurs due to chance and leads to the effect estimate (e.g. relative risk in cohort studies) being equally likely to be higher or lower than the true value. It is caused by inherently unpredictable variations in the reading of a measurement tool, the investigator's inability to make the same measurement in exactly the same way in each subject or by chance variations between subjects. Statistical measures such as confidence intervals and *P*-values (discussed in Chapter 3) are used to assess the role of random error on the effect estimate.
- Systematic error is called bias, and like random error, can lead to the effect estimate being over- or underestimated compared to the true value. Bias is anything that produces systematic variation in a research finding. As a result, the association between an exposure and outcome may be inaccurate if bias has affected the selection or measurement processes involved in the study. In general:
  - Bias usually occurs due to poor study design or poor data collection.
  - Unlike confounding, little can be done to control for bias when analysing the data.

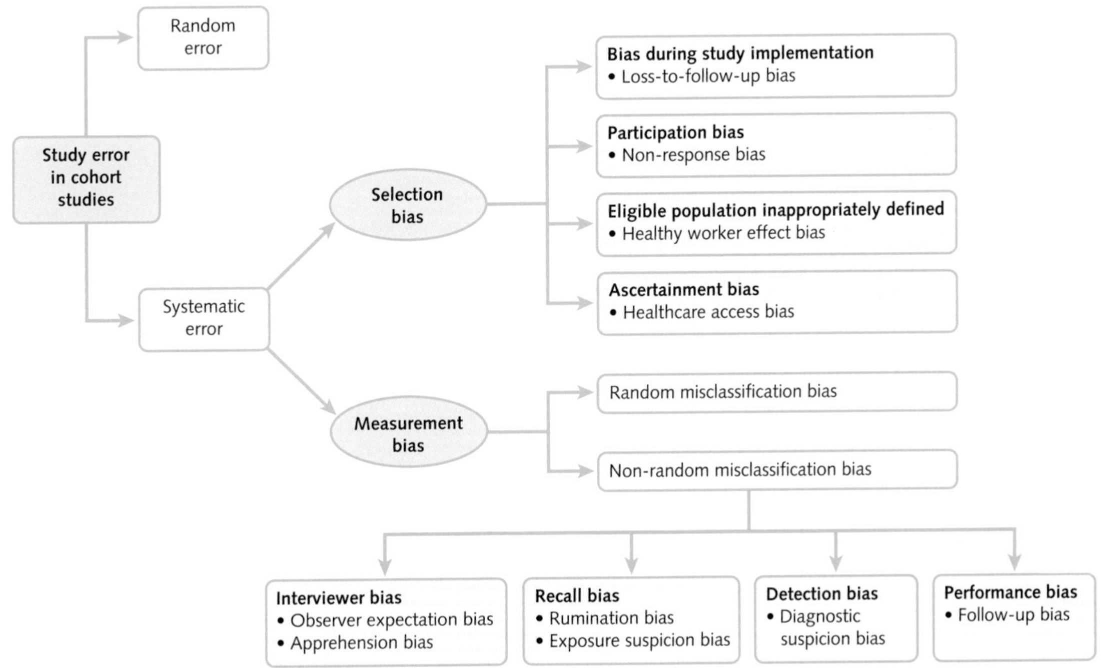

Fig. 7.5 Study error in cohort studies.

- Bias limits the conclusions that can be drawn from the study outcome.
- Systematic error can be divided into selection bias and measurement bias.

Selection bias

Selection bias occurs when the association between an exposure and disease is different for those who complete the study, compared with those who are in the target population. Selection bias may exist when procedures for subject selection or factors that influence subject's participation affect the outcome of the study. The main types of selection bias that may occur in cohort studies include:

- Bias during study implementation
  - Loss-to-follow-up bias
- Participation bias
  - Non-response bias
- Eligible population inappropriately defined
  - Healthy worker effect bias
- Ascertainment bias
  - Healthcare access bias.

Bias during study implementation: loss-to-follow-up bias

Loss-to-follow-up bias reflects the differences in the number of subjects who are lost to follow-up between the exposed and unexposed groups. This is a particular issue in prospective cohort studies as subjects, who are followed up until the outcome occurs or the study ends, may lose contact with the investigators, move out of the area, die, etc. Loss-to-follow-up bias may be an issue if the reasons why patients are lost to follow-up are associated with *both the exposure and outcome*, e.g. associated with exposed cases. With differences in loss to follow-up between the exposed and unexposed groups, bias can occur if the subjects lost to follow-up are more (or less) likely to have developed the outcome.

The association between an exposure and outcome, and therefore the risk, may be over- or underestimated compared to the true risk. If the proportion of subjects lost is substantial (e.g. 20% lost to follow-up), this will affect the validity of the study, can lead to data misinterpretation and limit the generalisability of the study results. It is important to note that if subjects are lost randomly in both the exposed and unexposed groups, loss-to-follow-up bias should not be an issue.

Consider a cohort study investigating whether the incidence of lung cancer is different between smokers (exposed group) and non-smokers (non-exposed group). During the multi-year follow-up, exposed subjects may be at greater risk of developing co-morbid conditions and becoming unwell, compared to unexposed subjects, thus discontinuing study participation. The fact that some of them subsequently develop lung cancer will not be known to the investigators.

HINTS AND TIPS

Those subjects with multiple symptoms may be more likely to drop out of a study. If these symptoms are related to the exposure status, it is unfair to compare the outcome measurement between the exposed and unexposed subjects. Plans should be made at the start of the study to track those lost to follow-up.

Participation bias: non-response bias

This may be an issue if non-response (i.e. not participating in the study) is associated with *both* the exposure and the outcome. It is important to determine whether there are any similarities or differences between the participants and the non-participants. A sample of those not participating among the source population (or target population) should be reviewed to ensure that the study participants are a truly representative sample. Non-response bias behaves similarly to loss-to-follow-up bias. For example, as described under the loss-to-follow-up bias section above, consider a cohort study investigating the association between smoking and lung cancer. Due to similar reasons contributing to loss to follow-up, exposed subjects (i.e. smokers) are at greater risk of having co-morbid conditions and are generally more unwell than unexposed subjects, and thus are less likely to participate in the study in the first place.

Eligible population inappropriately defined: healthy worker effect bias

Healthy worker effect bias leads to an underestimation of the morbidity/mortality related to occupational exposures. In general, working individuals are healthier than the general population, which includes people who are unemployed because they are too unwell to work. Therefore, in cohort studies investigating the effect of occupational exposures, the unexposed group should *not* be chosen from the general population. Instead, the unexposed comparison group should consist of subjects from within the workforce (who are unexposed!). This will prevent the association between the exposure and outcome from being biased towards the null.

HINTS AND TIPS

Any excess risk of exposure (associated with an occupation) is likely to be underestimated if the unexposed group includes subjects from the general population. The relative risk of the occupational exposure on the disease outcome will therefore be underestimated.

Ascertainment bias: healthcare access bias

Healthcare access bias is a type of ascertainment bias in which the patients included in the study do not represent the cases arising in the target population. Healthcare access bias may be an issue when the members of the public who have been admitted to hospital (who are subsequently enrolled into the study) do not represent the cases that arise in the community. This may arise if:

- certain wards are very specialist and are only interested in treating particular kinds of cases.
- there are geographical, cultural or economical reasons associated with access to particular hospitals.
- the public visit a particular hospital (even if it means travelling further), knowing that they would be seen by a world renowned clinician.
- more unwell patients are referred to a tertiary hospital for their care.

Measurement bias

Measurement bias occurs when the information collected for the exposure and/or outcome variables is inaccurate. This type of bias can be divided into random or non-random misclassification bias (Fig. 7.5).

Random misclassification bias

Random misclassification bias (also known as non-differential misclassification bias) can occur when either the exposure or outcome is classified incorrectly (with equal probability) into different groups. The misclassification is random if the errors in exposure classification have occurred independent of the disease outcome. Similarly, any misclassification of disease outcome in the study participants should be independent of the exposure status.

Non-validated questionnaires are especially prone to this type of bias. For example, if investigating smoking status, we normally classify subjects into groups based on the number of cigarettes smoked per day. However, to avoid measurement bias, it is important to ask about:

- cigarette brand (and therefore nicotine content)
- whether they normally take deep breaths whilst smoking
- whether each cigarette is smoked to the end.

If the above details are not sought, some subjects will be misclassified into the wrong smoking status group. This is only considered *random* misclassification bias if the probability of being classified in the wrong group is the same for subjects who do and do not go onto develop the disease outcome of interest.

When random misclassification bias occurs, the exposed and unexposed groups seem more similar than they actually are, thus leading to an underestimation (dilution) of the true effect of the exposure on the disease outcome. In other words, the effective sample size is reduced and the estimates of effect are biased towards the null hypothesis, therefore, the observed risk ratio will be closer to 1 than the true risk ratio. The risk of random misclassification bias can be dealt with, in part, by increasing the sample size of a study. However, using high-quality validated methods to measure an exposure or outcome status can help minimise the risk of random misclassification bias from occurring.

Non-random misclassification bias

Non-random misclassification bias (also known as differential misclassification bias) can lead to the effect of the exposure on the disease outcome being biased in either direction. This type of misclassification occurs only when the exposure measurement is related to the disease outcome status or vice versa. As the misclassification is different in the groups being compared, this can lead to the effect of the exposure on the disease outcome being biased in either direction. The main types of non-random misclassification bias that may occur in cohort studies include:

- Performance bias
  - Follow-up bias
- Detection bias
  - Diagnostic suspicion bias
- Recall bias
  - Rumination bias
  - Exposure suspicion bias
- Interviewer bias
  - Observer expectation bias
  - Apprehension bias.

Performance bias: follow-up bias

If one exposure group is followed up more closely than the other exposure group, the outcome could be diagnosed more often in the more closely followed-up group. This is known as follow-up bias. In prospective cohort studies, it is important to ensure that follow-up and data collection are equally thorough, exhaustive and accurate for both the exposed and unexposed groups, thus preventing follow-up bias. This may only be possible if the study investigators involved in follow-up surveillance are kept 'blind' to the exposure status of all study participants.

Detection bias: diagnostic suspicion bias

Please refer to Chapter 6 for a discussion on detection bias.

Recall bias: rumination bias and exposure suspicion bias

Recall bias may arise in studies in which subjects are asked to recall whether they were exposed to certain factors in the past. There are two main types of recall bias that may occur in retrospective cohort studies (but also in case–control and cross-sectional studies):

- *Rumination bias*: When exposure status is recalled by subjects who know their disease status, those with the disease may put in extra effort (ruminate) into recalling their exposure status. In other words, compared to control subjects, those with the disease outcome may have a greater incentive (due to personal concern) to recall any past exposure events.

- *Exposure suspicion bias*: Knowledge of the subject's disease status may have an influence on how rigorous the investigators are in searching for an exposure event to the putative cause.

In an attempt to minimise the amount of recall bias, information from medical records (or other independent sources) should be reviewed, i.e. using objective records rather than relying on recall.

Interviewer bias: observer expectation bias and apprehension bias

Interviewer bias (or observer bias) may arise in studies in which subjects are interviewed! The study investigator may inadvertently 'coach' subjects when:

- questioning about their exposure history, e.g. in retrospective cohort studies (but also in case–control studies and cross-sectional studies).
- questioning about their disease status, e.g. in both prospective and retrospective cohort studies (but also in randomised controlled trials, case–control studies and cross-sectional studies).

This type of bias is known as observer expectation bias, as the study investigator (observer) may put varying emphasis or use different gestures when asking different questions. Apprehension bias is a particular type of interviewer bias, in which certain measures alter systematically from their usual levels if the subject is apprehensive at the time of interview, e.g. white coat hypertension when measuring blood pressure during a medical interview. Interviewer bias may be minimised if:

- the investigator is 'blind' to the outcome status when gathering data on the exposure status.
- the investigator is 'blind' to the exposure status when gathering data on the outcome status.
- different investigators are used to collect information on a subject's exposure and outcome status, especially if blinding is not possible.
- well-standardised data collection protocols are used.
- the investigators conducting the interview are trained to collect data using a standardised approach.
- the same information is sought from two different sources.

ADVANTAGES AND DISADVANTAGES

What are the advantages and disadvantages of cohort studies? Figure 7.6 highlights the key points that apply to prospective cohort studies, retrospective cohort studies or both types of studies.

KEY EXAMPLE OF A COHORT STUDY

We all know that smoking is bad for your health. However, what is the evidence base behind this well-recognised fact? In October 1951, postal questionnaires were sent out to all doctors on the British medical register who resided in the United Kingdom. In addition to their name, age and address, questions were asked about their smoking habits. Replies were received from 34,439 male and 6194 female doctors. The relatively few female smokers had not, in general, smoked as intensively or for as long as the male smokers, and thus were excluded from analysis. Observations on mortality from any cause began on November 1951 and continued until 2001. Let's look at the data collected in October 1991, the 40-year follow-up point. Figure 7.7 shows the risk of death by cause and smoking habit.

There appears to be a trend of increasing mortality risk with a higher smoking status for both lung cancer- and ischaemic heart disease-related deaths. Using the data presented in Fig. 7.7, we can calculate the risk ratio and risk difference for current smokers as compared to non-smokers for:

(a) Lung cancer-related deaths:

$$\text{Risk ratio} = \frac{\text{Risk of mortality for current smokers}}{\text{Risk of mortality for non-smokers}} = \frac{209}{14} = 14.93$$

$$\begin{aligned}\text{Risk difference} &= \text{Risk of mortality for current smokers} \\ &\quad - \text{Risk of mortality for non-smokers} \\ &= 209 - 14 \\ &= 195 \text{ per } 100\,000\end{aligned}$$

(b) Ischaemic heart disease-related deaths:

$$\text{Risk ratio} = \frac{\text{Risk of mortality for current smokers}}{\text{Risk of mortality for non-smokers}} = \frac{892}{572} = 1.56$$

$$\begin{aligned}\text{Risk difference} &= \text{Risk of mortality for current smokers} \\ &\quad - \text{Risk of mortality for non-smokers} \\ &= 892 - 572 \\ &= 320 \text{ per } 100\,000\end{aligned}$$

The results for the above calculations are displayed in Fig. 7.8.

The risk ratio and risk difference are two different measures of association, both of which have equal importance when analysing the data. Using the data in Fig. 7.8, we can conclude that:

- smokers are nearly 15 times more likely to die from lung cancer (risk ratio 14.93) than non-smokers.

Fig. 7.6 Advantages and Disadvantages of Cohort Studies.

Advantages	Disadvantages
Prospective • The time sequence between exposure and disease is clear as exposure status is measured before disease onset (preventing reverse causality). • The exposure can be measured at various time points, thus establishing any changes in exposure status during follow-up. • Exposure is measured before disease onset, thus minimising bias in exposure measurement.	**Prospective** • As the length of follow-up increases, the study is more prone to selection bias as subjects migrate or leave the study. • Following up subjects for disease occurrence is time consuming, therefore costly. • Not suitable for rare diseases as the length of follow-up may be considerable to get enough incident cases of the disease outcome. • Not suitable for rare diseases as very large sample sizes are required. • Prone to surveillance bias. • Unsuitable if there is a long time lag between exposure and outcome.
Retrospective • It is possible to measure long-term effects of exposure as the follow-up period has already occurred. • Useful for rare outcomes (diseases with low incidence), as the outcome has already happened. • Less expensive than prospective cohort studies because outcome and exposure have already occurred. • Useful if there is a long time lag between exposure and outcome.	**Retrospective** • Prone to recall bias (unlike prospective cohort studies). • Reverse causality may be an issue, as the temporal sequence of exposure and outcome was not observed.
Prospective and Retrospective • Information on exposure to a wide range of factors can be assessed (cohort studies are useful if little is known about the effect of an exposure). • They can provide information on associations between an exposure and *multiple* outcomes (retrospective studies are better for this). • It is possible to directly measure the incidence/risk of disease in the exposed and unexposed groups. • It is possible to investigate the effect of *rare* exposures (frequency less than 20%) on disease outcome.	**Prospective and Retrospective** • Disease outcome or the aetiology of disease may change over time. • Prone to interviewer bias.

Fig. 7.7 Annual risk of death by cause and smoking habit.

Cause of death	Number of deaths	Annual mortality risk per 100 000 men, standardised for age		
		Non-smokers	Former smokers	Current smokers
Lung cancer	893	14	58	209
Ischaemic heart disease	6438	572	678	892

(Data from Doll R et al. (1994) BMJ 309: 901–911.)

- smokers are at 56% increased risk of dying from ischaemic heart disease (risk ratio 1.56) than non-smokers.

Fig. 7.8 Association between smoking and male mortality.

Cause of death	Risk ratio	Risk difference (per 100 000)
Lung cancer	14.93	195
Ischaemic heart disease	1.56	320

- for every 100 000 male smokers, there will be 195 extra lung cancer-related deaths per year (risk difference 195 per 100 000).
- for every 100 000 male smokers, there will be 320 extra ischaemic heart disease-related deaths per year (risk difference 320 per 100 000).
- ischaemic heart disease is a *more common* cause of death than lung cancer (the risk difference is greater for ischaemic heart disease-related deaths than for lung cancer-related deaths).

Case–control studies

Objectives

By the end of this chapter you should:

- Be able to identify case–control studies.
- Know the steps involved in carrying out a case–control study.
- Understand the difference between incident cases and prevalent cases.
- Understand the difference between population controls and hospital controls.
- Be able to calculate and interpret the odds ratio and its 95% confidence interval.
- Know the difference between the odds ratio and risk ratio.
- Understand the terms confounding and causality in relation to case–control studies.
- Be able to define the term bias and understand the different types of bias implicated in case–control studies.
- Be able to list the advantages and disadvantages of case–control studies.

A methodological checklist on how to critically appraise case–control studies is provided in Chapter 19.

STUDY DESIGN

- A case–control study is a form of observational study that aims to identify risk factors for developing the outcome of interest.
- Subjects with the outcome (cases) and without the outcome (controls) are selected and risk factor exposure measurements are collected retrospectively in both groups either from the subject or from any available records (Fig. 8.1).
- Case–control studies simply tell us whether any exposure factors occurred more or less frequently in cases than in controls.
- If a particular exposure is more common in cases, it is associated with an increased risk of the outcome and may be a causal factor.
- If the exposure is less common in cases than in controls, it may be a protective factor.
- Case–control studies give us insight into which factors increase or decrease the risk of developing the outcome of interest.
- Unlike cohort studies, case–control studies do not usually give us information on the incidence or prevalence of disease (please refer to Chapter 7 for a discussion on cohort studies).

COMMUNICATION

What research questions are best answered with a case–control study design?

Like cohort studies, case–control studies are useful when investigating causes of disease, or factors associated with a particular condition. However, specifically, the case–control study design is best suited to answering research questions investigating:

- the causes for an acute outbreak (e.g. of legionnaire's disease or gastroenteritis).
- the risk factors for a *rare* disease (e.g. certain types of leukaemia). A prospective study, i.e. cohort studies, would take too long to identify a sufficient number of cases.
- the aetiology of a disease where there is a long time-lag between an exposure and disease outcome.

Case definition

The case definition of the outcome:

- Should be clearly defined at the start of the study to ensure that all cases chosen satisfy the same diagnostic criteria.
- Is usually based on:
    - clinical findings, e.g. cases with acute appendicitis diagnosed by patient history and examination findings made by a surgeon.

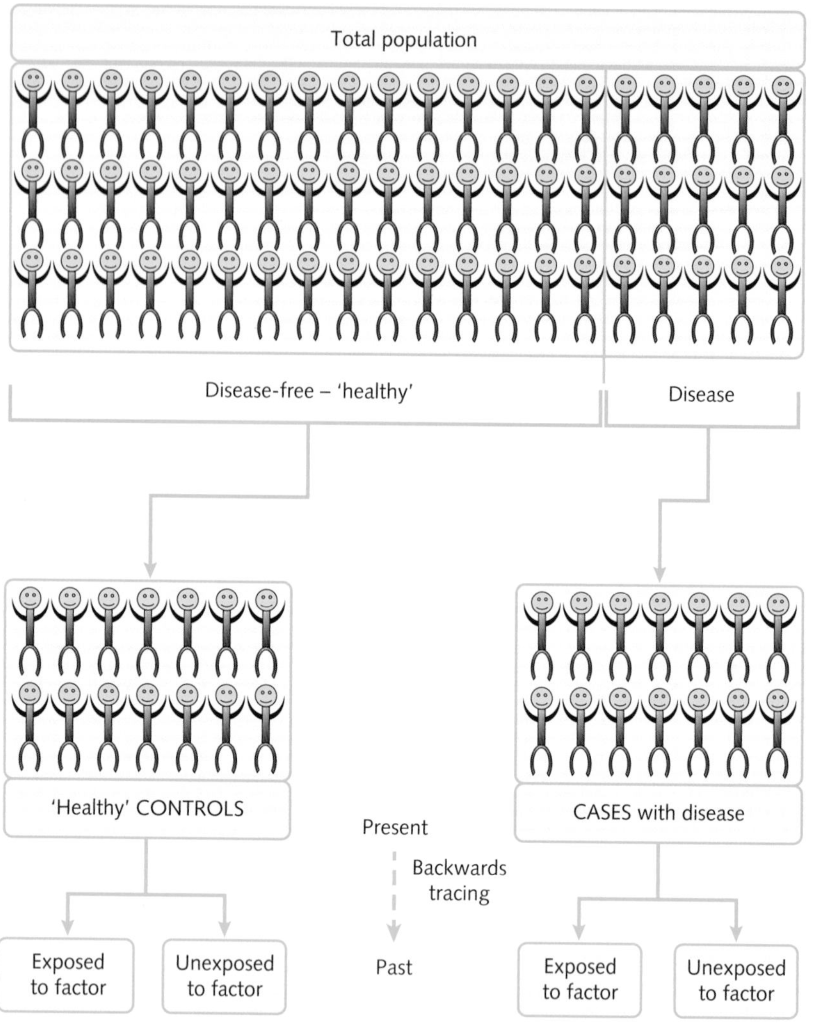

Fig. 8.1 Study design – case–control study.

- radiological findings, e.g. cases with a pulmonary embolism diagnosed with a CT pulmonary angiography scan.
- pathological findings, e.g. cases with a histological diagnosis of cervical cancer.
- microbiological findings, e.g. cases with stools positive for *Clostridium difficile* infection.

Case selection

- Case–control studies may use incident cases or prevalent cases when recruiting subjects with the outcome of interest.
- In general, incident cases are preferred to prevalent cases when recruiting subjects for a case–control study investigating the possible causes of a disease outcome (Fig. 8.2).
- However, when investigating the causes of insidious diseases (whose exact onset is difficult to determine), we may have no choice but to rely on information from prevalent cases. For a more general discussion on prevalence and incidence please refer to Chapter 9.
- As case–control studies are prone to various types of bias (discussed in detail underneath), it is especially important in this type of study design to recruit a large number of cases to increase the power of the study (discussed in Chapter 3).
- The cases selected should ideally be representative of all cases of the outcome in the population. Typical sources for identifying cases include:
    - hospital in-patients
    - out-patient clinics
    - GP registers
    - death certificates
    - disease registries.

Fig. 8.2 Incident cases vs prevalent cases in case–control studies.

Incident cases	Prevalent cases
Incident cases are recruited at the time of diagnosis of the outcome.	Prevalent cases are subjects who have already been diagnosed with the outcome.
Recollection of past exposure(s) will be relatively accurate, as cases have been newly diagnosed with the outcome.	Prone to recall bias as prevalent cases may be less likely to accurately recollect past exposure(s).
Temporal sequence of exposure and outcome is easier to assess.	Difficult to ensure that reported exposure(s) occurred before the development of the outcome rather than as a consequence of the outcome itself (or a combination of both).
The exposure factor(s) identified are more likely to be those that are involved in the aetiology of the outcome rather than those that affect the duration (prognosis) of the outcome.	Impossible to determine the extent to which the exposure factor(s) identified are involved in the aetiology of the outcome, its prognosis or both.

- The process of enrolling cases in the study should be accurate and efficient so as to identify a sufficient number of cases as quickly and cheaply as possible.

Control selection

- Controls should:
  - ideally be selected from the same source as cases, i.e. cases and controls both being selected from the same GP register.
  - be sampled independently of the exposure status; i.e. unexposed and exposed controls should have the same probability of selection.
  - meet all the selection criteria for cases, apart from not having the disease outcome of interest; i.e. if the cases are men aged between 40 and 50 years old with lung cancer, the controls should be (1) male (2) aged between 40 and 50 years old, who do *not* have lung cancer.
- Selecting up to four controls per case may improve the statistical power of the study (please refer to Chapter 3 for a discussion on power) to detect a difference between cases and controls.
- Including more than four controls per case does *not* generally increase the power of the study much further.
- Similar to the methods involved in case selection, typical sources for identifying controls include:
  - hospital in-patients
  - out-patient clinics
  - death certificates
  - relatives or friends to cases
  - general population; voter registration lists, GP registers, telephone directories, random digit dialling of telephone numbers from a defined geographic area.
- Controls should not have an outcome related to the exposure being investigated. This is usually an issue when controls are selected from a hospital population. For an in-depth discussion on selection bias in case–control studies, please refer to the 'Bias' section below.
- Population controls are therefore usually selected when the cases are chosen from a well-defined population such as those living in a particular neighbourhood.
- The advantages and disadvantages of using either population or hospital/clinic controls are summarised in Fig. 8.3.

Matching

- Many case–control studies have a matched design when selecting cases and controls to ensure that the two groups are as similar to each other as possible. For example, cases and controls can be matched for gender and age, i.e. male subjects aged within 3 years of each other. However, due to this matched design, the effect of the matching variables on the disease outcome cannot be investigated when analysing the study results.
- If there are missing data for the case or control in a matched pair, the data from both subjects are excluded from the statistical analysis.

Measuring exposure status

- The exposure status to possible risk factors for the outcome is measured retrospectively for all cases and controls.
- Data on a wide variety of exposures are usually collected, including those related to:
  - occupation
  - diet
  - lifestyle
  - genes
  - medications.
- The methods used to measure the exposure status should be the same for all cases and controls.

Fig. 8.3 Advantages and disadvantages of population controls vs hospital/clinic controls.

	Population controls	Hospital/clinic controls
Advantages	• Have similar demographics and characteristics to cases, i.e. age and gender. • As subjects are generally healthy, the prevalence of exposure is less likely to be biased by the presence of another disease.	• Comparable demographics and characteristics to cases if they are selected from the same source population. • Easy to recruit, therefore cheaper to identify subjects. • More likely to be motivated to participate in the study. • As subjects are generally in poor health, they may be as motivated as the cases in being able to recall prior exposure(s).
Disadvantages	• Time consuming and therefore expensive to identify subjects. • Less likely to be motivated to participate in the study. • As subjects are generally healthy, their recall of prior exposure(s) may be less accurate (recall bias).	• Higher risk of selection bias. • Based on current knowledge, medical problems in controls should be unrelated to the exposure.

- Various sources can be used to obtain data on exposure status, including:
  - telephone or in-person interviews with subjects or family members
  - standardised questionnaires
  - pharmacy records
  - medical records
  - employment records
  - biological specimens.
- The accuracy, availability, cost and logistics of data collection should be taken into account when considering which sources should be used to ascertain the exposure status.
- While collecting data on exposure status is relatively quick (no follow-up period required), the data collected may be inaccurate and susceptible to recall bias (discussed below).

COMMUNICATION

What are the differences between case–control studies and retrospective cohort studies?

Distinguishing between case–control studies and retrospective cohort studies can be very difficult. The key differences include:

- In case–control studies, we categorise subjects according to *outcome status* and then trace subjects backwards to record exposure status.
- In retrospective cohort studies, we categorise subjects according to *exposure status* (based on historical records) and then measure outcome status in the present time.
- The incidence of a disease outcome can be measured in cohort studies, but not in case–control studies.
- A diagrammatic representation of the time sequence for exposure and outcome measurements in case–control studies and cohort studies can be found in Chapter 5 (Fig. 5.2).

INTERPRETING THE RESULTS

We can use a 2 × 2 table to summarise the number of cases and controls who were exposed to the risk factor being investigated (Fig. 8.4).

		Exposure		
		Yes	*No*	*Total*
Disease	*Yes (Case)*	d_1	d_0	$d_1 + d_0$
	No (Control)	h_1	h_0	$h_1 + h_0$
	Total	$d_1 + h_1$	$d_0 + h_0$	$n = d_1 + d_0 + h_1 + h_0$

d = disease *h* = healthy 1 = exposed 0 = unexposed

Fig. 8.4 Observed frequencies.

Odds and odds ratio

Calculating the odds ratio

In case–control studies, the odds ratio is used to measure the strength of the association between the exposure and outcome of interest. To calculate the odds ratio, we must first determine the odds of exposure in both cases and controls. An odds is defined as the probability of an 'event' occurring, divided by the probability of it not occurring:

$$\text{Odds of exposure in cases} = \frac{\text{Probability of being exposed amongst all cases}}{\text{Probability of being unexposed amongst all cases}}$$

$$= \frac{\frac{d_1}{d_0 + d_1}}{\frac{d_0}{d_0 + d_1}} = \frac{d_1}{d_0}$$

$$\text{Odds of exposure in controls} = \frac{\text{Probability of being exposed amongst all controls}}{\text{Probability of being unexposed amongst all controls}}$$

$$= \frac{\frac{h_1}{h_0 + h_1}}{\frac{h_0}{h_0 + h_1}} = \frac{h_1}{h_0}$$

The odds ratio is a measure of the difference in odds of exposure between the case and control groups:

$$\text{Exposure odds ratio} = \frac{\text{Odds of exposure in cases}}{\text{Odds of exposure in controls}}$$

$$= \frac{d_1/d_0}{h_1/h_0} = \frac{d_1 \times h_0}{d_0 \times h_1}$$

The odds ratio can also be calculated by comparing the odds of disease in the exposed subjects with the odds of disease in the unexposed subjects:

$$\text{Disease odds ratio} = \frac{\text{Odds of disease amongst exposed subjects}}{\text{Odds of disease amongst unexposed subjects}}$$

$$= \frac{d_1/h_1}{d_0/h_0} = \frac{d_1 \times h_0}{d_0 \times h_1}$$

As demonstrated, the right-hand formula for both the exposure odds ratio and disease odds ratio is the same and is known as the cross-product ratio.

Interpreting the odds ratio

The odds ratio indicates the increased (or decreased) odds of the disease being associated with the exposure of interest. The odds ratio can take any value between 0 and infinity, for example:

- If the odds ratio is 1, the odds of disease is the same in the exposed and unexposed groups.
- If the odds ratio is 2, the exposure of interest doubles the odds of disease.
- If the odds ratio is 0.5, the exposure of interest halves the odds of disease.
- If the odds ratio is 0.25, the exposure of interest reduces the odds of disease by 75%.

Confidence interval for an odds ratio

The statistical methods used when calculating the 95% confidence interval for an odds ratio are similar to those for a risk ratio. The 95% confidence interval for an odds ratio is calculated using an error factor with the following two formulae

$$\text{Error factor} = \text{exponential}\ (1.96 \times \text{standard error}\ (\text{log odds ratio}))$$

where,

$$\text{the SE of log OR} = \sqrt{\frac{1}{d_1} + \frac{1}{h_1} + \frac{1}{d_0} + \frac{1}{h_0}}$$

95% confidence interval for an odds ratio =

$$\frac{\text{Odds ratio}}{\text{Error factor}}\ \text{to Odds ratio} \times \text{Error factor}$$

The error factor is defined as the 95th percentile divided by the median. It is a measure of the spread of the distibution, and is usually denoted by 'EF'. For the purposes of your undergraduate training, you do not need to understand the formula for the confidence interval for an odds ratio.

The example at the end of this chapter demonstrates the application of these formulae in a real case-control study investigating the association between smoking and lung cancer.

HINTS AND TIPS

If you're still not sure how to calculate the odds ratio or the confidence interval for an odds ratio, try using an online calculator that walks you through the basic steps. One example, accessible online, is www.hutchon.net/confidOR.htm

Odds ratio versus risk ratio

- In case–control studies, the incidence rate of disease (and hence the risk and risk ratio) cannot be calculated, as we don't know the size of the population from which the cases were drawn. However, in cohort studies, a set number of 'healthy' individuals susceptible to the disease are recruited at the start of the study period. These subjects are then followed up longitudinally over time, and new cases of disease recorded, thus allowing us to calculate the incidence rate and risk ratio.

- In case–control studies, provided the outcome event is rare, the odds is approximately the same as the risk and so the odds ratio is an estimate of the risk ratio, and is interpreted in a similar way (please refer to the case study below).
- The prevalence and incidence (and hence the risk ratio) of a disease can only be calculated in a case–control study if the study is population-based and *all cases* in a *defined population* (which means knowing the total number of subjects disease-free (controls) in the population) are selected.

Case Study: Risk of constrictive pericarditis after acute pericarditis

This cohort study demonstrates how the risk ratio and odds ratio can be very similar in those studies where the outcome is rare.

Sudden and short-lived inflammation of the membranous sac surrounding the heart, the pericardium, is known as acute pericarditis. Pericarditis often causes central chest pain which worsens on inspiration or lying supine. A possible rare complication of acute pericarditis is when the pericardium becomes thick and rigid, making it hard for the heart muscle fibres to relax after each contraction. This is known as constrictive pericarditis. In a cohort study carried out by Imazio and colleagues in 2011, 500 consecutive cases with a first episode of acute pericarditis were recruited and followed up to evaluate the risk of developing constrictive pericarditis as a complication of acute pericarditis. During a median follow-up of 72 months, only 9 out of the 500 subjects developed constrictive pericarditis (Fig. 8.5).

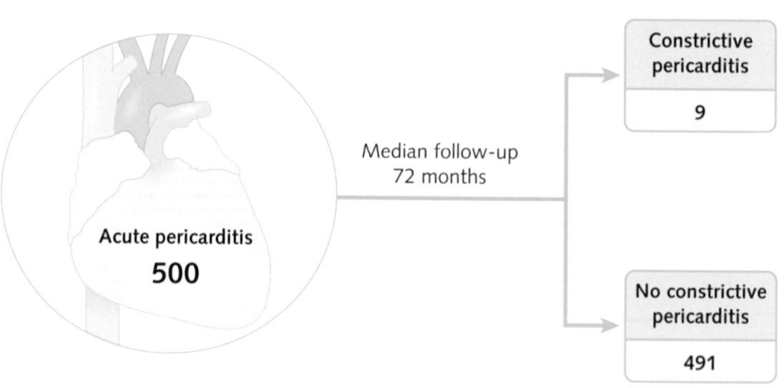

Fig. 8.5 Observed frequencies of constrictive pericarditis.

$$\text{The risk of constrictive pericarditis} = \frac{\text{Number of new cases of constrictive pericarditis over study period}}{\text{Total number of subjects initially disease-free}} = \frac{9}{500} = 0.018$$

$$\text{The odds of constrictive pericarditis} = \frac{\text{Probability of constrictive pericarditis}}{\text{Probability of not developing constrictive pericarditis}} = \frac{9/500}{491/500} = \frac{9}{491} = 0.183$$

As constrictive pericarditis is a *rare* complication of acute pericarditis, the number of subjects who do not develop constrictive pericarditis ($n = 491$) is approximately the same as the total number of individuals initially disease-free ($n = 500$). When calculating the risk and odds of developing constrictive pericarditis, the values of the denominator for both formulae are therefore approximately equal and so the odds is approximately the same as the risk.

COMMUNICATION

What is the difference between the odds ratio and risk ratio?

- Odds and odds ratio are calculated in case–control studies.
- Risk and risk ratio are calculated in cohort studies.
- When the disease is rare, the odds ratio is approximately equal to the risk ratio.
- When the disease is not rare, the odds ratio can overestimate the risk ratio.
- The odds ratio is interpreted in the same way as the risk ratio.

CONFOUNDING, CAUSALITY AND BIAS

Due to the methodology involved, there are three general issues that must be addressed when appraising observational studies:

1. Confounding
2. Causality
3. Bias.

Confounding

- Confounding occurs when the exposure of interest is not only associated with the risk of disease but also associated with a third variable that provides an alternative explanation for any association measured between the exposure and disease (please refer to Chapter 13 for an in-depth discussion on confounding).
- Provided the confounding factors are recognised and measured at the start of the study, they may be controlled for at the study design level or when analysing the results of the case-control study (discussed in Chapter 13).

Causality

In case–control studies, the temporal relationship between an exposure and outcome is not clear-cut as the exposure status is measured after the outcome has occurred. For a more in-depth discussion on causality, please refer to the Bradford-Hill criteria, which is discussed in Chapter 5.

Bias

Study error can broadly be categorised into two main groups: random error and systematic error. For an in-depth discussion on the difference between random error and systematic error, please refer to the Chapter 7 section 'Bias'. Systematic error can be divided into selection bias and measurement bias (Fig. 8.6).

Selection bias

Selection bias occurs when the association between exposure and disease is different for those who complete the study, compared with those who are in the target population. Selection bias can exist when procedures for subject selection or factors that influence a subject's participation affect the outcome of the study. The main types of selection bias that may occur in case–control studies include:

- Eligible population inappropriately defined
  - Hospital admission rate bias
  - Exclusion bias
  - Inclusion bias
  - Overmatching bias
- Participation bias
  - Non-response bias
- Detection bias
  - Diagnostic suspicion bias
  - Unmasking-detection signal bias
- Ascertainment bias
  - Incidence–prevalence bias
  - Healthcare access bias
  - Migration bias.

Eligible population inappropriately defined: hospital admission rate bias

Hospital admission rate bias may be an issue in hospital-based studies, especially in case–control studies. Considering hospitalised patients are more likely to suffer from many illnesses and engage in less healthy behaviours, they are probably not representative of the target population. Berkson's bias, one form of hospital admission bias, may be an issue if controls are selected from the same hospital where cases were recruited.

Consider a case–control study investigating the association between alcohol consumption and ischaemic heart disease. Hospitals contain a higher proportion of heavy drinkers than the general population, with admissions due to conditions such as mental illness, gastrointestinal bleeding, liver disease or pancreatitis, as well as ischaemic heart disease. How does this affect the odds ratio for an association between alcohol consumption and ischaemic heart disease? If controls are chosen from:

- the general population, the strength of the association between alcohol consumption and ischaemic heart disease will be overestimated.
- the hospital in-patient population, the strength of the association between alcohol consumption and ischaemic heart disease will be underestimated.

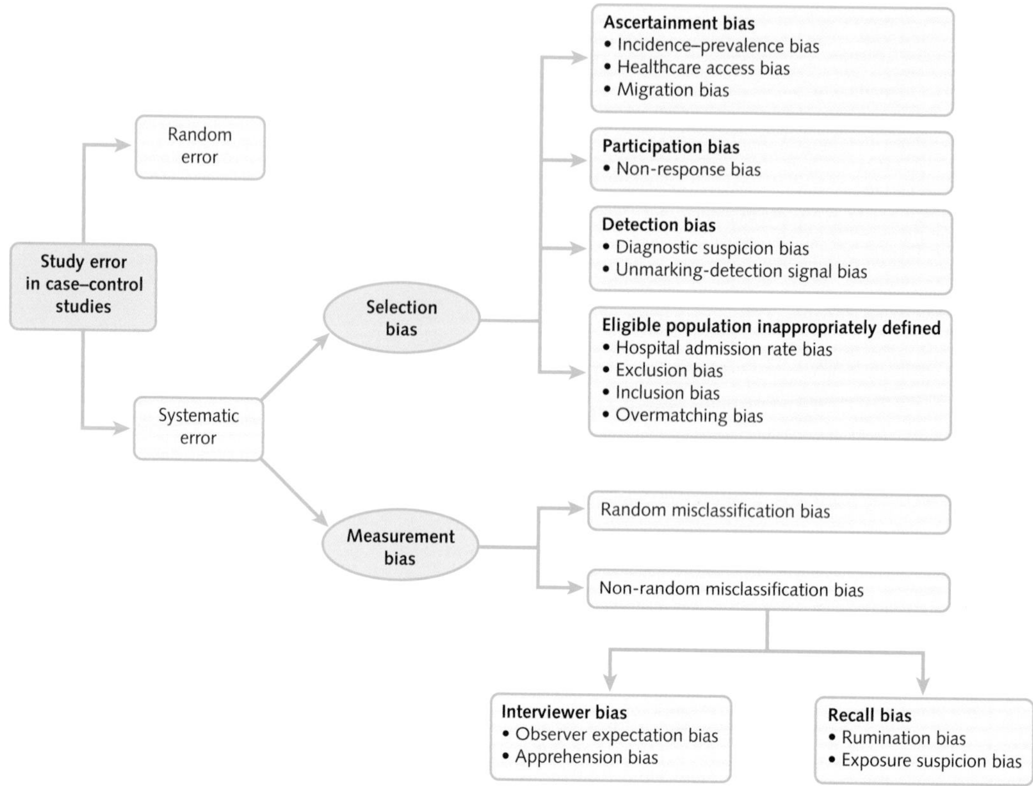

Fig. 8.6 Study error in case–control studies.

If choosing hospital controls, one way of minimising this type of bias is to select controls with different conditions so that biases introduced by specific diseases will tend to cancel each other out.

COMMUNICATION

Selection bias of cases

If exposure to the factor of interest is associated with an increased risk of being admitted to hospital, and the cases (but not the controls) for the case–control study are selected from a hospital in-patient population, the effect of the exposure on the outcome will be overestimated.

Selection bias of controls

As hospital in-patients are more likely to have been exposed to various risk factors compared to the general population, selecting hospital in-patients as cases and controls will underestimate the effect of the exposure on the outcome.

Eligible population inappropriately defined: exclusion bias and inclusion bias

When control subjects with conditions related to the exposure are excluded, whereas cases with these conditions (as co-morbidities) are included in the study, exclusion bias will occur.

If control subjects have one or more conditions related to the exposure being investigated, inclusion bias will occur. This may be an issue when controls are selected from a hospital in-patient population. The frequency of the exposure will be higher than that expected in the control group; therefore, the association between the exposure and outcome will be biased towards the null.

Eligible population inappropriately defined: overmatching bias

As discussed above, many case–control studies have a matched design when selecting cases and controls to ensure that the two groups are as similar to each other as possible. If the investigators match cases and controls by a non-confounding variable, which is associated with the exposure but not with the disease outcome, overmatching bias may be an issue and can underestimate the association between an exposure and outcome.

Participation bias: non-response bias

A separate participation rate should be calculated for both cases and controls using the formula:

$$\frac{\text{Number of study participants}}{\text{Number of people eligible to participate}}$$

There may be differences between the participants and non-participants if:

- the participation rate is low
- there is a large difference in participation rate between cases and controls

It is important to determine whether there are any similarities or differences between the participants and the non-participants. A sample of those not participating among the source (or target) population should be reviewed to ensure that the study participants are a truly representative sample. It is important to note that case or controls may differ from other members of the target population even if the participation rates are relatively high and comparable.

In particular, non-response bias is an issue if participation in the study is *related to the exposure status*. In case–control studies, it is sometimes very difficult to identify a sufficient number of control subjects; for example, some people cannot be contacted or the exposure status cannot be determined. We assume that the non-respondents have the same history of exposure as those controls who respond. However, if the non-respondents have different exposures (or outcomes) to those controls who respond, the odds of exposure amongst the controls may be over- or underestimated. Consider a case-control study investigating whether an association exists between smoking and lung cancer. If non-response is higher amongst the exposed than unexposed lung cancer cases, this will lead to an underestimation of the odds ratio between smoking and lung cancer.

Detection bias

If an exposure influences the *diagnosis* of the outcome, detection bias will occur. Detection bias may be an issue if:

1. the diagnostic approach (i.e. outcome determination) is related to knowledge of the subject's prior exposure status (diagnostic suspicion bias). In other words, knowledge of the subject's prior exposure status to a putative cause may have an influence on the intensity (and possibly the outcome) of the diagnostic process.
2. the exposure triggers the search for the outcome.

Consider a case–control study investigating the association between taking oral contraceptive pills (OCPs) and breast cancer. Cases of breast cancer are compared with a random sample of the general population (the controls), with regards to having taken OCPs in the past. However, some cases of breast cancer were diagnosed as a result of the subject visiting the GP for an OCP prescription. Therefore, exposed cases (i.e. those on OCPs) would have a greater likelihood of being diagnosed with breast cancer, compared with unexposed cases. This will result in an overestimation of the odds ratio.

Detection bias may also have occurred in this study if more thorough follow-up examinations were performed on those individuals on OCPs: for example, if OCPs were suspected of being harmful on the basis of animal experiments, preliminary case reports, etc. In conclusion, OCPs may be associated with breast cancer detection, rather than causing the cancer itself.

3. the exposure produces a symptom or sign that favours outcome diagnosis (unmasking-detection signal bias).

Consider a case–control study investigating the association between OCPs and endometrial cancer. As OCPs are associated with side effects such as breakthrough bleeding, it is possible that those subjects who were taking the OCP were more likely to be offered screening for endometrial cancer than those subjects who were not taking the OCP. The likelihood of detecting endometrial cancer would therefore be higher amongst the exposed subjects (i.e. those on OCPs) than the unexposed subjects. This will result in an overestimation of the odds ratio. Therefore, OCPs may be associated with endometrial cancer detection, rather than causing the cancer itself.

HINTS AND TIPS

While detection bias is a type of selection bias in case–control studies, it is a type of measurement bias in randomised controlled trials and prospective cohort studies as the outcome is measured during the follow-up period in the latter study designs.

Ascertainment bias: incidence–prevalence bias

Incidence–prevalence bias (also known as survival bias or Neyman bias) is a type of ascertainment bias where the patients included in the study do not represent the cases arising in the target population.

Incidence–prevalence bias may be an issue if the *survivors* of a lethal disease are more likely to enrol in the case–control study than the other cases. This may be because the serious cases have already passed away and are therefore unavailable (with the same frequency) as the mild cases.

Referring to Fig. 8.7, consider a hypothetical case-control study in which 50 potential subjects with the disease have been identified in a hospital. Out of all those with the disease, 10 cases agree to participate

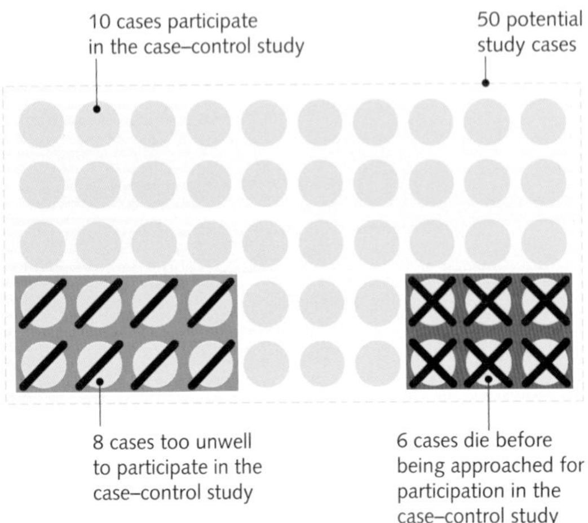
10 cases participate
in the case–control study
50 potential
study cases
8 cases too unwell
to participate in the
case–control study
6 cases die before
being approached for
participation in the
case–control study

Fig. 8.7 Survival bias when recruiting cases in case–control studies.

in the study. These 10 subjects may represent a biased sample as those who are unwell with severe disease (8 cases) or those who die (6 cases) before being approached to participate in the case-control study are not represented. Please refer to Chapter 9 on cross-sectional studies for a further discussion on incidence-survival bias.

It is important to note that in incidence–prevalence bias, the sample of cases enrolled has a distorted frequency of exposure if:

- the exposure itself determines the prognosis (e.g. mortality) of the outcome (e.g. disease).
- the exposure is related to the prognostic factor(s) of the outcome.

Consider a case–control study investigating the association between smoking and myocardial infarction (MI). If cases (i.e. those who have had a MI) who were smokers die more frequently, there will be a lower frequency of smokers amongst the remaining cases. This will underestimate the association between smoking and MI.

Ascertainment bias: healthcare access bias

Please refer to Chapter 7 for a discussion on healthcare access bias.

Ascertainment bias: migration bias

Please refer to Chapter 9 for a discussion on migration bias, which may be an issue in case–control studies dealing with prevalent cases.

Measurement bias

Measurement bias occurs when the information collected for the exposure and/or outcome variables is inaccurate. This type of bias can be divided into random or non-random misclassification.

Random misclassification bias

Random misclassification bias (also known as non-differential misclassification bias) can occur in case–control studies when either the exposure or outcome is classified incorrectly (with equal probability) into different groups. The exposed and unexposed groups therefore seem more similar than they actually are, leading to an underestimation (dilution) of the true effect of the exposure on the disease outcome. Random misclassification bias is discussed in further detail in Chapter 7.

Non-random misclassification bias

Non-random misclassification bias (also known as differential misclassification bias) occurs only when the exposure measurement is related to the disease outcome status or vice versa. As the misclassification is different in the groups being compared, this can lead to the effect of the exposure on the disease outcome being biased in either direction. The main types of non-random misclassification bias that may occur in case–control studies include:

- Recall bias
  - Rumination bias
  - Exposure suspicion bias
- Interviewer bias
  - Observer expectation bias
  - Apprehension bias.

Please refer to Chapter 7 for a discussion on these types of measurement bias.

ADVANTAGES AND DISADVANTAGES

What are the advantages and disadvantages of case–control studies (Fig. 8.8)?

KEY EXAMPLE OF A CASE–CONTROL STUDY

A classic case–control study investigating the effect of smoking on lung cancer was published by Doll and Hill in 1950. Cases with lung cancer were identified in 20 London hospitals and an equal number of controls were selected among in-patients of the same age range with diagnoses other than lung cancer. Figure 8.9 summarises the frequencies of lung cancer amongst the male smokers and non-smokers in the study.

Using the data presented in Fig. 8.9, we can calculate the odds of exposure (smoking) in cases (lung cancer)

Fig. 8.8 Advantages and disadvantages of case–control studies.

Advantages	**Disadvantages**
Efficient for studying the effect of exposures on *rare diseases*.	Reverse causality may be an issue, as the temporal sequence of exposure and outcome was not observed.
Efficient for studying the effect of exposures on *disease outcomes with long latency periods*.	A retrospective study, therefore particularly prone to recall bias and interviewer bias.
Useful for studying the effect of *multiple exposures* on disease outcome.	Can be prone to selection bias when choosing cases or controls.
A retrospective study; therefore there are no long periods of follow-up as the investigator does not need to wait for incident cases.	Limited to investigating the effect of exposures on only *one outcome*.
As cases are identified at the beginning of the study, there is no loss to follow-up.	Not suitable when investigating the effect of *rare exposures* on disease outcome.
Relatively quick, cheap and easy to perform.	The incidence rate of disease outcome cannot be estimated (unless the case–control study is population based).

Fig. 8.9 Frequencies of lung cancer amongst male smokers and non-smokers.

	Cases (lung cancer)	**Controls (no lung cancer)**
Exposed (smoker)	647	622
Unexposed (non-smoker)	2	27
Total	649	649

(Data from Doll R and Hill AB. (1950) Br Med J. 1950 2(4682): 739–748.)

and controls (no lung cancer), and therefore, the exposure odds ratio:

Odds of exposure in cases

$$= \frac{\text{Probability of being exposed amongst all cases}}{\text{Probability of being unexposed amongst all cases}}$$

$$= \frac{647/649}{2/649} = 323.50$$

Odds of exposure in controls

$$= \frac{\text{Probability of being exposed amongst all controls}}{\text{Probability of being unexposed amongst all controls}}$$

$$= \frac{622/649}{27/649} = 23.04$$

$$\text{Exposure odds ratio} = \frac{\text{Odds of exposure in cases}}{\text{Odds of exposure in controls}}$$

$$= \frac{323.50}{23.04} = 14.04 \text{ (2 dp)}$$

In order to calculate the 95% confidence interval for the odds ratio, we must first determine the value for the 'error factor':

Error factor (EF) =

exponential (1.96 × standard error (log odds ratio))

where,

$$\text{the SE of log OR} = \sqrt{\frac{1}{d_1} + \frac{1}{h_1} + \frac{1}{d_0} + \frac{1}{h_0}}$$

$$= \sqrt{\frac{1}{647} + \frac{1}{622} + \frac{1}{2} + \frac{1}{27}}$$

$$= \sqrt{0.54}$$

$$= 0.73 \text{(2 dp)}$$

therefore,

$$\text{EF} = \exp(1.96 \times 0.73) = 4.22 \text{ (2 dp)}$$

95% confidence interval for an odds ratio

$$= \frac{\text{Odds ratio}}{\text{Error factor}} \text{ to Odds ratio} \times \text{ Error factor}$$

$$95\% \text{ CI OR} = (14.04/4.22) \text{ to } (14.04 \times 4.22)$$

$$= 3.3 \text{ to } 59.3$$

The calculated odds ratio is 14, meaning that male smokers have a 14 times greater chance/odds of having lung cancer than male non-smokers. With 95% confidence, the odds of lung cancer in male smokers compared to male non-smokers lies between 3.3 and 59.3.

In order to make the move from an 'association' between cigarette smoking and lung cancer to a 'causal relationship', Doll and Hill immediately followed up their retrospective study with a large prospective cohort study, which is discussed in Chapter 7.

Measures of disease occurrence and cross-sectional studies

Objectives

By the end of this chapter you should:

- Be able to calculate and interpret the prevalence, incidence risk and incidence rate of a disease.
- Understand the interrelationship between the incidence rate and prevalence of a disease.
- Be able to identify and critically appraise cross-sectional studies.
- Understand the difference between descriptive cross-sectional studies and analytical cross-sectional studies.
- Know the steps involved in carrying out a cross-sectional study.
- Be able to calculate and interpret the prevalence ratio and prevalence odds ratio.
- Understand the terms confounding and causality in relation to cross-sectional studies.
- Be able to define the term bias and understand the different types of bias implicated in cross-sectional studies.
- Be able to list the advantages and disadvantages of cross-sectional studies.

A methodological checklist on how to critically appraise cross-sectional studies is provided in Chapter 19.

MEASURES OF DISEASE OCCURRENCE

The prevalence and incidence are both measures of the extent of disease in a defined population. There are key differences in the characteristics of both these measures.

Prevalence

- Prevalence:
  - is a static measure of the proportion of a disease in a defined population at a particular point in time.
  - includes both new cases and those diagnosed with the disease in the past who are still alive.
  - is calculated using the formula:

$$\text{Prevalence} = \frac{\text{Number of new and old cases of the disease at a single point in time}}{\text{Total number of people in the population at the same point in time}}$$

  - has the units 'cases/total population'.
- For example, as part of the Quality and Outcomes Framework (introduced in 2004 to provide financial incentives to general practices for the provision of high-quality care), most general practices across England provide annual data on the number of people with diabetes registered at their practice. Among the 44,653,400 people registered at general practices across England, 2,455,937 of them had a diagnosis of diabetes in 2011. Therefore, the prevalence of diabetes in England, in 2011, was:

$$\frac{2{,}455{,}937}{44{,}653{,}400} = 0.055 = 5.5\%$$

Incidence risk

- The incidence risk (also known as the cumulative incidence):
  - reflects the number of new cases of a disease in a 'population-at-risk' during a specified time period. The 'population-at-risk' defines the number of people in the population who are disease-free at the beginning of the observation period, but who are at risk of developing the disease of interest.
  - is calculated using the formula:

$$\text{Incidence risk} = \frac{\text{Number of new cases of the disease in a given time period}}{\text{Population at risk (initially disease-free)}}$$

  - has the units 'cases/population-at-risk'.
- For example, if a population initially contains 10 000 non-diabetic people and 480 of them develop diabetes over 2 years of observation, the incidence risk of diabetes over the 2-year period was:

$$\frac{480}{10\,000} = 0.048 = 4.8\%$$

HINTS AND TIPS

The denominator of both the prevalence and incidence risk formulae consists of the number of subjects in the population (e.g. country, county, town or city) from which cases of disease arise.

HINTS AND TIPS

Both the incidence risk and incidence rate are stated in relation to time. However, the units for the incidence risk are 'percentage of cases per unit time', while the units for the incidence rate are 'number of cases per person-year'.

Incidence rate

- The incidence RISK formula does *not* take into account the duration of time over which new cases have been identified. On the other hand, the formula for the incidence RATE does take the 'observation time' into account:

Incidence rate =

$$\frac{\text{Number of new cases of the disease}}{\text{Population at risk (initially disease-free)} \times \text{Time interval}}$$

- The units for the incidence rate are 'person-time'.
- In the same example used to demonstrate incidence risk, the incidence rate of diabetes is

$$\frac{480}{(10\,000 \times 2)} = 0.024 \text{ cases per year, or}$$

24 cases per 1000 person-years.

- The incidence rate calculated using this method implies that the rate of new cases of disease occurrence is constant over different periods of time such that, for an incidence rate of 24 cases per 1000 person-years:
  - 24 cases would be expected for 1000 persons observed for 1 year
  - 24 cases would be expected for 250 persons observed over 4 years, and so on.

Calculating person-time

- In certain types of studies, people are followed up for different lengths of time, as some individuals will remain disease-free for longer than others.
- Each subject contributes to the denominator of the incidence rate formula (person-time) so as long as the individual remains disease-free and, therefore, still at risk of being diagnosed with the disease of interest.
- This approach allows us to accurately calculate how quickly people are being diagnosed with a disease. For example, suppose we are investigating the incidence of hydrocephalus (a condition that occurs when there is too much cerebrospinal fluid in the ventricles of the brain) in patients admitted with a haemorrhagic stroke. We follow 10 subjects from baseline (i.e. those with a haemorrhagic stroke) for 15 weeks to investigate the incidence of hydrocephalus in these subjects (Fig. 9.1).

The bar graph shown in Fig. 9.1 illustrates the number of days each of the 10 subjects remained in the study during its 15-week (105-day) duration. The person-time is the sum of the total time contributed by all 10 subjects. The unit for person-time is person-days in this study.

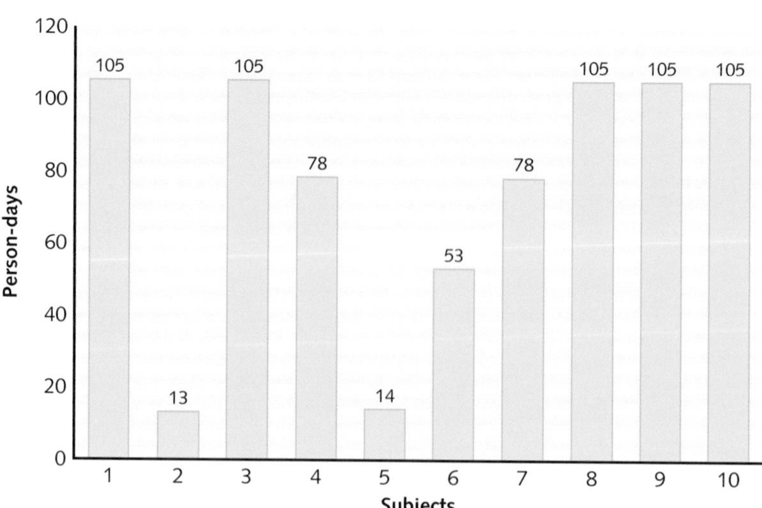

Fig. 9.1 Cases of hydrocephalus secondary to haemorrhagic stroke.

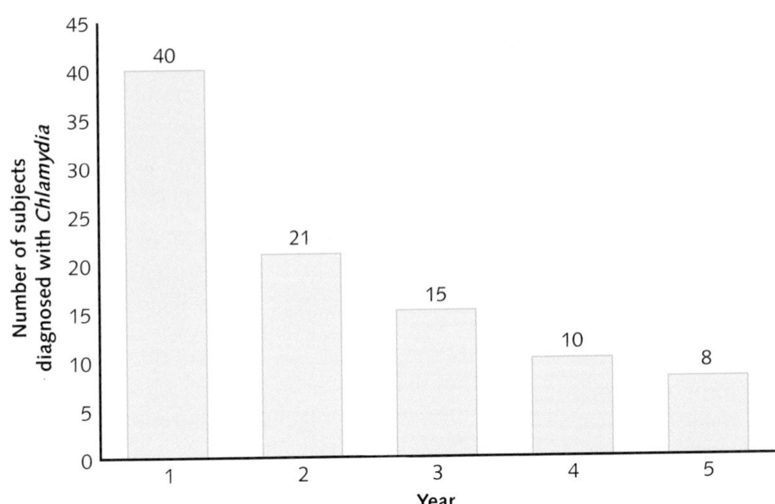

Fig. 9.2 Number of subjects diagnosed with *Chlamydia* on a yearly basis.

- The total person-days in this study is 761 person-days (105 + 13 + 105 + 78 + 14 + 53+78 + 105 + 105 + 105), which becomes the denominator of the incidence rate formula.
- The total number of subjects with haemorrhagic stroke who develop hydrocephalus is 5 (subjects 2, 4, 5, 6 and 7), which becomes the numerator of the incidence rate formula.
- Therefore, the incidence rate of hydrocephalus secondary to haemorrhagic stroke is:

$$\frac{5}{761 \text{ person-days}} = 0.00657 \text{ cases per person-day}$$

- By multiplying the numerator and denominator by 10 000, the incidence rate becomes 65.7 cases per 10 000 person-days.
- As highlighted above, the units for person-time can also be expressed as person-years or person-months, but other time units are possible.

For example, 0.00657 cases per person-day,
= 2.40 cases per person-year (= 0.00657 × 365)
= 0.079 cases per person-month (= 0.00657 × 12)

When does a person become a case?

- In some studies, subjects are only examined at specific time intervals during the observation period. It is therefore unknown when subjects develop the outcome of interest and the person-time cannot be accurately calculated. We therefore assume that the outcome develops at the halfway point between intervals when calculating the person-time.
- For example, suppose we are investigating the incidence rate of *Chlamydia* in a sample population of 200 medical students. Subjects are examined once a year for up to 5 years.
- The graph shown in Fig. 9.2 illustrates the number of students diagnosed with their first attack of *Chlamydia* when subjects were examined on a yearly basis. The person-time is the sum of the total time contributed by all 200 subjects. The unit for person-time is person-years in this study. Therefore the person-time contributed by all subjects is:
  - At 1 year, there were 40 new cases, and we assume they all developed *Chlamydia* at 0.5 years, thus contributing (40 × 0.5) = 20 person-years.
  - At 2 years, there were 21 new cases, and we assume they all developed *Chlamydia* at 1.5 years, thus contributing (21 × 1.5) = 31.5 person-years.
  - At 3 years, there were 15 new cases, and we assume they all developed *Chlamydia* at 2.5 years, thus contributing (15 × 2.5) = 37.5 person-years.
  - At 4 years, there were 10 new cases, and we assume they all developed *Chlamydia* at 3.5 years, thus contributing (10 × 3.5) = 35 person-years.
  - At 5 years, there were 8 new cases, and we assume they all developed *Chlamydia* at 4.5 years, thus contributing (8 × 4.5) = 36 person-years.
  - Accounting for the 106 people who never developed *Chlamydia* over the 5-year study period, they contributed (106 × 5) = 530 person-years.
- The total time-years contributed by all subjects is 690 person-years (= 20 + 31.5 + 37.5 + 35 + 36 + 530).
- The incidence rate of *Chlamydia* in medical students is:

$$\frac{94}{690 \text{ person-years}} = 0.136 \text{ cases per person-year}$$

- By multiplying the numerator and denominator by 1000, the incidence rate becomes 136 cases per 1000 person-years. In other words, if you were to follow 1000 medical students for one year, you would see 136 new cases of *Chlamydia*!

HINTS AND TIPS

Mortality is a type of incidence in which the events measured are deaths rather than the occurrence of a new disease. Mortality can be reported as a risk (e.g. 10-year mortality) or as a rate.

Prevalence versus incidence

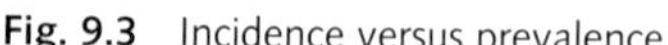

- We can use the concept of tap water running into a sink to demonstrate the relationship between incidence and prevalence (Fig. 9.3).
- Prevalence can be considered as the proportion of a sink (total population) filled with water (prevalent cases).
- Flow of the tap water into the sink represents incident cases.
- Drainage of water down the sink drainpipe represents prevalent cases leaving the prevalence pool due to recovery (cure), death or emigration.
- Using this model, we can conclude that the prevalence increases if:
  - the rate of new cases arising increases (more tap water runs into the sink).
  - the number of cases who recover, die or emigrate decreases (less water drains from the sink).
- A successful treatment that improves survival rates (without curing the disease) will increase the prevalence of the disease.
- The interrelationship between prevalence and incidence can be mathematically expressed as:

$$\text{Prevalence} = \text{Incidence rate} \times \text{Average duration of the disease}$$

- We assume that the prevalence of the disease in the population is low, i.e. less than 0.10, when using this formula.
- This formula can only be used under certain conditions, known as the 'steady state', which implies that:
  1. the length of time from diagnosis to recovery or death is stable.
  2. the incidence rate of the disease has been stable over time, i.e. no marked reduction of the disease or recent epidemics.

HINTS AND TIPS

The prevalence of a disease can increase, either because the disease prevalence has increased or because the average duration of the disease has increased.

Fig. 9.3 Incidence versus prevalence.

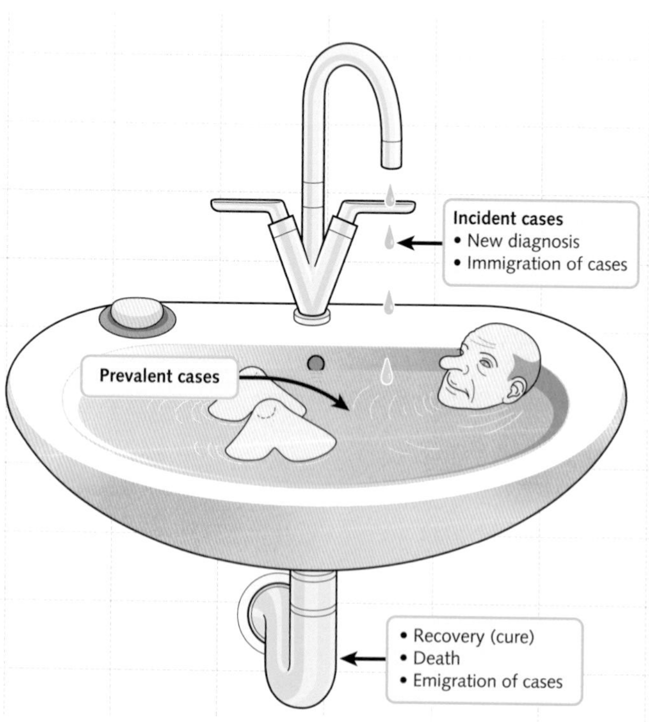

STUDY DESIGN

- A cross-sectional study is a form of observational study that involves collecting data from a target population at a single point in time.
- This methodology is particularly useful for assessing the true burden of a disease or the health needs of a population. Cross-sectional studies are therefore useful for planning the provision and allocation of health resources. Most government surveys conducted by the National Centre for Health Statistics are cross-sectional studies.
- Compared to information from routine hospital or primary care health records, the data collected from cross-sectional studies are systematically collected and less subject to measurement bias.
- Data collection methods include questionnaires, medical examinations, and interviews. While questionnaires are cheaper than interviews the response rate is usually lower; thus a large study sample size is required when using questionnaires.
- Cross-sectional studies are good at discovering people with a disease who have not previously sought any medical advice. Healthcare professionals are usually only aware of the relatively small proportion of individuals that present to them with an illness. There is often more disease in the community, irrespective of whether individuals are symptomatic (e.g. stable angina) or asymptomatic (e.g. asymptomatic HIV infection). This phenomenon is known as the 'clinical iceberg' (Fig. 9.4). Cross-sectional studies are able to uncover the iceberg of disease.

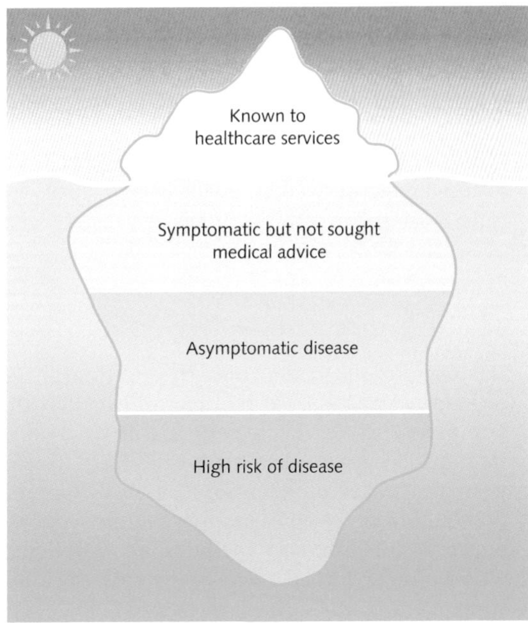

Fig. 9.4 The clinical iceberg.

Descriptive cross-sectional studies

- Descriptive cross-sectional studies are used to measure the prevalence and distribution of a disease in a defined population.
- Prevalence can be assessed at a single point in time (point prevalence). For example, a random sample of medical schools across London were selected to measure the prevalence or burden of depression amongst medical students.
- Prevalence can also be assessed over a defined period of time (period prevalence). The period prevalence is usually determined if it takes time to gather sufficient information on the outcome in the population. For example, a random sample of movement disorder clinics across London were selected to measure the prevalence of Meige's syndrome, a rare form of dystonia, in patients referred to the clinic over 10 months.

Analytical cross-sectional studies

- Analytical cross-sectional studies are used to investigate the interrelationship between any variables of interest. For example, a target population could be sampled to determine the characteristics (age, sex, ethnicity, etc.) of those people with ischaemic heart disease.
- However, valid conclusions about the strength of the association between putative risk factors and a particular disease outcome are limited. This is primarily because the disease status is measured at the same time as the exposure status (discussed below).

HINTS AND TIPS

While cross-sectional studies aim to provide data from the entire population under study, case-control studies usually only include a *sample* of subjects from the population.

COMMUNICATION

What research questions are best answered with a cross-sectional study design?

A cross-sectional study design is best suited when:

- carrying out surveys on the prevalence of a disease (or other health-related characteristics) in order to assess its burden in a defined population (and for planning the allocation of health resources accordingly).

- carrying out surveys of views or attitudes, such as studies on smoking behaviour, alcohol consumption or patient satisfaction.
- studying the association between an exposure and disease onset for a *chronic disease* (where there is limited information available on the time of onset of the disease).

Selecting a representative sample

- Having formulated the research question(s), the *target population* should be determined. It is this population to which the results will be generalised. A *study population* is then randomly selected from the target population. The study population should be a representative sample from the target population and includes all individuals who are invited to take part in the cross-sectional study.
- The sample size should be large enough to ensure that the prevalence calculated has adequate precision.
- Having excluded all individuals from the study population who are non-responders, we are left with the *study sample* (Fig. 9.5).
- If a high response rate is achieved (the study sample is a high proportion of the study population), the findings from the study can be generalised back to the target population with a high degree of validity.

Repeated cross-sectional studies

- Cross-sectional studies may be repeated at different:
  - places, i.e. to look for variability in the study findings.
  - time points, i.e. to assess for trends in data over time. However, changes in findings can be difficult to assess as the results may simply reflect a different population of individuals being studied.

HINTS AND TIPS

In a cross-sectional study, data are collected on each subject at one point in time. This does not necessarily imply that all data are collected at exactly the same time point for each subject! For example, when collecting data on cholesterol levels from patients of African descent enrolled at a GP practice, blood tests may be taken from the study sample over the course of 2 weeks.

INTERPRETING THE RESULTS

We can use a 2 × 2 table to summarise the number of exposed and unexposed subjects who do or do not have the disease of interest (Fig. 9.6).

Prevalence

The main outcome measure estimated from a cross-sectional study is the prevalence of a disease in the population:

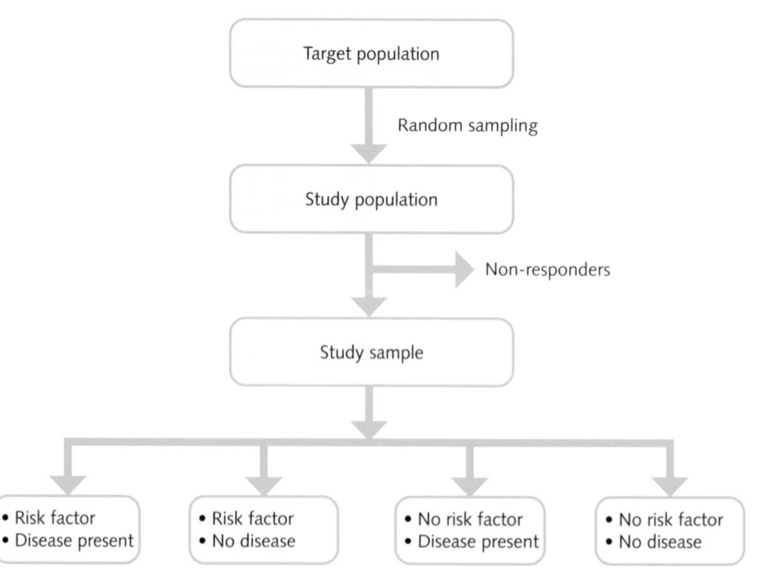

Fig. 9.5 Study design – cross-sectional studies.

		Exposure		Total
		Yes	No	
Disease	Yes	d_1	d_0	$d_1 + d_0$
	No	h_1	h_0	$h_1 + h_0$
	Total	$d_1 + h_1$	$d_0 + h_0$	$n = d_1 + d_0 + h_1 + h_0$

d = disease h = healthy 1 = exposed 0 = unexposed

Fig. 9.6 Observed frequencies in analytical cross-sectional studies.

$$\text{Prevalence} = \frac{\text{Number of cases of the disease in the study sample at a single point in time}}{\text{Total number of people in the the study sample at the same point in time}}$$

As discussed at the start of this chapter, the prevalence is defined as the proportion of cases with a disease at a particular point in time in a defined population. Both old and new cases of the disease are included in the numerator of the formula.

HINTS AND TIPS

The incidence of a disease cannot be calculated using a cross-sectional study design as healthy individuals are not being followed up over time to identify new cases of the disease.

Prevalence odds ratio

- The prevalence odds ratio is a measure of the association between the exposure and outcome, analogous to the odds ratio:

$$\text{Prevalence odds ratio} = \frac{\text{Odds of the disease amongst the exposed subjects at a single point in time}}{\text{Odds of the disease amongst the unexposed subjects at the same point in time}}$$

$$= \frac{d_1/h_1}{d_0/h_0} = \frac{d_1 \times h_0}{d_0 \times h_1}$$

- It is interpreted in the same way as the odds ratio calculated in case–control studies. For example, if the prevalence odds ratio is 4, the odds of having the disease are 4 times higher in the exposed group than in the unexposed group.
- If the duration of the disease is the same in both the exposed and unexposed groups (i.e. the duration is not affected by the exposure status), and exposure to the risk factor occurs over an extended period of time, the prevalence odds ratio provides an estimate for the risk ratio.
- Additionally, as in case–control studies, provided the outcome is rare, the odds is approximately the same as the risk and so the odds ratio is an estimate of the risk ratio, and is interpreted in a similar way.

Prevalence ratio

- The prevalence ratio is another measure of association between the exposure and outcome. It is analogous to the risk ratio:

$$\text{Prevalence ratio} = \frac{\text{Probability of the disease amongst the exposed subjects at a single point in time}}{\text{Probability of the disease amongst the unexposed subjects at the same point in time}}$$

$$= \frac{d_1/(d_1 + h_1)}{d_0/(d_0 + h_0)}$$

- It is interpreted in the same way as the risk ratio in cohort studies. For example, if the prevalence ratio is 2, the exposed subjects are twice as likely as the unexposed subjects to have the disease.

Prevalence odds ratio versus prevalence ratio

- If the outcome measured is a chronic disease or if the period of exposure to a potential risk factor is long-lasting, the prevalence odds ratio is the preferred measure of association in a cross-sectional study (Fig. 9.7).
- On the other hand, the prevalence ratio is calculated when the outcome occurs over a relatively short period of time (days to weeks).
- The lower the prevalence of a disease in both the exposed and unexposed groups, i.e. 15% or less, the closer the values of the prevalence odds ratio and the prevalence ratio will be.

Fig. 9.7 Prevalence odds ratio versus prevalence ratio.

Prevalence odds ratio	Prevalence ratio
A prevalence measure of association between an exposure and outcome	
Provides an estimate of the odds ratio as in case–control studies	Provides an estimate of the risk ratio as in cohort studies
Preferable for chronic diseases (months to years)	Preferable for acute diseases (days to weeks)

- Since cross-sectional studies are particularly useful for investigating chronic diseases, the prevalence odds ratio is usually the preferred measure of association.

CONFOUNDING, CAUSALITY AND BIAS

Due to the methodology involved, there are three general issues that must be addressed when appraising observational studies:

1. Confounding
2. Causality
3. Bias.

Confounding

- Confounding occurs when the exposure of interest is not only associated with the risk of disease but also associated with a third variable that provides an alternative explanation for any association measured between the exposure and disease (please refer to Chapter 13 for an in-depth discussion on confounding).
- Provided the confounding factors are recognised and measured at the start of the study, they may be controlled for at the study design level or when analysing the results of the cross-sectional study (discussed in Chapter 13).

Causality

In cross-sectional studies, the temporal relationship between an exposure and outcome is not clear-cut as the exposure status is measured at the same time as the outcome. For a more in-depth discussion on causality, please refer to the Bradford-Hill criteria, which are discussed in Chapter 5.

Bias

Study error can broadly be categorised into two main groups: random error and systematic error (Fig. 9.8). For an in-depth discussion on the difference between random error and systematic error, please refer to the Chapter 7 section 'Bias'. Systematic error can be divided into selection bias and measurement bias.

Selection bias

Selection bias occurs when the association between an exposure and disease is different for those who complete the study, compared with those who are in the

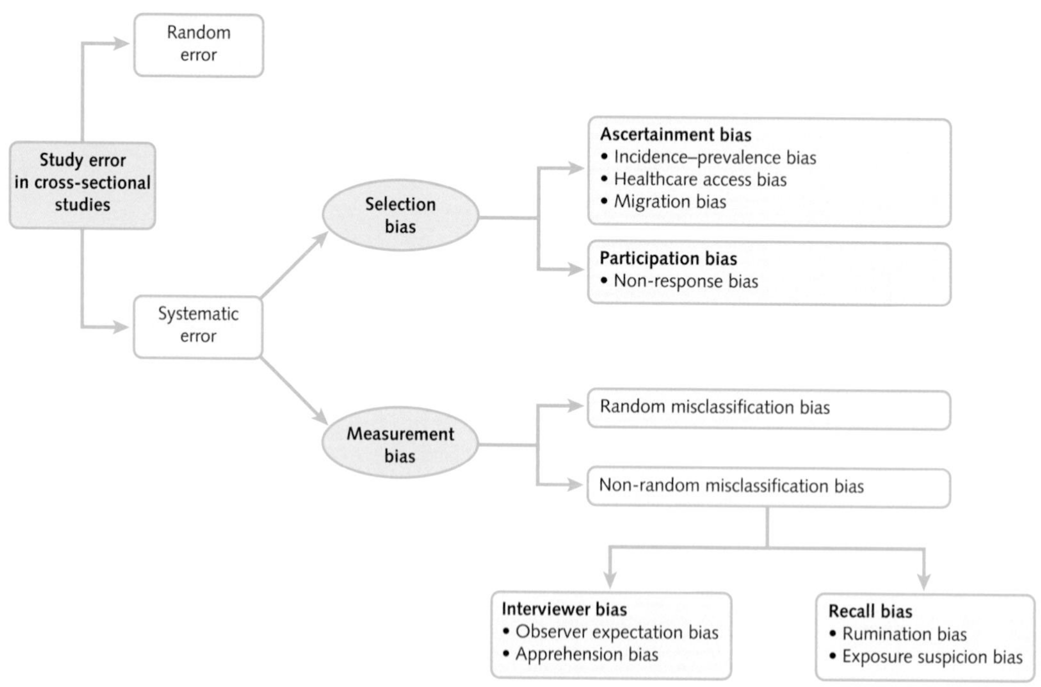

Fig. 9.8 Study error in cross-sectional studies.

target population. Selection bias can exist when procedures for subject selection or factors that influence a subject's participation affect the outcome of the study. It can occur if the exposure status of cases or controls has an influence on whether subjects are selected for study participation. The main types of selection bias that may occur in cross-sectional studies include:

- Participation bias
  - Non-response bias
- Ascertainment bias
  - Incidence–prevalence bias
  - Healthcare access bias
  - Migration bias.

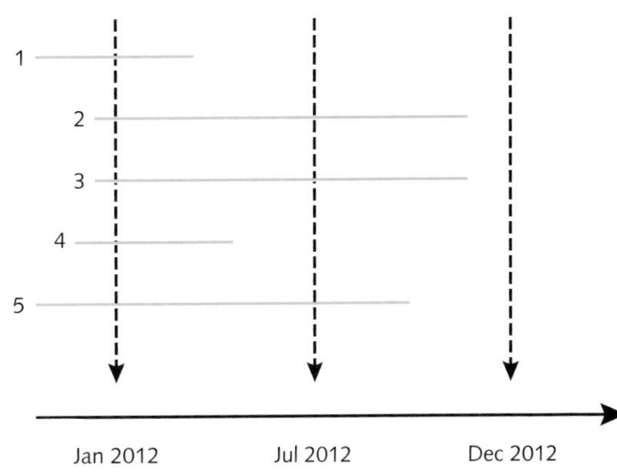
1
2
3
4
5
Jan 2012
Jul 2012
Dec 2012
If the cross-sectional study was carried out in July 2012 cases 1 and 4 would be missed.

Fig. 9.9 Incidence–prevalence bias.

Participation bias: non-response bias

While participation in cross-sectional studies never reaches 100%, it has been recognised that the decision for individuals in the study population to take part (or not take part) in a study is not random. Factors associated with low response rates include:

- Younger age
- Male sex
- Alcohol or drug misuse
- Lower socioeconomic status
- More unwell.

If there is an association between the exposure or outcome with any of the factors associated with a low response rate, the study sample will not be representative of the target population. Additionally, as non-responders are more likely to be unwell than those who participate in the study, most surveys will underestimate the prevalence of disease in the target population.

Strenuous efforts must be made to ensure that the response rates are as high as possible. To determine whether there are systematic differences between the group of responders and the group of non-responders, as much information should be recorded from the non-participants as is deemed feasible, therefore allowing for comparisons to be made between the two groups.

Ascertainment bias: incidence–prevalence bias

As discussed above, in a steady state, the prevalence of a disease is influenced by both its duration and incidence rate. In cross-sectional studies where the duration of the disease outcome (or survival with the disease) is different in both the exposed and unexposed groups being compared, the prevalence odds ratio and the prevalence ratio will not provide a valid estimate of the odds ratio and risk ratio, respectively.

If studies are performed late in the disease process, asymptomatic or mild cases that have been successfully treated, as well as severe or fatal cases, will be missed. Prevalent cases are likely to include long-term survivors, who will have a better average survival than that of incident cases. The numerator of the disease prevalence formula is therefore dependent on when the cross-sectional study is being conducted (Fig. 9.9). Please refer to Chapter 8 on case–control studies for a further discussion on incidence–prevalence bias.

Ascertainment bias: healthcare access bias

Please refer to Chapter 7 for a discussion on healthcare access bias.

Ascertainment bias: migration bias

Outmigration of cases from an environment perceived as causing the disease of interest can bias measures of prevalence. Selective migration may occur if the disease itself, or the threat of developing the disease may cause cases to leave the environment under investigation. For example, if the prevalence of lung cancer in people who live within a five mile radius of a nuclear power plant is studied, selective migration of people living near the power plant will result in migration bias.

Measurement bias

Measurement bias occurs when the information collected for the exposure and/or outcome variables is inaccurate. This type of bias can be divided into random or non-random misclassification.

Random misclassification bias

Random misclassification bias (also known as non-differential misclassification bias) can occur in cross-sectional studies when either the exposure or outcome is classified incorrectly (with equal probability) into different groups. The exposed and unexposed groups therefore seem more similar than they actually are, leading to an underestimation (dilution) of the true effect of the exposure on the disease outcome. Non-validated questionnaires are especially prone to this type of bias. Random misclassification bias is discussed in further detail in Chapter 7.

Non-random misclassification bias

Non-random misclassification bias (also known as differential misclassification bias) occurs only when the exposure measurement is related to the disease outcome status or vice versa. As the misclassification is different in the groups being compared, this can lead to the effect of the exposure on the disease outcome being biased in either direction. The main types of non-random misclassification bias that may occur in cross-sectional studies include:

- Recall bias
  - Rumination bias
  - Exposure suspicion bias
- Interviewer bias
  - Observer expectation bias
  - Apprehension bias

Please refer to Chapter 7 for a discussion on these types of measurement bias.

ADVANTAGES AND DISADVANTAGES

What are the advantages and disadvantages of cross-sectional studies (Fig. 9.10)?

Fig. 9.10 Advantages and disadvantages of cross-sectional studies.

Advantages	Disadvantages
Useful for measuring the prevalence of a disease in a defined population and for planning the allocation of health resources accordingly.	Usually cannot test epidemiologic hypotheses as cross-sectional studies are low on the hierarchy of evidence.
Able to measure the prevalence of a disease for all the exposure factors under investigation.	Not useful for studying rare diseases or diseases with a short duration.
Multiple exposures and outcomes can be measured at the same time in the same cross-sectional study.	Cannot usually discern a temporal relationship between an exposure and disease outcome.
Useful for generating hypotheses by studying the association between exposure and disease onset for chronic diseases.	The incidence rate of a disease outcome cannot be estimated.
Generally quick (no long periods of follow-up) and cheap to conduct.	Can be prone to selection bias due to poor study participation response rates.
As routinely collected, readily available data are commonly used, fewer resources are required to run the study.	Susceptible to measurement bias, including survival and migration bias.

KEY EXAMPLE OF A CROSS-SECTIONAL STUDY

Thyroid hormones are known to regulate cardiac function and cardiovascular haemodynamics. In 2005, Walsh and colleagues carried out a cross-sectional study examining the prevalence of coronary heart disease in subjects with and without subclinical hypothyroidism (increased serum thyrotropin concentration and normal serum thyroxine levels). Data were collected from the community health survey carried out in Busselton, Western Australia, in 1981. Figure 9.11 summarises the frequency of coronary heart disease according to thyroid status.

Fig. 9.11 Frequencies of coronary heart disease according to thyroid status.

	Coronary heart disease	No coronary heart disease	Total
Subclinical hypothyroidism	18	101	119
Euthyroidism (normal)	154	1752	1906
Total	172	1873	2025

(Data from Walsh JP et al. (2005) Arch. Intern. Med. 165: 2467–2472.)

Using the data presented in Fig. 9.11, we can calculate the prevalence of coronary heart disease in subjects with subclinical hypothyroidism and in subjects who are euthyroid:

$$\text{Prevalence} = \frac{\text{Number of cases of the disease in the study sample at a single point in time}}{\text{Total number of people in the study sample at the same point in time}}$$

Prevalence of coronary heart disease in subjects with subclinical hypothyroidism (exposed group):

$$= \frac{\text{Number of cases of coronary heart disease amongst those subjects with subclinical hypothyroidism}}{\text{Total number of subjects with subclinical hypothyroidism}}$$

$$= \frac{18}{119}$$

$$= 15.1\%$$

Prevalence of coronary heart disease in subjects who are euthyroid (unexposed group):

$$= \frac{\text{Number of cases of coronary heart disease amongst those subjects who are euthyroid}}{\text{Total number of subjects who are euthyroid}}$$

$$= \frac{154}{1906}$$

$$= 8.1\%$$

We can calculate the prevalence odds ratio and the prevalence ratio to measure the association between having subclinical hypothyroidism and coronary heart disease:

Prevalence odds ratio

$$= \frac{\text{Odds of the disease amongst the exposed subjects at a single point in time}}{\text{Odds of the disease amongst the unexposed subjects at a single point in time}}$$

$$= \frac{\text{Odds of having coronary heart disease amongst those subjects with subclinical hypothyroidism}}{\text{Odds of having coronary heart disease amongst those subjects who are euthyroid}}$$

$$= \frac{d_1/h_1}{d_0/h_0} = \frac{d_1 \times h_0}{d_0 \times h_1}$$

$$= \frac{18/101}{154/1752} = \frac{18 \times 1752}{154 \times 101}$$

$$= 2.0$$

Prevalence ratio

$$= \frac{\text{Probability of the disease amongst the exposed subjects at a single point in time}}{\text{Probability of the disease amongst the unexposed subjects at the same point in time}}$$

$$= \frac{\text{Probability of having coronary heart disease amongst those subjects with subclinical hypothyroidism}}{\text{Probability of having coronary heart disease amongst those subjects who are euthyroid}}$$

$$= \frac{d_1/(d_1 + h_1)}{d_0/(d_0 + h_0)}$$

$$= \frac{18/(18 + 101)}{154/(154 + 1752)} = \frac{18/119}{154/1906}$$

$$= 1.9$$

Using the data calculated above, we can conclude that:

- The prevalence of coronary heart disease was higher in those subjects with subclinical hypothyroidism (15.1%) than in the euthyroid subjects (8.1%).
- The odds of having coronary heart disease were 2 times higher in those subjects with subclinical hypothyroidism than in the euthyroid subjects (prevalence odds ratio = 2.0).
- The subjects who had subclinical hypothyroidism were 1.9 times more likely than the euthyroid subjects to have coronary heart disease (prevalence ratio = 1.9).
- As the prevalence of coronary heart disease in both the exposed (subclinical hypothyroidism) and unexposed (euthyroid) groups is relatively low, and nearly equal, the values for the prevalence odds ratio and the prevalence ratio are similar.
- As coronary heart disease is a chronic disease and the period of exposure (to the biochemical abnormalities associated with subclinical hypothyroidism) is long lasting, the prevalence odds ratio is the preferred measure of association in this particular cross-sectional study.

Ecological studies

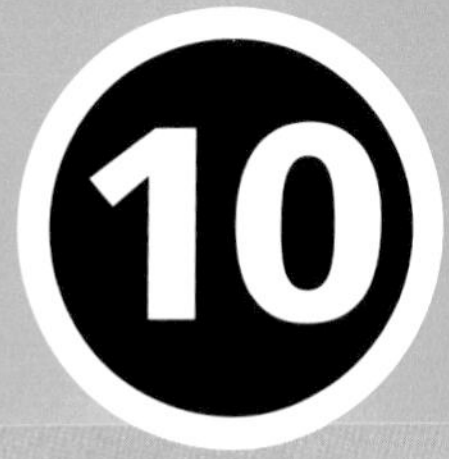

Objectives

By the end of this chapter you should:

- Be able to identify and critically appraise the different types of ecological studies.
- Know the steps involved in carrying out an ecological study.
- Understand the difference between biologic and ecologic inferences.
- Know the steps involved in analysing and interpreting the results of an ecological study.
- Understand the limitations commonly faced when using ecological studies to make causal inferences.
- Be able to define the term ecological fallacy.
- Be able to list the advantages and disadvantages of ecological studies.

STUDY DESIGN

- An ecological study is an observational study in which the units of observation and analysis are at a group level, rather than at an individual level.
- Ecological studies are near the bottom of the hierarchy of what counts as reliable evidence for clinical decision-making (Fig. 1.5).
- Using aggregate data, they examine the association between exposures and outcomes.

Levels of measurement

- In 1995, H. Morgenstern published a paper (see 'Further Reading') which highlighted that there are three types of ecologic measures:
  1. *Aggregate measures*: These combine data from individuals, summarised regionally or nationally, e.g. the percentage of smokers in a city.
  2. *Environmental measures*: These are physical characteristics of a place in which members of each group work or live, e.g. air-pollution level, temperature or climate of a country. Environmental measures have an analogue at the individual level; however, they are not easy to measure. In other words, there may be heterogeneity of the exposure level within groups. For example, the average temperature of the UK during the summer months may be 40°C (I wish!); however, not all populations in the UK will have been exposed to such a heatwave. The capacity of the urban land surface (e.g. roads, pavements, buildings etc.) to absorb and trap heat is higher than that in rural areas. Furthermore, not all individuals embrace the sun! This is why we measure the impact of environmental measures on the whole group by using an ecological study design.
  3. *Global measures*: These are attributes of places or groups for which there is no obvious individual analogue. Examples include contextual variables such as laws restricting smoking in public places, the population density of a country, or policies to improve equity in access to health care.

Levels of inferences

- The goal of an ecological study may be to make:
  - biologic inferences about effects on individual risks. For example, if the objective of a study is to estimate the biologic effect of having the measles, mumps and rubella (MMR) vaccine on the risk of getting autism, the target level of causal inference is biologic.
  - ecologic inferences about effects on group rates. For example, the causal inference is ecologic if the objective of a study is to investigate whether the rates of autism vary across different countries, each with their specific national health guidelines on MMR vaccination.
- It is important to note that the magnitude of the ecologic effect depends not only on the biologic effect of the MMR vaccination but also on the pattern and degree of compliance with the health guidelines in each country.

- On top of this, there may be individual-level confounders such as the age of the subject when the vaccine was given, which may affect the validity of the ecologic-effect estimate.
- Sometimes we are interested in making cross-level inferences. For example, interpreting ecologic effects, which are based on aggregate measures, as individual effects. However, such inferences are particularly vulnerable to bias.

Types of ecological studies

The grouping used in ecological studies may be by time or place.

Time trend studies

- If grouping is by time, the study is known as a time trend study; for example, investigating whether changes in the incidence of lung cancer over time correlate with changes in smoking habit over time (in the same population).
- Risk factor or disease frequencies may decrease, increase or stay constant over time. These trends between risk factors and disease outcomes can assist us in determining whether:
    - a certain risk factor might be causing a particular disease.
    - attempts at risk factor (or disease prevention) have been successful.

Geographical studies

- If grouping is by place, the study is known as a geographical study (or multiple-group study); for example, investigating the association between smoking and lung cancer in different countries.
- Disease occurrence in a defined population can be compared either within a country (e.g. between cities or regions), or between countries (during the same time period).

Mixed design

- Sometimes, you may combine a time trend and geographical study design.
- We are particularly interested in whether temporal patterns of a particular disease or risk factor vary between different geographical areas. For example, while there has been a trend toward increasing life expectancy in Western Europe since 1990, this has been paralleled by a decreasing trend in life expectancy in Russia and portions of Eastern Europe.

COMMUNICATION

What research questions are best answered with an ecological study design?

Ecological studies may be used:

- to investigate possible correlations between changes in risk factor profiles and disease rates over time.
- to monitor the effectiveness of health interventions.
- for the surveillance of communicable and non-communicable diseases.
- to explore the inequalities in care; e.g. is the incidence rate of hospital admissions for community-acquired pneumonia higher in deprived areas?
- to explore the quality of care, e.g. comparing mortality rates between different hospitals or geographical regions.
- to inform resource allocation or health promotion programmes.
- to generate hypotheses about what factors (e.g. environmental) may be involved in preventing or causing a disease.
- to investigate the physical characteristics of a place in which members of each group work or live, e.g. air-pollution level, temperature or climate.

Data collection

- The data collected on the exposure and outcome variables should be at the same level of aggregation (e.g. time period, city, region, country, continent).
- The studies often use data previously collected for an alternative purpose:
    - Primary care data
    - Secondary care (hospital) data
    - Mortality and census data
    - Infectious disease notification data
    - National survey data, e.g. population registries or the census.
- While using routinely collected data makes ecological studies less time consuming and less expensive than if the data was systematically collected, the data often has less accuracy and may be of poor quality.

INTERPRETING THE RESULTS

- While a variety of methods can be used to analyse the results of the various types of ecological study designs that exist, we will focus on how to interpret the results of a geographical (multiple-group) study, one of the more common types of ecological studies. We will assume that the measures of exposure and outcome are continuous variables (discussed in Chapter 2), which is typical in ecological studies.

Scatter plots and correlation coefficients

- The results of a geographical study are usually analysed initially by looking at the strength of the association between the exposure and outcome variables.
- Typically, we construct a scatter plot and calculate an overall measure of correlation.
- The Pearson correlation coefficient (r) measures the degree of linear association between two continuous variables, i.e. the exposure and outcome variables:
  - If $r = 1$, this indicates a perfect positive linear relationship, i.e. a straight line with a positive gradient.
  - If $r = -1$, this indicates a perfect negative or inverse linear relationship, i.e. a straight line with a negative gradient.
  - If $r = 0$, this indicates there is no linear relationship.
- Therefore, the closer the value of r is to 1, the stronger the relationship between the two continuous variables.
- Each point on the scatter plot represents one unit of analysis, e.g. a city or country.
- For example, the scatter plot in Fig. 10.1A displays the hypothetical results of a geographical study investigating the relationship between cholesterol level and the stroke mortality rate. Each point plotted on Fig. 10.1A represents a country. The scatter shows a strong positive linear relationship between cholesterol level and the stroke mortality rate.

Regression analysis

- The relationship between an exposure (i.e. the hypothesised cause of an effect) and outcome (i.e. the actual effect) is also commonly quantified using regression analysis.
- When there is one independent variable (the exposure) and one dependent variable (the outcome), simple linear regression analysis can be used.
- When there is more than one independent variable but still one dependent variable, multiple linear regression analysis can be used.

Discussing the findings of a mixed design study

- If there is a temporal pattern of disease outcome that varies between groups, it is important to consider the following reasons for your findings:
  - *Demographic variables*: The age and sex distribution of different groups/populations may vary. Using statistical tests, disease rates can be standardised to take into account age and sex differences between and within populations.
  - *Coding*: There may be variations in the way diseases are coded between populations.
  - *Ascertainment*: Diagnostic techniques may vary between populations; e.g. some regions may have more sensitive imaging techniques for diagnosing certain types of malignancies.
  - *Changes in incidence rates*: There may be a true change in the incidence of the disease if there is a corresponding change in the risk factor profile for the disease.

HINTS AND TIPS

While scatter plots give us a graphical display of the degree of association between two continuous variables, r-values quantify this degree of association.

SOURCES OF ERROR IN ECOLOGICAL STUDIES

- Despite having many advantages (which will be covered in the following section), there are several methodological issues in the design of an ecological study. These issues may have an impact on the causal inferences (especially biologic inferences) we can draw from our data.
- The major source of error in ecological studies is the error that exists between groups, often causing ecological fallacy.
- Issues regarding confounding (discussed in Chapter 13) and bias (discussed in the Chapter 7 section 'Bias') will be raised during our discussion.
- The usual sources of bias that exist when carrying out an individual-level analysis still occur during an ecological study.

Ecological fallacy

- A limitation commonly faced when using ecological studies to make causal inferences between an exposure and outcome, is ecological fallacy, which is a type of bias.
- Ecological fallacy is the failure of an expected ecologic effect estimate to reflect the biologic effect that exists at the individual level. In other words, ecological fallacy occurs when correlations based on grouped data are incorrectly assumed to hold at the individual level.
- Let's refer to the scatter plots in Fig. 10.1, which display the hypothetical results of a geographical study investigating the relationship between cholesterol and the stroke mortality rate in four different countries.

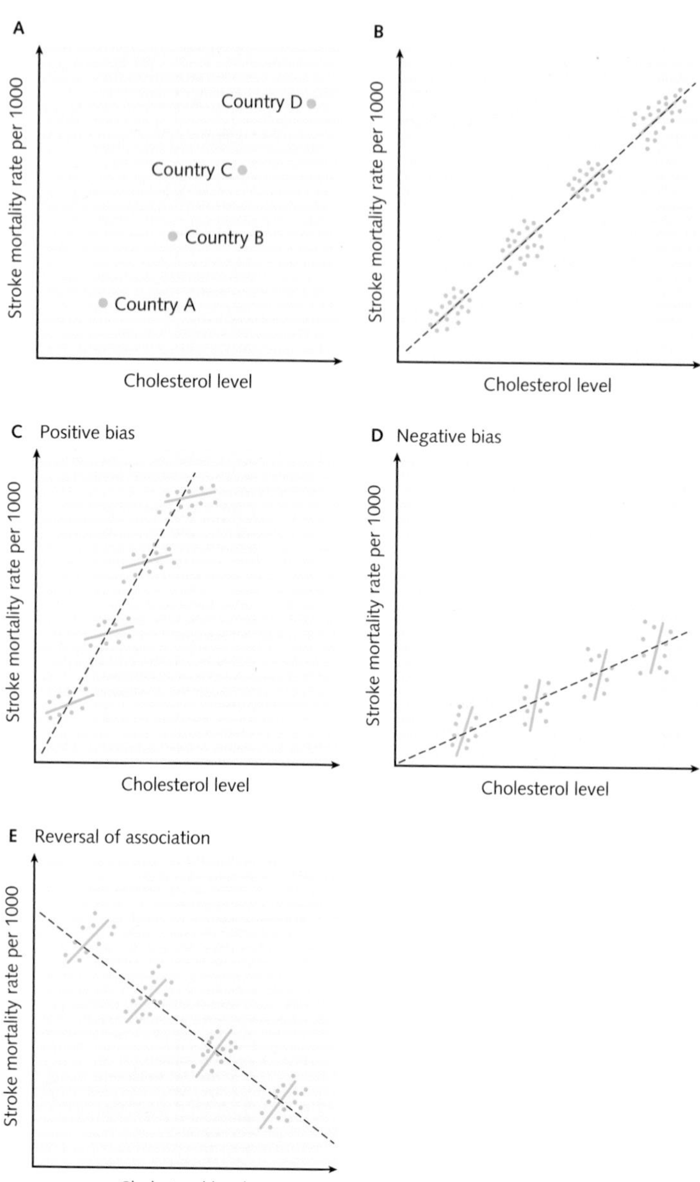

Fig. 10.1 Graphical representation of ecological fallacy (see text).

- The scatter in Fig. 10.1A shows a strong positive linear relationship between cholesterol level and the stroke mortality rate. However, it is people, not countries, who have strokes! Figures 10.1B–E display the association between cholesterol level and the stroke mortality rate at an individual level for each country.
- Referring to Fig. 10.1B, individual-level studies confirm this association as subjects with higher cholesterol levels also have a higher stroke mortality rate (represented by the solid orange line for each country). Furthermore, the degree of association has been correctly quantified using the ecological study, as the dotted line (representing the association between the two variables on a group level) has the same gradient as the solid orange line.
- Referring to Fig. 10.1C, the same conclusions about our association would have been reached with our ecological study. However, the importance of cholesterol in this relationship would have been overestimated as the dotted line is steeper than the solid orange line. This is referred to as positive bias.

- Referring to Fig. 10.1D, the same conclusions about our association would have been reached with our ecological study. However the importance of cholesterol in this relationship would have been underestimated as the dotted line is less steep than the solid orange line. This is referred to as negative bias.
- Lastly, referring to Fig. 10.1E, our ecological study would have reached the opposite conclusion, in that higher cholesterol levels are associated with a lower stroke mortality rate. However, at an individual level, there is still a positive association between these two variables. This is referred to as a reversal of association.

- Ecologic bias can result from three main sources:
  1. Within-group bias
  2. Confounding by group
  3. Effect modification by group.

Within-group bias

- Heterogeneity of the exposure level may exist within groups. For example, suppose we carry out an ecological study to investigate whether there is an association between the prevalence of *Plasmodium falciparum* and the rate of malaria. Heterogeneity in exposure occurs due to some individuals being bitten more frequently than others. There is evidence to show that this between-individual variation in biting rate may be related to differences in age, human sweat components, proximity to larval breeding sites and in-house design!
- If there is a negative net bias in every group, the ecologic estimate will be biased as well.

Confounding by group

- Confounding exists when the background rate of disease in the unexposed population (e.g. the stroke mortality rate in the normal cholesterol level population, in the example above) varies between the different groups. In other words, the exposure prevalence in each group correlates with the disease rate in the *unexposed* population in the same group.
- To demonstrate this difficult concept, let's look at the sample data shown in Fig. 10.2. You can see that there is no association between the exposure and the disease outcome as the relative rate (i.e. the ratio of the rate of disease in the exposed population to that in the unexposed population) in each group is equal to one. However, in an ecological analysis, correlating the exposure prevalence with the rate of disease does show a positive correlation.
- Confounders are not necessarily associated with exposure of the individual, as is the case for confounders in individual-level analyses.

Fig. 10.2 Confounding by group.

Group	Exposure prevalence	Disease rate in the unexposed population	Disease rate in the exposed population	Relative rate
A	5%	4%	4%	1.0
B	10%	5%	5%	1.0
C	15%	6%	6%	1.0

Effect modification by group

- Effect modification may be an issue when the rate difference for the exposure effect (at the individual level) varies across groups.
- Effect modification is different from confounding as instead of 'competing' with the exposure as an aetiological factor for the disease, the effect modifier identifies subpopulations (or subgroups) that are particularly susceptible to the exposure of interest. Effect modifiers are therefore not in the causal pathway of the disease process.
- Ecological fallacy may be an issue if these covariate levels exist within groups.
- To demonstrate this concept, let's look at the effect of smoking on the risk of developing lung cancer. It is well known that smoking and asbestos exposure are both risk factors for lung cancer.
  - People who smoke cigarettes have a risk of developing lung cancer that is 20–25 times greater than that in non-smokers.
  - Non-smokers exposed to asbestos have a three- to five-fold increased risk of developing lung cancer than those not exposed to asbestos.
  - However, people who chronically inhaled asbestos fibres (e.g. shipyard workers) and also smoked cigarettes had about a 64-fold increased risk of developing lung cancer.
- Therefore, the effects of smoking and asbestos exposure are not additive, but multiplicative. There seems to be an interaction whereby the effects of smoking on the risk of developing lung cancer are magnified in people who have also been exposed to asbestos. In this example, asbestos exposure is the effect modifier.

HINTS AND TIPS

Unlike confounding, effect modification is a biological phenomenon whereby the effect modifier identifies subpopulations that are particularly susceptible to the exposure of interest.

Confounders and modifiers

- Confounding and effect modification can arise in three distinct ways:
  - The ecologic exposure variable has an effect on risk which is distinct from the effect of its individual-level analogue, e.g. living in a country with national health guidelines favouring MMR vaccination versus actually having the MMR vaccine (in the autism example discussed above).
  - The confounders and effect modifiers may have different patterns of distribution across the groups.
  - The risk of the disease outcome may depend on the prevalence of that disease in the rest of the population in the group. This usually holds true for many infectious diseases.
- These scenarios cannot be observed in ecologic data and the degree of association between the exposure and outcome gives no indication of the presence, direction or magnitude of ecologic bias.
- In an attempt to reduce the risk of ecological fallacy, some researchers use smaller geographical catchment areas (e.g. cities instead of countries) in order to make the groups more homogeneous in terms of exposure level.
- However, this strategy has its disadvantages:
  - There is a greater chance of migration of individuals between groups. This can lead to migration bias as the migrants and non-migrants may differ on both exposure prevalence and disease risk. Studies have shown that migration can also contribute to ecological fallacy.
  - Sufficient data may not be available.

HINTS AND TIPS

Ecologic associations can differ from the corresponding associations at the individual level within groups of the same population. This underpins the reason behind ecological fallacy.

Causality

- In ecological studies, the temporal relationship between the exposure and the outcome is not clear-cut as the exposure status is measured at the same time as the outcome.
- For a more in-depth discussion on causality, please refer to the Bradford-Hill criteria, which are discussed in Chapter 5.

ADVANTAGES AND DISADVANTAGES

- What are the advantages and disadvantages of ecological studies (Fig. 10.3)?

Individual-level studies versus group-level studies

- It is important to understand that group-level study designs sometimes surpass individual-level study designs for one of the following reasons.

Design limitations of individual-level studies

- If a particular exposure varies little within a study area, individual-level studies may not be suitable

Fig. 10.3 Advantages and disadvantages of ecological studies.

Advantages	Disadvantages
Can investigate whether differences in exposure between areas are bigger than at the individual level.	Associations cannot be confirmed at the individual level.
Utilise routinely collected health data; therefore, may be relatively cheap and quick to conduct.	There is potential for ecological fallacy when applying grouped results to the individual level.
Generate hypotheses which can be investigated at the individual level using studies higher up in the hierarchy of evidence.	There is lack of available data on confounding factors.
Can investigate the effect of exposures that are measured over groups or areas, e.g. diet, air pollution and temperature.	There is potential for systematic differences between areas in how disease frequency is measured, e.g. differences in disease classification and coding.
Can search for associations in large populations.	There is potential for systematic differences between areas in how exposures are measured.

for estimating the exposure effects. On the other hand, ecological studies may be able to measure significant variations in mean exposure across different geographical areas.

Measurement limitations of individual-level studies

- With limited time and resource availability, we often cannot accurately measure relevant exposures at the individual level for large numbers of subjects. This usually holds true when investigating apparent clusters of disease in small areas.
- On some occasions, individual-level exposures cannot be measured accurately due to considerable person-to-person variability, e.g. when measuring dietary factors. In such situations, ecologic measures might accurately reflect group averages.

KEY EXAMPLE OF AN ECOLOGICAL STUDY

- There is increasing evidence to suggest that determinants such as an individual's educational background or socioeconomic status may have a profound effect on their health status. However, gathering data on socioeconomic status at an individual level has proven to be very difficult as:
  - it is a sensitive issue to discuss with members of the public.
  - the socioeconomic status varies dramatically depending on the life course of the subject. For example, if someone has recently retired, they may have a low annual income, yet have a relatively high socioeconomic status based on income acquired during their working life.
- Due to these challenges faced, ecological studies have been utilised to investigate the effect of socioeconomic status on various health outcomes. In these studies, we assume that the region where people live is a reflection of their socioeconomic status. These regions are usually defined using postcodes, which are linked to census information on the median household income within a given area. This approach makes the assumption that all individuals living within a defined geographical area have a similar socioeconomic status.

Relationship between socioeconomic status and mortality after an acute myocardial infarction

- Alter and colleagues conducted a well-known ecological study investigating the relationship between a patient's socioeconomic status (along with access to cardiac procedures such as angioplasty and cardiac bypass grafting surgery) and mortality after an acute myocardial infarction, in Ontario, Canada.
- Patients were categorised into five income quintiles from the lowest to the highest using the strategy described above.
- The research group found that patients living in higher-income neighbourhoods had the highest rates of cardiac procedure use and the lowest one-year mortality rates.
- However, this finding alone does *not* provide us with evidence that the socioeconomic status, the degree of access that an individual has to a cardiac procedure and the mortality after an acute myocardial infarction are *Causally Related.*
- A follow-up study was therefore conducted at the individual level using clinical and socioeconomic status data.
- The research group showed that much of the acute myocardial infarction mortality gradient was associated with differences in the patient's baseline cardiovascular risk factor profile (and not associated with discrepancies in the degree of access that the patients had to a cardiac procedure).
- Consequently, we can conclude that universal healthcare for all individuals, regardless of socioeconomic status, cannot eliminate health disparities on its own.
- Instead, policy-makers should focus on improving the resources available to healthcare professionals to reduce the cardiovascular risk factor profile of their patients, especially among those who have a lower socioeconomic status.

HINTS AND TIPS

An association between a particular exposure and outcome (observed in an ecological study) can stimulate the need for an individual-level study in order to determine the mechanisms involved for this association.

Case report and case series

Objectives

By the end of this chapter you should:

- Understand the importance of case reports and case series as providing evidence for clinical decision-making.
- Be able to identify and critically appraise case reports and case series.
- Be able to conduct your own case report or case series.
- Be able to list the advantages and disadvantages of case reports and case series.

BACKGROUND

According to NHS Centre for Reviews and Dissemination, case reports and case series are near the bottom of the hierarchy (Fig. 1.5) of what counts as reliable evidence for clinical decision-making.

- A case report (or case study) usually describes a single unique case or finding of interest.
- A case series (or clinical series):
  - is a descriptive study that reports on data from a group of individuals who have a similar disease or condition.
  - is a type of observational study useful for identifying similar or differing characteristics between selected cases.
  - can be prospective or retrospective and usually involves only a small number of individuals.
  - can include either non-consecutive (a selection of cases) or consecutive individuals (all cases) with the same condition or disease.
- The information gained from a case series can be used to generate hypotheses.
- Case series studies are commonly used to report on a consecutive series of patients with a defined disease who have been treated in a similar manner (without a control group).

COMMUNICATION

The role of case reports and case series

Most case reports and case series cover one of six topics:

1. Identifying and describing new diseases.
2. Identifying rare or unique manifestations of known diseases.
3. Audit, quality improvement and medical education.
4. Understanding the pathogenesis of a disease.
5. Detecting new drug side effects, both beneficial and adverse.
6. Reporting unique therapeutic approaches.

CONDUCTING A CASE REPORT

Preparation

- Identify an interesting case in a clinic or on the ward, with guidance and advice from a senior colleague.
- Having identified a suitable case, carry out a literature review to explore the uniqueness of the case. Have similar cases already been published?
- Discuss the case with senior doctors who have been looking after the patient in order to gain permission and support.
- Gain written consent from the patient, especially if there may be patient identifiers in the report, including medical pictures and specific clinical details.
- Some journals require patient consent regardless of whether or not patient identifiers are included in the report, so read the journal guidelines carefully!
- Having successfully completed the above, relevant information should be gathered about the case from the patient notes, available imaging, laboratory results and other relevant sources.

Structuring a medical case report

The following guideline for writing a case report manuscript can also be used as a checklist when critically appraising case studies already published.

Abstract

- There is usually a strict word limit for the abstract, so carefully read the journal guidelines before you begin!
- The abstract will help readers discern whether they are interested (or not interested) in reading the case report.
- The abstract should include all the sections included in the main text of the case report, including the introduction and objective(s), case presentation, discussion and conclusion.
- The abstract should be engaging and to the point, highlighting the key details from the main text of the case report.

Introduction

- The opening sentence should be catchy and attract the attention of the reader.
- The subject matter of interest should be introduced with background information on the topic.
- The search strategy for the literature review, including the search terms used, should be described with enough detail to allow the reader to easily reproduce the search.
- The purpose and merit of the case report should be highlighted using the literature identified in the search.
- The patient case should be introduced to the reader with a one- or two-sentence description.
- There should not be more than three or four concise paragraphs for the introduction of the case report.

Case presentation

- The case should be described in enough detail to allow readers to make their own conclusions about the case.
- Patient identifiers such as precise dates and the patient's date of birth should be avoided.
- A narrative description of the case should be written with significant events discussed in chronological order (headings for each part of the patient history should not be used).
- The patient information described should be relevant and may include details on:
    - Patient demographics – age, sex, race, height and weight.
    - Presenting complaint.
    - Past medical history.
    - Drug history before and during the admission (include over-the-counter medications, recreational drugs, vaccines and herbal remedies) – the name, dose, route, times of administration and compliance rates of all medications should be listed.
    - Renal and hepatic function – allows assessment of the appropriateness of the medication doses used.
    - Drug allergies – including the name of culprit medications, the date and type of drug reactions.
    - Family history.
    - Social history – diet, occupation, smoking and alcohol status.
    - Important physical examination findings.
    - Relevant (not routine) laboratory data.
    - Differential diagnoses and the diagnostic procedure.
    - Report the results of any diagnostic tests.
    - Therapeutic effects and side effects of any treatments on the disease outcome.
    - Potential causal relationships between an exposure and outcome.
    - Current status of the patient case and future treatment plans.
- Relevant figures should be used, including electrocardiograms (ECGs), radiological images, blood films and photographs of skin manifestations.

Discussion

- What new information has been learnt from the case report?
- Comment on how unique the case is by comparing and contrasting it to other cases already published in the literature.
- Are there any inaccuracies in the data that would question the validity of the case report?
- What are the limitations of the case report?
- Summarise the key points raised from the case report.

Conclusion

- A justified, sound and brief conclusion should be written based on information reviewed as part of the discussion.
- Any recommendations should be evidence-based rather than based on speculation.
- Describe whether any new findings from the case will have an impact on clinical practice.
- Has the case report generated any novel hypotheses that could be investigated using a study higher up in the hierarchy of evidence?

References

- Whether other articles are quoted or paraphrased, it is essential that all sources of information referred to in the case report are acknowledged in the reference section at the end of the paper.
- The Harvard Referencing System is a collection of rules that standardises the format in which articles are referenced (please refer to Chapter 5 for an in-depth discussion on how to reference articles using the Harvard Referencing System).
- Citations should be included in parentheses in the main text of the case report.

CONDUCTING A CASE SERIES

Guidelines similar to those outlined for case reports should be followed when conducting a case series. However, specifically for case series, it is important to consider the following:

- Is the case series prospective or retrospective? Prospective case series are less prone to bias.
- Case series should be carried out according to a predefined protocol, which clearly defines all stages of the study, including patient selection, measures, data collection, analysis and reporting.
- Inclusion and exclusion criteria should be clearly defined, with all eligible patients selected in order to avoid selection bias.
- Are non-consecutive or consecutive cases selected? Recruiting consecutive cases is preferable in order to avoid selection bias.
- Are patients recruited over a fixed time period or (preferably) until a sufficient number of cases are identified? Formal sample size calculations could be used if a particular change in measure is worth demonstrating.
- The diagnostic process should be clearly documented for all patients.
- Details of baseline information, and pre- and post-treatment measures should be recorded.
- The outcome for all study participants should be measured in the same way according to the predefined protocol.
- Outcomes should be measured objectively, wherever possible, in order to minimise measurement bias.
- Measurements made should be valid and reliable.
- Differences in treatment effects should be compared and contrasted between cases.
- Quantitative data should be statistically analysed, for example, by calculating the average value (the mean) and the degree of spread of the data set (e.g. the standard deviation or interquartile range).
- The 'flow of patients' should be described, accounting for anyone who dropped out of the study, therefore avoiding selection bias (please refer to Chapter 7 for a discussion on selection bias).
- An intention-to-treat analysis should be considered, where appropriate (please refer to Chapter 6 for a discussion on how to calculate and interpret the intention-to-treat analysis).

CRITICAL APPRAISAL OF A CASE SERIES

Key methodological issues should be considered when critically appraising a case series:

1. Was there a well-defined study protocol with a clear objective or research question?
2. Were consecutive cases within a specified time interval enrolled?

If non-consecutive cases were enrolled, the study results are subject to selection bias.

3. Were explicit inclusion and exclusion criteria stated for the selection of study participants?

If the study population was too restrictive, the generalisability of the results to more representative populations will be limited.

4. Were relevant exposure variables measured accurately?
5. Were potential confounding factors measured?

If confounding factors were not taken into account, a potential relationship between the exposure and outcome may be biased.

6. Were the outcome measures clinically relevant and measured accurately?
7. Was outcome measure data collected prospectively?

Prospective data collection will improve the accuracy of the data collected.

8. Was there a high loss to follow-up?

The study findings are less valid if a considerable number of participants dropped out of the study (loss-to-follow-up bias).

ADVANTAGES AND DISADVANTAGES

What are the advantages and disadvantages of case reports and case series? Figure 11.1 highlights the key points that apply to case reports, case series or both types of papers.

KEY EXAMPLES OF CASE REPORTS

The first cardiac transplantation

In 1967, Christiaan Barnard, a surgeon from South Africa, published a case report on the first human heart transplant. While the transplant operation was only temporarily successful, this was an important historical event. Within one year of this publication, surgeons from the Texas Heart Institute had performed 20 heart transplant operations. The first human heart transplantation and subsequent research at the Univeristy of Cape Town (and in other specialist surgical centres) over the following 15 years laid the foundation for heart transplantation to become a well-established surgical option for end-stage cardiac disease.

Figure 11.1 Advantages and disadvantages of case reports and case series

Advantages	Disadvantages
Case Reports and Case Series • Useful for describing clinical experience, including identifying new diseases and reporting unique therapeutic approaches to known diseases. • Relatively easy and inexpensive to conduct. • Information gained can help provide suggestions for generating clinical hypotheses, which can be tested using stronger study designs. • Allows junior doctors and students to apply new knowledge and skills.	***Case Reports and Case Series*** • At the bottom of the hierarchy of evidence due to the lack of scientific rigour (compared to larger observational and experimental study designs). • Cannot usually be used to establish cause-and-effect relationships. • If the case(s) chosen are not representative of the wider population, the findings may not be generalisable.
Case Reports • Many different aspects of the patient's medical situation, including patient history, physical examination, diagnosis, social issues and follow-up can be detailed. • Relatively quick to complete.	***Case Series*** • Prone to selection, measurement and attrition bias.

Multiple myeloma

Multiple myeloma is a disorder of plasma cell proliferation in the bone marrow that is associated with skeletal destruction. The first well-known case of multiple myeloma was described by Dr William MacIntyre, who published a case report on the features of multiple myeloma proteinuria based on a urine sample produced by Thomas Alexander McBean, a 45-year-old grocer from London. These urine specimens were subsequently studied in detail by Henry Bence Jones, a chemical pathologist from London, who identified the protein as a 'hydrated deutoxide of albumin' and commented on its importance in diagnosing multiple myeloma. These findings accredited him with the discovery of Bence Jones protein in the urine!

KEY EXAMPLE OF A CASE SERIES

Thalidomide and congenital abnormalities

Thalidomide, a sedative drug first synthesised in 1953, was widely prescribed for the morning sickness often experienced by pregnant women. By 1958, thalidomide was being promoted as an anti-emetic in many countries around the world. However, in 1961, William McBride, an obstetrician from New South Wales, published a famous case series to alert healthcare professionals of the dangers of thalidomide:

> Congenital abnormalities are present in approximately 1.5% of babies. In recent months I have observed that the incidence of multiple severe abnormalities in babies delivered of women who were given the drug thalidomide ('Distaval') during pregnancy, as an anti-emetic or as a sedative, to be almost 20%.
>
> These abnormalities are present in structures developed from mesenchyme – i.e., the bones and musculature of the gut. Bony development seems to be affected in a very striking manner, resulting in polydactyly, syndactyly, and failure of development of long bones (abnormally short femora and radii).
>
> Have any of your readers seen similar abnormalities in babies delivered of women who have taken this drug during pregnancy?

Following this publication, the drug was eventually withdrawn and countless babies were saved from the teratogenic effects of thalidomide.

Qualitative research

Objectives

By the end of this chapter you should:

- Be able to identify and critically appraise qualitative research studies.
- Know the steps involved in carrying out qualitative research.
- Understand the differences between quantitative and qualitative research.
- Know about the different methods of data collection: participant observation, in-depth interviews and focus groups.
- Understand the different sampling methods commonly used in qualitative research.
- Know the steps involved in organising qualitative data using a standardised approach.
- Know how to assess the validity, reliability and transferability of the findings of a qualitative study.
- Be able to list the advantages and disadvantages of qualitative research.

A methodological checklist on how to critically appraise qualitative studies is provided in Chapter 19.

STUDY DESIGN

What is qualitative research?

- Qualitative research shares all the characteristics of scientific research; however, it does not currently have a universally accepted position in the hierarchy of evidence (Fig. 1.5).
- It seeks to understand the research question or topic from the perspectives of the local population involved.
- Additionally, it allows us to obtain information on the actions, behaviours, values and opinions of different groups in the population, e.g. from different cultures, socioeconomic classes or genders.
- Qualitative research can be used in combination with quantitative research to help us interpret and better understand the various stages of a quantitative research study:
  - *Designing the quantitative research study:* Qualitative research can assist us in:
    - generating hypotheses.
    - designing and validating questionnaires.
  - *During the quantitative research study:* Qualitative research can assist us in:
    - measuring subjective outcomes.
  - *Following the quantitative research study:* Qualitative research can assist us in:
    - exploring and making sense of any unexpected findings.

> COMMUNICATION
>
> **What research questions are best answered with a qualitative study design?**
>
> In addition to being used alongside quantitative methods, qualitative research is useful in its own right, for instance, to:
> - investigate the perceptions that healthcare professionals have of national healthcare guidelines.
> - understand how the healthcare organisation works and identify those areas where there is scope for improvement.
> - explore patients' views, experiences and understandings of illness and the quality of care received.
> - explore carers' feelings about their caring role.
> - understand the behaviour of individuals with certain illness, e.g. their help-seeking behaviour and reasons for lack of medication compliance.

Qualitative versus quantitative research methods

- What are the key differences between quantitative and qualitative research methods?
- As described in Fig. 12.1, the main difference between qualitative and quantitative methods is in their degree of flexibility.
- Despite qualitative methods being more flexible, the degree of flexibility is not an indication of how scientifically rigorous a method may be.

Fig. 12.1 Qualitative versus quantitative research methods.

	Qualitative	Quantitative
Framework	• Inductive. • Explores a topic to generate a hypothesis. • Semi-structured methods are used. • Based on participant response, interview questions may be added, removed or altered during the study to improve study design. • Questions asked by the researcher depend on participant responses.	• Deductive. • Tests a hypothesis about a topic. • Structured methods are used from beginning to end. • Questions asked by the researcher are not influenced by participant responses.
Aim	• To explain why certain relationships may exist. • To explore the values and opinions of different groups. • To explore individual experiences. • To *describe* the variation that exists.	• To predict a casual relationship between an exposure and outcome. • To use sample data to make inferences about the characteristics of a population. • To *quantify* the degree of variation that exists.
Participant responses to questions are:	Open-ended	Closed-ended
Sampling	Usually small scale	Usually large scale
Data	Written or spoken language	Numerical values are assigned to responses

Methods of data collection

- The three most commonly used qualitative research methods, each suited for obtaining a specific type of data, are:
  1. Participant observation
  2. In-depth interviews
  3. Focus groups.

Participant observation

- Participant observation is suitable when collecting data on naturally occurring behaviours of participants in their usual setting.
- This method is based on traditional ethnographic research, whose objective is to understand perspectives held by study populations.
- Participant observation involves understanding the life and customs of people living in various cultures.
- The objective is not only to identify the multiple perspectives that exist within a given population but also to understand the interplay among them.
- Ethnographic research methods may include both observing people/processes and participating, to various degrees, in the day-to-day activities in the community setting.
- The community setting chosen should have some relevance to the research question, and may include hospital wards, general practice, etc.
- The researchers make objective notes about what they see whilst in the community setting.
- All accounts and observations are recorded as field notes in a field notebook.
- The field notes should also include details on all interactions that the researcher has with members of the study population, including informal conversations.
- While this method of data collection is time consuming, it allows:
  - the researcher to overcome the discrepancy between what people say they do and what they actually do.
  - for insight into contexts, relationships and behaviour.

In-depth interviews

- In-depth interviews are suitable when collecting data on the participants' perspectives and experiences in relation to the research topic.
- The researcher should pose questions in a neutral manner and ask follow-up questions based on participant response.
- The questions should be unbiased and open-ended (not leading or closed questions).
- The interviews are usually carried out on a one-to-one basis, giving the participants an opportunity to talk about their personal feelings, experiences

and opinions. They are therefore useful for learning about the perspectives of individuals, as opposed to exploring group norms.

- In particular, one-to-one interviews are useful for exploring sensitive topics that would be difficult to discuss in a group setting.
- Observations during the interview are noted and the interview tape-recorded.

Focus groups

- Focus groups are suitable when collecting data on the cultural norms of various groups.
- There are usually one or two researchers and several participants who meet as a group in order to discuss a particular research topic.
- Due to the dynamic discussions that take place, focus groups are particularly useful for exploring how people express, debate and on some occasions, modify their opinions.
- Focus group sessions are usually tape-recorded and on some occasions, video-taped.
- Similar to the type of questions asked during an in-depth one-to-one interview, open-ended, unbiased questions should be used.

Sampling

- It is not necessary to collect data from large samples in order to achieve valid findings.
- Qualitative research is usually based on selecting small samples (i.e. a subset of the population) to investigate a particular topic in depth and detail.
- The sample size and type of sample selected are determined by the research objectives and the study population characteristics.
- Rather than being calculated and fixed, the sample size is flexible and purposeful.

Purposive sampling

- Purposive sampling (also known as purposeful or target sampling) involves choosing participants with a purpose!
- Participants are grouped according to predefined criteria; i.e. they have particular characteristics that will allow the researcher to investigate the research topic as fully as possible; for example, men with ischaemic heart disease living in London.
- Sample sizes:
  - depend on the study objectives, as well as the time and resources available.
  - are often determined by the saturation point. This is the point in data collection where interviewing new people will no longer bring additional insights to the research question. This theoretical saturation point can only be determined if data review and analysis are done in conjunction with data collection. This process is known as iteration, i.e. moving back and forth between sampling and analysis.
- The four most common types of purposive sampling are:
  - Quota sampling
  - Snowball sampling
  - Maximum variation sampling
  - Negative sampling.

Quota sampling

- Quota sampling is sometimes considered a type of purposive sampling.
- The decision on how many people with certain characteristics to include as study participants is made during the design phase of the study. These characteristics include gender, age, socioeconomic class, marital status, profession, disease status, etc.
- The characteristics chosen are to identify people most likely to have insight or have experienced the research topic.
- Individuals from the community are then recruited until the predefined quota is satisfied.

HINTS AND TIPS

What is the difference between purposive and quota sampling?

While the aim of both purposive and quota sampling is to identify study participants who satisfy predefined criteria, quota sampling is more specific with regards to sample size. For example, you may be interested in investigating gender-specific responses to a new diagnosis of colon cancer. Assuming there is a 1:1 gender ratio in the population, the aim of a quota sample would be to identify an equal number of men and women with colon cancer in the population. On the other hand, purposive sampling would involve setting a target for the number of participants in each group, rather than a strict quota.

Snowball sampling

- Snowball sampling (also known as chain referral sampling) involves using study participants as informants to identify other people who could potentially participate in the study.
- The study participants, with whom contact has already been made, use their social networks to identify groups not easily accessible to researchers, such as the homeless.

Maximum variation sampling

- Maximum variation sampling involves selecting people to obtain a broad range of perspectives on the research topic. In other words, the aim of maximum variation sampling is to increase the diversity of the perspectives obtained.
- For example, you may be interested in investigating patient responses to a new diagnosis of cancer. Maximum variation sampling would involve recruiting patients with different demographic profiles, e.g. age, ethnicity, gender, as well as including patients who have different types of cancer.

Negative sampling

- Negative sampling (also known as deviant case sampling) involves searching for unusual or atypical cases of the research topic of interest.
- For example, you may be interested in interviewing women who had a positive cervical screen for cervical intraepithelial neoplasia. Negative sampling would also involve interviewing those women who tested negative to see whether their views about the cervical screening process differ.

ORGANISING AND ANALYSING THE DATA

Organising the data

- Organising data in a standardised way is essential to ensure the validity of the study results.
- Despite being a challenging process, qualitative data needs to be systematically compared and analysed in its raw form.
- Soon after collecting the data:
  - the field notes should be expanded into a descriptive narrative of what was observed. The narrative is usually typed into computer files.
  - tape recordings should be transcribed.
- Any initial observations should be elaborated in as much detail as possible, describing what happened, and what was learnt from:
  - the setting and study population (during participant observation).
  - the interview content, the participant(s) and the context (during one-to-one interviews and focus groups).
- Narrative accounts and typed transcripts are subsequently coded according to the particular responses to each question and/or to common emerging themes.

Analysing the data

- Following the research question as a guide, every line of text is coded for relevant themes.
- Coding is the process of collecting observations into groups that are like one another, and assigning a symbol, known as a code, as a name for the group.
- As themes/categories are developed, the researcher assigns a working definition to each code. This definition is continually being challenged when going through the text. Using this process, new codes are developed when the properties of the current codes do not fit the text. Furthermore, codes that are rarely used are dismissed.
- As highlighted previously, there is usually a constant cycle of collecting data, analysing that data, generating codes and themes/categories and then collecting more data to refine our understanding of the topic until saturation is achieved. This 'constant comparison' approach is therefore iterative (moving back and forth) and inductive (a type of reasoning that involves extrapolating patterns from the data in order to form a conceptual category/theme).
- The analysis is 'grounded' in the categories or theories generated from the data.
- Software data management packages are available to assist with the analysis.
- The ultimate goal of the analysis is to generate analytical concepts that can be used to generate new hypotheses.

VALIDITY, RELIABILITY AND TRANSFERABILITY

- There are three key concepts that need to considered when appraising a qualitative paper:
  1. *Validity*: The degree to which the findings accurately represent the specific concept that the researcher is attempting to measure.
  2. *Reliability*: Would another researcher be able to reproduce the same data and interpret it in the same way?
  3. *Transferability*: Are the findings applicable to other patients and/or settings?

Validity

- The setting and method used for data collection should be justified. For example, if investigating how patients with breast cancer want their doctors to communicate with them, study participants should be interviewed, on a one-to-one basis, but not on hospital premises. Carrying out interviews away from the hospital, for example, at the patient's

home, will allow study participants to feel more at ease, thus giving them an opportunity to discuss any negative feelings that they may have.
- All the data collected should be analysed, even if negative attitudes are portrayed. The final report should include quotes which highlight both positive and negative experiences.
- The researcher should reflect on whether his or her values and attributes may have influenced (or biased) any stages of the study. This is often referred to as 'reflexivity'. For example, an 18-year-old man and a 50-year-old woman are likely to elicit different responses to questions about sexual health when interviewing a group of teenagers. The values and attributes considered may include:
  - ethnicity
  - gender
  - age
  - whether the researcher has the same condition as the one being investigated.
- The findings from the study (i.e. analytical categories/themes) should be well 'grounded' in the data. Did the researchers use the constant comparison method to clarify the emerging themes? Sufficient raw data should be included in the final report to enable the reader to draw the same conclusions as the researchers. The report should therefore include direct quotes from the study participants.
- Some studies show evidence of triangulation, which involves cross-verifying the research findings by using more than one research method. The major types of triangulation involve:
  - having multiple researchers in the study.
  - using more than one method to gather data.
  - recruiting a range of patients from different backgrounds.
- You would be more confident with a research finding if various methods lead to the same finding.

Reliability

- Similar to our discussion for validity, the setting and method used for data collection should be justified.
- If the issue of reflexivity has not been considered, another researcher might obtain different findings if the research study was repeated.
- The codes and themes should be derived from the data, i.e. using the actual words of the participants. Otherwise, if they were derived from the researcher's own beliefs, other researchers might obtain different codes and themes if they tried to replicate the research study.
- In an attempt to ensure that the codes and themes are derived from the data, some research groups get a second researcher to independently code the data, thus checking for inter-rater reliability.

Transferability

- After ensuring that the study findings are valid and reliable, the final step is to consider whether they can be applied to other patients and settings.
- Assessing transferability doesn't involve carrying out statistical calculations, as is the case for quantitative research. Instead, you must assess whether the nature of the sample and the study setting have been described in enough detail to allow readers to determine whether the findings can be applied to their patients and settings.

ADVANTAGES AND DISADVANTAGES

What are the advantages and disadvantages of qualitative research (Fig. 12.2)?

KEY EXAMPLE OF QUALITATIVE RESEARCH

- Research has shown that doctors often communicate poorly with patients who have cancer.
- Systematic research into patients' perspectives can guide future development of communication training for clinicians specialising in cancer.
- In 2004, Emma Wright and her colleagues carried out a qualitative study to determine how patients with breast cancer want their doctors to communicate with them.
- Thirty-nine women with primary breast cancer were consecutively selected from surgery and oncology clinics.
- Clinical consultations were audiotaped and semi-structured interviews carried out in the patient's own home, thus making the participants feel more at ease.
- In an attempt to minimise idealised or generalised accounts, the semi-structured interviews were carried out within 1–5 days of the patient's consultation. Considering there are two sources for data collection (audiotaped consultations and semi-structured interviews), there is evidence of triangulation.
- Importantly, the interviewer explained that she was a researcher, independent of the clinical team.
- The transcript from the patient's clinical consultation was shown to the patient during the interview to help her describe those aspects of the doctor-patient communication that she valued or deprecated.
- The interviewer used open-ended questions, prompts and reflection during the interview.

Fig. 12.2 Advantages and disadvantages of qualitative research.

Advantages	Disadvantages
Can use a personal approach to investigate sensitive issues, e.g. mental health, sexual health.	Researcher bias is inherent in this type of study design and is sometimes unavoidable.
Can investigate the views of people usually excluded from surveys, e.g. individuals with dementia or learning difficulties.	Compared to quantitative studies, it is more difficult to determine the validity and reliability of qualitative research data.
Can investigate processes by exploring answers to how and why questions.	The study sample may not be representative of the larger population.
Can discover issues that are important from the perspective of those being studied, e.g. patients, healthcare professionals.	It takes time for the researcher to build trust with the study participants in order to facilitate full self-representation.
Can investigate behaviours, opinions, beliefs, experiences and emotions of individuals.	Data collection using 'participant observation' is time-consuming and potentially expensive, and requires a well-trained researcher.
Can investigate how an individual's social environment influences behaviour.	Transcribing recorded findings is time-consuming and labour intensive.
	Using an in-depth, comprehensive approach to gathering data limits the scope of the findings.

- Anonymised interview transcripts were analysed inductively, in parallel with the interviews, using a constant comparison approach.
- By cycling between data collection and data analysis, recurrent patterns were identified.
- The transcripts were reviewed by two researchers, thus taking into account inter-rater reliability.
- The study ended when the saturation point was achieved.
- Using the constant-comparison approach, the codes and categories derived from the data were well-grounded.
- Some of the codes identified for the category, 'Ways in which doctors could communicate expertise', include:
    - Demonstrate a tangible skill.
    - Display confidence and efficiency and make things happen.
    - Answer all questions without hesitation.
    - Do not mislead.
    - Tell the patient you will be open.
- Furthermore, the paper presented sufficient raw data to enable the reader to generate similar codes.
- Overall, as highlighted, this study addresses issues regarding the validity and reliability of the findings.
- Are the findings applicable to other patients/settings? To address issues regarding the transferability of the findings, the research group presented a table that summarising the characteristics of the patients and doctors whose consultations were recorded.

Confounding 13

Objectives

By the end of this chapter you should:

- Understand what confounding is and why it is such as problem in observational studies.
- Know how to assess for potential confounding factors.
- Understand how potential confounding factors are controlled for at the design or analysis stages of a study.
- Be able to interpret the crude and adjusted measures of association between an exposure and outcome.

WHAT IS CONFOUNDING?

- Confounding:
    - occurs when the association between an exposure and disease outcome is distorted by a third variable, which is known as a confounder (Fig. 13.1).
    - is a form of bias as it can lead to an over- or underestimation of the observed association between an exposure and disease outcome.
    - may be an issue in both observational and experimental studies (randomised controlled trials).
    - is more likely to occur in observational studies than in randomised controlled trials.
- As subjects are randomly allocated to exposed and unexposed groups in experimental studies, both groups are expected to be comparable with regard to known and unknown confounding factors. However, there may be random differences between the exposed and unexposed groups, which may potentially lead to confounding.
- In observational studies, in addition to random differences between the exposed and unexposed groups, variables related to the exposure may confound the association between the exposure and disease outcome.
- Of all study designs, ecological studies are the most susceptible to confounding due to the difficulty in controlling for confounders at a group level.
- Provided the confounding factors are recognised and measured at the start of the study, they may be controlled for at the study design level or when analysing the results of the study.

HINTS AND TIPS

Confounding may be present when:

- Studying an exposure–disease association.
- Quantifying the degree of association between an exposure and disease outcome, e.g. calculating the odds ratio in a case–control study.
- A number of aetiological factors directly or indirectly cause the disease outcome.

ASSESSING FOR POTENTIAL CONFOUNDING FACTORS

Potential confounders should be working independently of the exposure–disease association pathway. To decide whether this is the case, there must be a social or biological mechanism to link the exposure to the disease outcome. These mechanisms are based on the available evidence from previous clinical or non-clinical findings.

HINTS AND TIPS

Whether a given variable is an intermediary step in the causal pathway between the exposure and disease outcome or whether it works independently of the pathway, and is therefore a confounder, depends on the research question. The research question should always be considered when deciding whether a variable is a confounder.

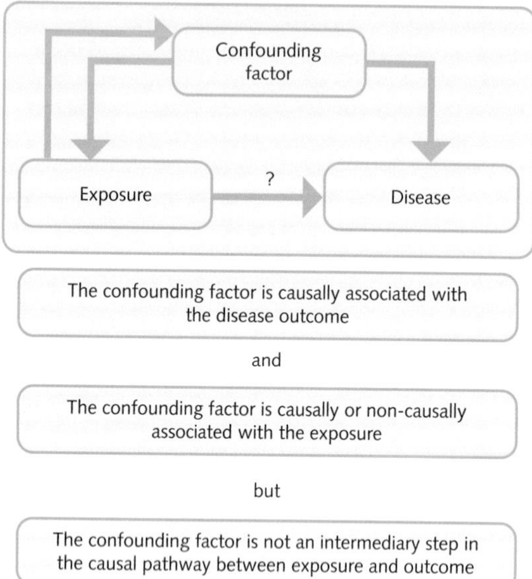

Fig. 13.1 Schematic of confounding.

Association with exposure

The confounding factor will be associated with the exposure with at least one of the following relationships.

The confounder causes the exposure

Research question: Is hypertension associated with mortality rates independent of levels of exercise?

Biological mechanism linking exposure to outcome: Hypertension increases mortality rate due to an increased risk of ischaemic heart disease.

Potential confounder: Physical inactivity

A person's level of physical activity may be a confounder in the relationship between hypertension and mortality, because physical inactivity is associated with both the exposure (hypertension) and the disease outcome (high mortality). Therefore, in this particular example, the confounder causes both the exposure and the outcome (Fig. 13.2A).

The confounder is a result from the exposure

Research question: Is low social class associated with ischaemic heart disease independent of smoking status?

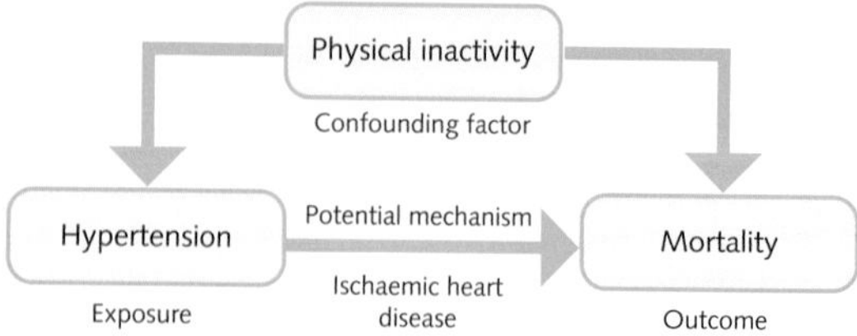

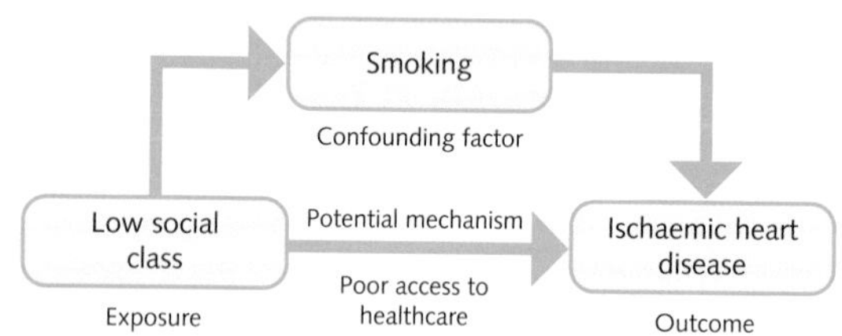

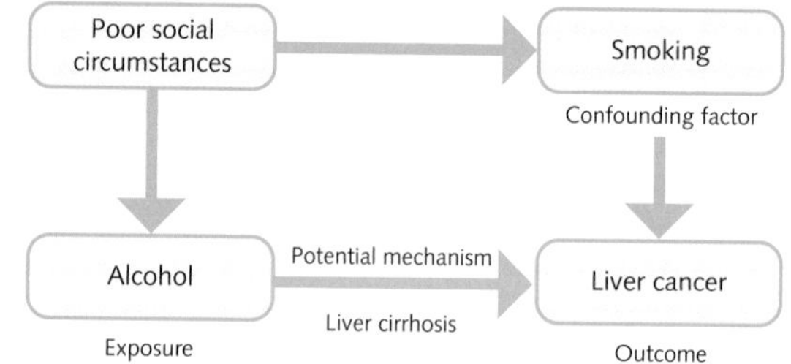

Fig. 13.2 Schematic of association between confounding and the exposure.

Social mechanism linking exposure to outcome: Lower social class groups have an increased risk of ischaemic heart disease due to poor access to healthcare.

Potential confounder: Smoking

A person's smoking status may be a confounder in the relationship between being a member of a low social class and ischaemic heart disease, because smoking is associated with both the exposure (low social class) and the disease outcome (ischaemic heart disease). Therefore in this particular example, the exposure causes the confounder while the confounder causes the outcome (Fig. 13.2B).

The confounder is related to the exposure with a non-causal association

Research question: Is alcohol associated with liver cancer independent of smoking?

Biological mechanism linking exposure to outcome: Excess alcohol is associated with primary liver cancer, through causing liver cirrhosis.
Potential confounder: Smoking.

A person's smoking status may be a confounder in the relationship between alcohol and liver cancer, via a non-causal relationship. In this example, poor social circumstances, such as poverty, may cause someone to both drink alcohol and smoke. Smoking has also been shown to be a risk factor for liver cancer. Therefore in this particular example, the confounder and the exposure are related via a non-causal separate pathway. As with all confounding factors, the confounder also causes the outcome (Fig. 13.2C).

Association with disease

In order to cause confounding, a factor must be causally associated with the disease outcome in both exposed and unexposed individuals. In all of the examples illustrated in Fig. 13.2, the confounding variables (physical inactivity and smoking) determine the likelihood of the outcome (mortality, ischaemic heart disease and liver cancer) to a certain degree.

CONTROLLING FOR CONFOUNDING FACTORS

Having identified the confounding factors that may exist in a study, the next step is to control for this confounding at either the study design level or when analysing the results of the study.

Design stage

It is sometimes important to control for very strong confounding factors at the design stage (provided the sample size is large) than at the analysis stage of a study. Several different methods may be used to minimise the degree of confounding in a study, including:

- Randomisation
- Restriction
- Matching

These methods are not exclusive to each other; therefore, more than one of these methods may be used in the same study.

Randomisation

- As mentioned above, randomly allocating subjects to the exposed and unexposed groups will control for both known and unknown confounders. For example, if individuals are randomly classified into two groups, the rules of probability state that both groups will have a similar distribution of confounders (especially when large sample sizes are used).
- Each study participant will have an equal chance of being allocated to either group. Therefore, in theory, each group will have an equal percentage of males, an equal percentage of overweight people, an equal number of women with red nail polish and so forth.
- The only difference between the two groups is therefore the exposure status. However, even if the sample size is large and the randomisation process is unbiased, there may be random differences between the exposed and unexposed groups, which may potentially lead to confounding.

HINTS AND TIPS

The randomisation process involves allocating study participants to either the exposed or unexposed group. However, in observational studies (e.g. cohort, case–control, cross-sectional and ecological), we observe subjects' exposure patterns without attempting to change them, so we cannot use randomisation to control for confounding in these study designs.

Restriction

- Restricting study participants to those people from the population who have not been exposed to one or more confounding factors will control for confounding caused by these variables. For example, in a study investigating whether alcohol use is associated with liver cancer independent of smoking (illustrated in Fig. 13.2C), the investigators could restrict the study population to non-smokers.
- When there are strong confounding factors distorting the association between an exposure and disease outcome, restriction is ideal as it can be a useful, inexpensive and efficient method of controlling for the confounder of interest.
- However, there are instances when restriction is logistically unfeasible as following exclusion of subjects with the confounding factor, the remaining study population from which cases are selected may be too small, thus reducing the power of the study. Unfortunately, the findings from a study using this method of control for confounding cannot be generalised to those who were left out by the restriction process, thus reducing the applicability of the findings.

Matching

- Matching on the confounding variable(s) is a statistical technique commonly used in observational studies, especially in case–control studies.

- Matching constrains subjects in both the exposed and unexposed groups to have the same value of potential confounders, such as sex and age. For example, in a study published in 2012, Driver and colleagues carried out a case–control study evaluating the relation between dementia and subsequent cancer. They matched each dementia case with up to three controls of the same sex and age who were free of dementia at the time of dementia diagnosis of the case.
- The cost of a study is usually lowered with matching, as a smaller sample size will be needed to carry out the study with the same degree of power.
- The feasibility and precision of carrying out a study can generally be increased with matching on the confounding variable(s).
- However, matching has certain disadvantages:
  - The more variables that are matched for, the more demanding it will be to identify a sufficient number of matched subjects.
  - The effect of the matching variables on the disease outcome cannot be investigated during the statistical analysis.
  - If there are missing data for the case or control in a matched pair, the data from both subjects are excluded from the statistical analysis.

Analysis stage

Once the study data have been collected, there are two options for controlling for confounding factors at the analysis stage:

1. Stratified analysis
2. Mathematical modelling.

Stratified analysis

- We can estimate the association between the exposure and disease outcome separately for different levels (strata) of the confounding variable (e.g. in the example illustrated in Fig. 13.2B, we would create two subgroups, smokers and non-smokers).
- The separate estimates of the measure of association for each subgroup are combined to calculate the 'adjusted' measure of association (e.g. risk ratio adjusted for confounding). Although there are many methods for calculating the 'adjusted' measure of association using stratified analysis, the Mantel–Haenszel method is the most commonly used pooling procedure.
- Stratified analysis is usually employed to control for confounding when there are only a few confounders, i.e. three confounders. However, stratified analysis may be problematic as the subgroups created may be too small and hence the power to detect a significant effect will be low. Furthermore, false-positive results may arise if multiple hypotheses are tested in each subgroup. In other words, the type 1 error rate (please refer to Chapter 3 for a discussion on type 1 error) increases as the number of comparisons made increases.

Mathematical modelling

- Mathematical modelling is useful when simultaneously adjusting for many confounding factors in a study (e.g. the odds ratio calculated in a case–control study investigating an association between drinking carbonated drinks high in aspartame and Parkinson's disease may be adjusted for age, social class, smoking and sex).
- Simultaneous control of two or more confounding factors can give different results from those calculated by controlling for each confounding factor individually.
- Calculating the 'adjusted' measure of association between an exposure and disease (by assessing the confounding factors simultaneously) better models the natural environment where the exposure, disease and confounding factors all coexist, than does controlling for each confounding factor individually.
- Although there are various types of mathematical models, the most commonly used model used to control for multiple confounders is logistic regression.

REPORTING AND INTERPRETING THE RESULTS

- When critically appraising any observational study, it is important to consider whether the investigators accounted for the effects of confounding at the design and/or analysis stage of the study.
- In those studies where confounding is controlled for at the analysis stage, it is usual to display the 'crude' measure of association (i.e. before potential confounding factors are taken into account) as well as the 'adjusted' measure of association (i.e. after correcting for distortions in the data caused by confounding).
- If the adjusted measure of association is significantly different from the crude measure of association, then confounding is present.
- It is useful to report the cut-off used to select which confounding factors are adjusted for (e.g. 10, 20 or 30% change from crude to adjusted).
- If the measure of association is adjusted by less than 10% after controlling for confounding, it would be unlikely that this influence would be taken into account. The more variables that are controlled

for, the wider the confidence interval will be for the measure of association (please refer to Chapter 3 for a discussion on confidence intervals), and therefore the less precise the study results will be.

- Age and sex are two confounding factors that are usually controlled for in every study due to the association of these variables with disease and mortality rate.

KEY EXAMPLE OF STUDY CONFOUNDING

Study type: Case–control study (hypothetical)

Research question: Does playing first-person shooter video games (for at least 15 hours per week) improve your ability in being able to successfully manage acute medical scenarios in an exam situation?

Biological mechanism linking exposure to outcome: Playing first-person shooters improves your ability in being able to successfully manage acute medical scenarios (and therefore pass the exam) as:

- Online play over the intercom with other players to decide the plan of attack on how to ambush the enemy will improve team-working, decision-making and delegating skills.
- Tapping the L1 button on the joystick as fast you can in order to sprint to help your team member will improve manual dexterity.

Potential confounder: Hours spent revising for the exam, age and sex.

The number of hours spent revising for the exam may be a confounder in the association between the exposure and outcome via a non-causal relationship. How active your social life is will affect the number of hours you play video games and the amount of time spent revising for the exam. Furthermore, as we all know, the more hours spent revising for an exam, the more likely you are to pass the exam! A person's age and sex may also influence both the exposure and outcome (Fig. 13.3).

Figure 13.4 summarises the crude and adjusted odds ratio for the association between playing video games and exam success. The following conclusions can be drawn from the data:

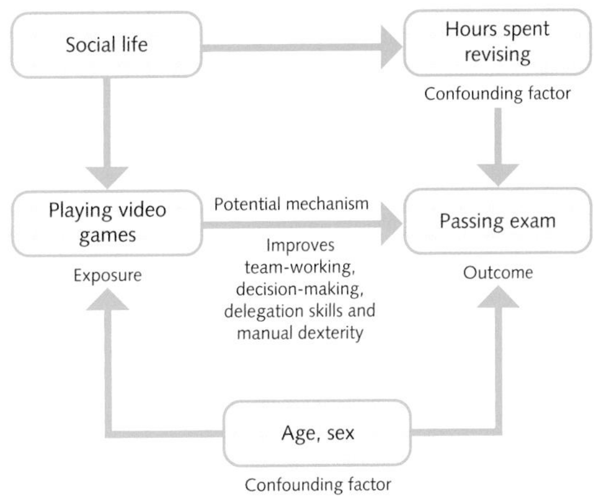

Fig. 13.3 Schematic of association.

Fig. 13.4 Crude and adjusted odds ratio.

Exposure	Crude odds ratio	Adjusted odds ratio
Playing video games	9.12	0.94

- The crude odds ratio of 9.12 suggests that people who played at least 15 hours of first-person shooter video games per week had an approximately 9 times greater chance/odds of passing the acute medical scenario exam.
- Before you head towards the games console, the adjusted odds ratio of 0.94 suggests that the apparent association between playing first-person shooter video games and exam success was explained by the confounding effects of the number of hours spent revising for the exam, sex and age.
- Those people who played at least 15 hours of first-person shooter video games per week must of course be playing hard, but the adjusted odds ratio of 0.94 suggests that they must also be revising hard!!!

HINTS AND TIPS

Work hard, play hard!

Screening, diagnosis and prognosis

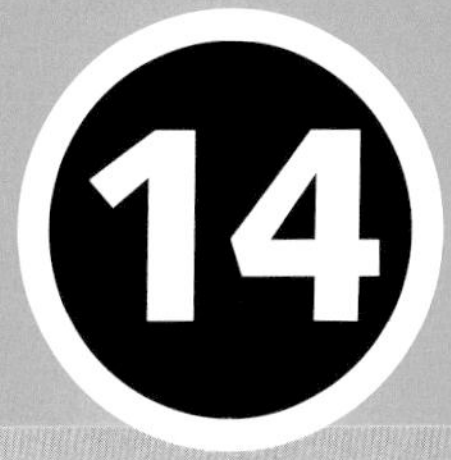

Objectives

By the end of this chapter you should:

- Know the reasons for carrying out a diagnostic test.
- Be able to define and calculate the sensitivity, specificity, positive predictive value and negative predictive value of a diagnostic test.
- Understand how predictive values can vary with disease prevalence.
- Be able to calculate the post-test probability of a diagnostic test using predictive values and the likelihood ratio.
- Understand how spectrum bias, verification bias, loss-to-follow-up bias and reporting bias are implicated when assessing the validity of a diagnostic study.
- Know the difference between diagnostic tests and screening tests.
- Be able to list the advantages and disadvantages of screening programmes.
- Understand how selection bias, length time bias and lead-time bias are implicated in studies investigating the effectiveness of screening tests.
- Be able to define the term prognosis and prognostic factor.
- Be able to describe the study methods used for investigating disease prognosis.

SCREENING, DIAGNOSIS AND PROGNOSIS

- Early diagnosis of a disease, prior to the patient experiencing any symptoms, may be through opportunistic tests (e.g. a bone scan on a patient who has fallen may detect metastatic bone disease) or *screening tests*.
- When a patient presents with symptoms, *diagnostic tests* may be used by the clinician to diagnose a particular disorder/disease in the patient.
- Once diagnosed with the disease, clinical guidelines, which are based on evidence from clinical trials, are used to initiate treatment (please refer to Chapter 1 for a discussion on clinical guidelines).
- Furthermore, a person who has just been diagnosed with a disease may be interested in knowing the *prognosis* of their disease, which may include recovery, disability or even death!
- The prognosis is affected by prognostic factors, which may depend on when the disease was diagnosed and when treatment was initiated.
- This overview of screening, diagnosis and prognosis has been illustrated in the time line shown in Fig. 14.1.

DIAGNOSTIC TESTS

- A diagnostic test can be used to determine whether a patient is likely to have:
    - a particular disease or condition (we will focus on this type of diagnostic test in this section).
    - a high risk of disease, e.g. checking the serum lipids in the assessment of cardiovascular disease risk.
    - been exposed to a particular factor, e.g. paracetamol levels in an individual suspected to have taken an overdose.
- Identifying new diagnostic tests may be necessary if the definitive gold standard test is expensive, invasive, risky, painful or time-consuming.
- Diagnostic tests are not always correct 100% of the time.
- As clinicians rely on these diagnostic tests to make decisions on which patients need treatment, the performance (or validity) of a new test must be properly assessed before implementing its use in the clinical setting. This assessment is usually made by comparing the results of the new diagnostic test to the patient's true disease status (as assessed using the 'gold standard' test). For example, how valid is an exercise stress test (also known as an exercise ECG)

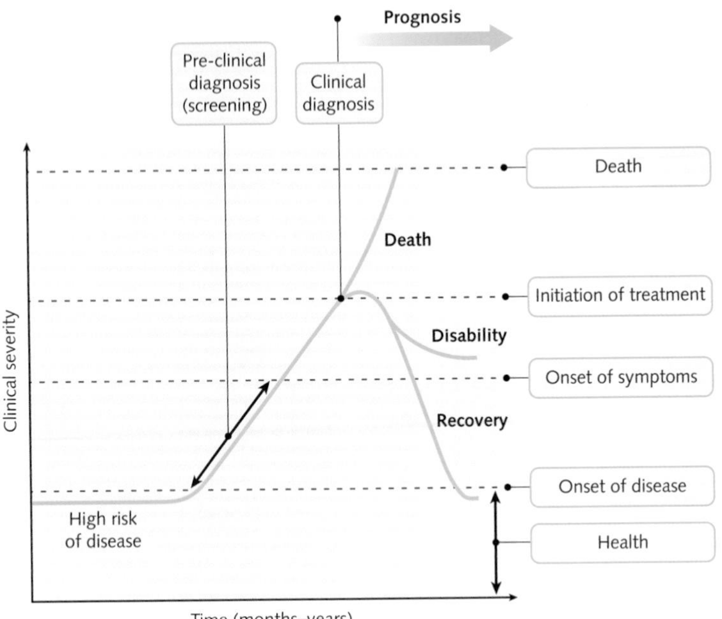

Fig. 14.1 Screening, diagnosis and prognosis of a disease.

for diagnosing coronary artery disease (usually > 50% fixed coronary artery stenosis) compared to the gold standard test used for cardiac testing, angiography?

- The four key measures used to evaluate the performance of a new test are:
  - Sensitivity
  - Specificity
  - Positive predictive value
  - Negative predictive value.

HINTS AND TIPS

The gold standard (or reference standard) is a term for the most definitive diagnostic procedure, which distinguishes people with disease from people without disease.

EVALUATING THE PERFORMANCE OF A DIAGNOSTIC TEST

Sensitivity and specificity

- Suppose we carry out a study to evaluate the performance of a new diagnostic test for a particular disease. Each person taking this test will either have or not have the disease. However, there are four possible types of outcomes of a diagnostic test:
  1. *True positive*: People with the disease who are correctly diagnosed as having the disease.
  2. *False positive* (also known as 'type I error'): People without the disease who are incorrectly identified as having the disease.
  3. *True negative*: People without the disease who are correctly identified as being disease-free.
  4. *False negative* (also known as 'type II error'): People with the disease who are incorrectly identified as being disease-free.
- Assuming the diagnostic test can only be positive or negative, indicating the presence or absence of disease, we can draw up a 2×2 table of frequencies for the different types of outcomes discussed above (Fig. 14.2).
- The sensitivity and specificity are measures that assess the validity of diagnostic tests.
- Sensitivity describes the ability of the test to correctly identify people *with* the disease, i.e. the percentage of individuals with the disease who have positive test results.
- The sensitivity of a test can be written as:

$$\text{Sensitivity} = \frac{\text{True positive}}{\text{True positive} + \text{False negative}} = \frac{\text{TP}}{\text{TP} + \text{FN}}$$

- Specificity describes the ability of the test to correctly identify people *without* the disease, i.e. the percentage of individuals without the disease who have negative test results.

Fig. 14.2 Table of frequencies for a diagnostic test.

		Disease status (according to gold standard test)	
		Disease (positive)	*No disease (negative)*
Test result	*Positive*	True positive	False positive (type 1 error)
	Negative	False negative (type 2 error)	True negative

- The specificity of a test can be written as:

$$\text{Specificity} = \frac{\text{True negative}}{\text{True negative} + \text{False positive}} = \frac{\text{TN}}{\text{TP} + \text{FP}}$$

- An ideal test would be both highly sensitive and highly specific, where disease would be correctly identified in 100% of those individuals who truly have the disease (100% sensitivity) and disease would be ruled out in 100% of those individuals who truly don't have the disease (100% specificity). However, it is often difficult in reality to have a diagnostic test that is high in both sensitivity and specificity.
- For any test, there is usually a trade-off between the sensitivity and specificity. Figure 14.3 demonstrates this point with the use of test result distribution curves.
- Referring to Fig. 14.3A, the two distributions represent the results of the diagnostic test (which consist of a continuous measurement) in individuals who do and do not have the disease.
- The threshold of the test is the cut-off used in declaring that the test is positive. The investigator can adjust the threshold (black vertical line in Fig. 14.3B), which will in turn alter the sensitivity and specificity of the test.
- Increasing the threshold (by shifting) the vertical line to the right increases the specificity, but decreases the sensitivity of the diagnostic test (Fig. 14.3C).
  - A diagnostic test with a high specificity (and therefore a low sensitivity) has a low false-positive rate (type I error).
- Reducing the threshold (by shifting the vertical line to the left) increases the sensitivity, but decreases the specificity of the diagnostic test (Fig. 14.3D).
  - A diagnostic test with a high sensitivity (and therefore a low specificity) has a low false-negative rate (type 2 error).

HINTS AND TIPS

Useful mnemonics

SpPin: A highly **S**pecific test with a **p**ositive result tends to rule **in** the diagnosis of the disease.
SnNout: A highly **S**ensitive test with a **n**egative result tends to rule **out** the diagnosis of the disease.

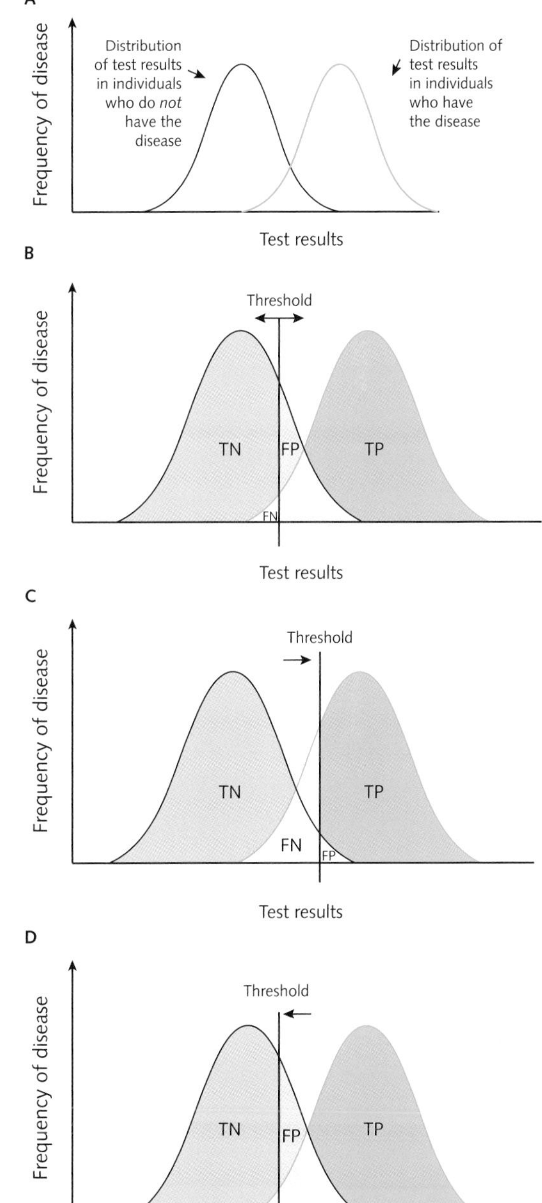

Fig. 14.3 Distribution curve: sensitivity and specificity (see text).

Using sensitivity and specificity to make clinical decisions

- As mentioned above, we gain sensitivity at the expense of specificity, and vice versa.
- Whether we decide to aim for a diagnostic test which has high sensitivity or high specificity (i.e. by decreasing or increasing the threshold, respectively), depends on:
  - the condition we are trying to diagnose.
  - the implications for the patient of either a false-negative or false-positive test result.
- A high sensitivity test is preferred if:
  - the disease is life-threatening if left untreated.
  - there is an improvement in survival rate if treatment is initiated early.
  - overdiagnosis is okay (if a screening test) because all those who screen positive will have further tests.
- For example, the absence of retinal vein pulsation for diagnosing of raised intracranial pressure, or screening programmes, such as for breast cancer or HIV.
- A high specificity test is preferred if:
  - the disease is *not* life-threatening if left untreated.
  - subsequent tests or treatments are invasive (e.g. prostate biopsy) or have severe side effects (e.g. chemotherapy).
  - treatment costs are high.
  - the pre-test probability of the condition is low.
- For example, screening tests for Down's syndrome during pregnancy are highly specific as the consequence of a wrong diagnosis is abortion!

HINTS AND TIPS

It is important in clinical decision-making to know the sensitivity and specificity of the test you are conducting.

Positive and negative predictive values

- The sensitivity and specificity are both characteristics of a diagnostic test but they don't inform us on how to interpret the results of the test for an individual patient. Therefore, in the clinical setting, we use positive and negative predictive values to indicate the probability that the patient has (or does not have) the disease, given a positive (or negative) test result.
- The positive predictive value (PPV) can be written as:

$$\text{PPV} = \frac{\text{True positive}}{\text{True positive} + \text{False positive}}$$
$$= \frac{\text{TP}}{\text{TP} + \text{FP}}$$

- A test with a high PPV means that there is only a small per cent of false positives within all the individuals with positive test results; i.e. the patient probably does have the disease.
- The negative predictive value (NPV) can be written as:

$$\text{NPV} = \frac{\text{True negative}}{\text{True negative} + \text{False negative}}$$
$$= \frac{\text{TN}}{\text{TN} + \text{FN}}$$

- A test with a high NPV means that there is only a small per cent of false negatives within all the individuals with negative test results; i.e. the patient probably does not have the disease.

HINTS AND TIPS

While the sensitivity and specificity are prevalence-independent tests, predictive values are dependent on the prevalence of the disease in the population being studied.

False positives and false negatives

- A false negative (type 2 error) is when an individual is incorrectly diagnosed as not having the disease, when in fact the person does have the disease.
- If you know the sensitivity of the test, the false negative rate is equal to:

$$\text{False negative } (\%) = 100\% - \text{Sensitivity } (\%)$$

- A false positive (type 1 error) is when an individual is incorrectly diagnosed as having the disease, when in fact the person is disease-free.
- If you know the specificity of the test, the false-positive rate is equal to:

$$\text{False positive } (\%) = 100\% - \text{Specificity } (\%)$$

Number needed to test

Another way of expressing the PPV is the number needed to test (NNTest). This is the number of patients with a specific symptom who would need to be tested in order to find one true positive. It is calculated as 1/PPV. For instance, if a patient presents in primary care with a new headache that is severe and of sudden onset, the PPV of that history for subarachnoid haemorrhage (SAH) is 25%. The NNTest is therefore 4 – only 4 such patients need to be tested for SAH in order to correctly diagnose one patient with the condition. Patients, and some doctors, find the NNTest easier to understand than the PPV.

THE DIAGNOSTIC PROCESS

- The positive and negative predictive values of a test (or a symptom or sign) are useful measures in clinical practice, especially when a patient wants the clinician to confirm that he doesn't have the disease when the test result is negative. Similarly, a patient may want the clinician to confirm that he definitely has the disease when the test result is positive.
- When a test is 100% specific, the positive predictive value is 100% as there are never any false-positive results (Fig. 14.4A).
- When a test is 100% sensitive, the negative predictive value is 100% as there are never any false-negative results (Fig. 14.4B).
- Unlike sensitivity and specificity, the positive and negative predictive values depend on the prevalence of disease in the population (as well as the sensitivity and specificity of the test).
- In the following section, we will discuss how knowing the disease prevalence in the population can assist us when deciding whether or not to order a particular diagnostic test for your patient.
- Figure 14.5 describes the process involved in deciding whether or not a test will alter the diagnosis of a disease in a specific patient.
- A test may range in complexity, from being something as simple as a physical examination to something complex like myocardial perfusion imaging.

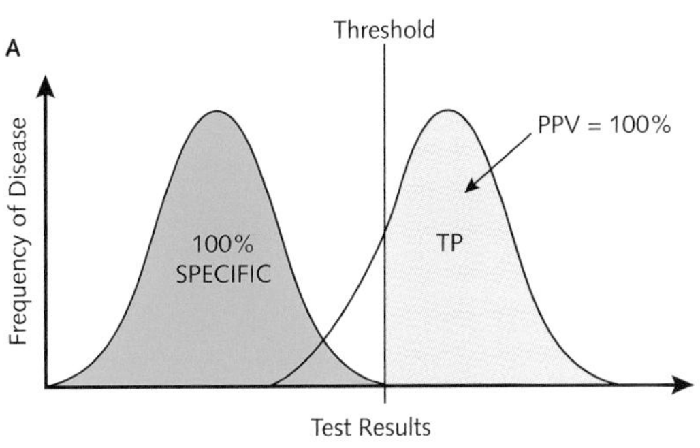

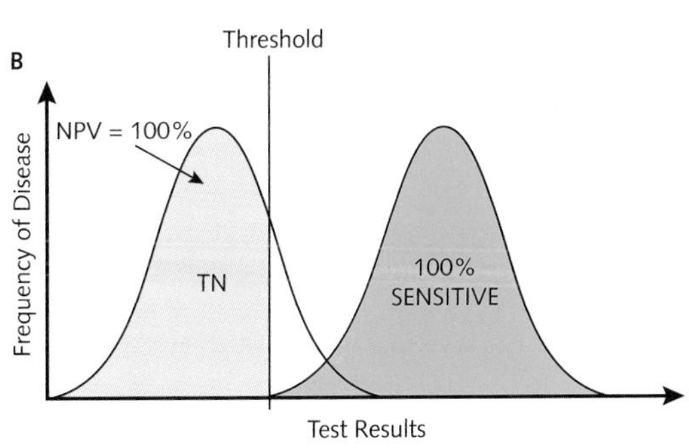

Fig. 14.4 Distribution curve: positive and negative predictive values.

Pre-test probability

- The first step of the diagnostic process is to determine the pre-test probability of the patient having the disease.
- The pre-test probability is the likelihood that the patient has the condition or disease before you know the result of the test.
- The pre-test probability of an individual can depend on:
    - the specific patient, including gender, risk factor profile and the presence of signs and symptoms.
    - the prevalence of the disease in the population.
    - the post-test probability of the disease resulting from one or more preceding tests.
- The pre-test probabilities have been described for a number of clinical presentations for various diseases, in the literature. For example, based on a report published by American College of Cardiology/American Heart Association, the pre-test probability for coronary artery disease can be estimated from the patient's age, sex and chest pain symptoms.
- In practice, clinicians use a more intuitive (i.e. quantitative but not explicit) approach when assessing the pre-test probability, based on previous experience of dealing with similar patients.

Post-test probability

- In the clinical setting, post-test probabilities are usually estimated based on clinical experience.
- Whether the doctor guesses the post-test probability or estimates it, as explained below, the probability is never 0 or 100%.
- The post-test probability can be estimated using predictive values or likelihood ratios.

Estimating the post-test probability using predictive values

- Positive and negative predictive values can be used to estimate the post-test probability of an individual having a condition or disease.
- Predictive values can only be used if the pre-test probability is the same as the prevalence of the disease in the reference (gold standard) group used to establish the positive predictive value of the test.
- If the test result has a binary classification (i.e. the result is either positive or negative), we can construct a frequency table as shown in Fig. 14.2.
- When using predictive values to estimate the post-test probability, the pre-test probability is equal to the prevalence of the disease:

Fig. 14.5 The diagnostic process.

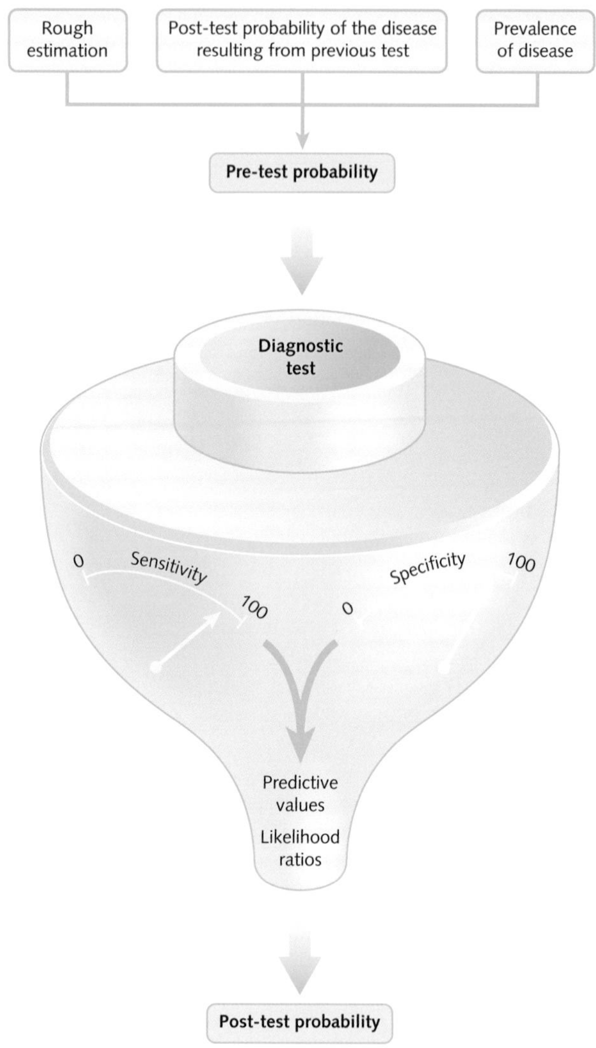

$$\text{Pre-test probability} = \frac{\text{True positive} + \text{False negative}}{\text{Total sample size}}$$
$$= \frac{\text{TP} + \text{FN}}{n}$$
$$= \text{Prevalence of disease}$$

- The positive post-test probability (i.e. the probability of having the disease if the result of the test is positive) is equal to the calculation for the positive predictive value (discussed above).
- The negative post-test probability (i.e. the probability of having the disease if the result of the test is negative) is equal to:

$$\text{Negative post-test probability } (\%) = 100\% - \text{Negative predictive value } (\%)$$

- However, these equations are only valid in the absence of bias (especially sampling bias) in the diagnostic studies used to obtain the frequencies shown in Fig. 14.2.

HINTS AND TIPS

It is only possible to use predictive values to calculate the post-test probability if the individual being tested does not have any additional risk factors that result in that individual have a different pre-test probability from the reference (gold standard) group used to calculate the positive and negative predictive values of the test.

Estimating the post-test probability using likelihood ratios

- If another test preceded the test we are planning on carrying out or if the individual being tested has a different pre-test probability to the reference (gold standard) group (for example, due to having different signs, symptoms or a higher/lower risk factor profile),
  - we can estimate the pre-test probability of the individual by making a rough estimation or by using the population prevalence of the disease (i.e. not the prevalence of the reference (gold standard) group, as discussed above) if this information is available.
  - we calculate the post-test probability by using a likelihood ratio for the test.
- The likelihood ratio:
  - is the probability that a given test result (i.e. positive or negative) would be expected in an individual with the disease compared to the probability that the same result would be expected in an individual without the disease.
  - is calculated from the sensitivity and specificity of the test.
  - does not depend on the prevalence of the reference (gold standard) group.
  - does not change if the pre-test probability changes for different individuals.
- There are two versions of the likelihood ratio, one for positive and one for negative test results. Respectively, they are known as the positive likelihood ratio (LR+) and negative likelihood ratio (LR–).
- A positive likelihood ratio (LR+) is a measure of how much we need to increase the pre-test probability of disease if the test result is positive:

$$\text{LR+} = \frac{\text{Probability (positive test result if disease is present)}}{\text{Probability (positive test result if disease is absent)}} = \frac{\text{Sensitivity}}{1 - \text{Specificity}}$$

- The higher the value for the LR+, the higher the probability that the individual has the disease.
- A negative likelihood ratio (LR–) is a measure of how much we need to decrease the pre-test probability of disease if the test result is negative:

$$\text{LR}- = \frac{\text{Probability (negative test result if disease is present)}}{\text{Probability (negative test result if disease is absent)}} = \frac{1 - \text{Sensitivity}}{\text{Specificity}}$$

- An LR– is associated with the absence of disease and will take a value < 1. The lower the value for the LR–, the lower the probability that the individual has the disease.
- We estimate the post-test probability using 'odds' rather than probabilities.
- We must first calculate the pre-test odds from the pre-test probability:

$$\text{Pre-test odds} = \frac{\text{Pre-test probability}}{1 - \text{Pre-test probability}}$$

- The post-test odds in a person with a positive result are:

$$\text{Post-test odds} = \text{Pre-test odds} \times \text{Positive likelihood ratio}$$

- The post-test odds in a person with a negative result are:

$$\text{Post-test odds} = \text{Pre-test odds} \times \text{Negative likelihood ratio}$$

- The post-test odds can be converted back into a probability:

$$\text{Post-test probability} = \frac{\text{Post-test odds}}{\text{Post-test odds} + 1}$$

- The Fagan nomogram (Fig. 14.6) is a graphical tool which converts pre-test probabilities into post-test probabilities for diagnostic test results with a known likelihood ratio. The nomogram therefore saves us from switching back and forth between probability and odds.

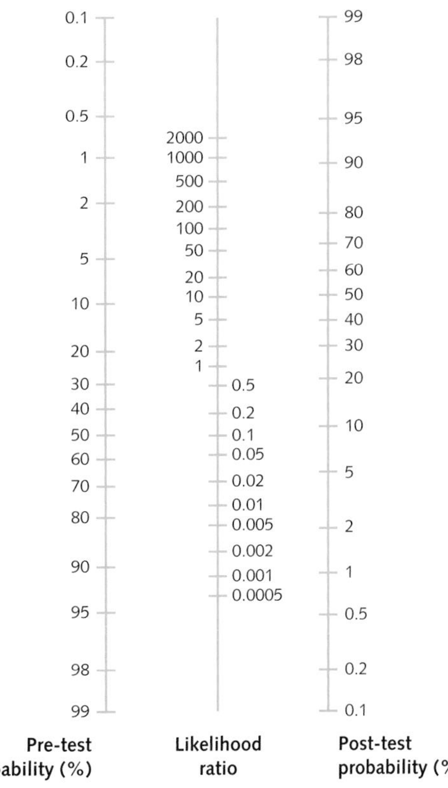

Fig. 14.6 Fagan nomogram.

- Referring to Fig. 14.6, the nomogram consists of three vertical axes which represent the pre-test probability, likelihood ratio and the post-test probability, from left to right.
- You can estimate the post-test probability using the Fagan nomogram by carrying out the following steps:
  1. Mark the pre-test probability on the left axis.
  2. Mark the likelihood ratio (positive or negative) on the middle axis.
  3. Draw a straight line between the two points marked on the nomogram, continuing the line to the post-test probability axis on the right.
  4. Where the line intersects the vertical post-test probability axis is the post-test probability.

HINTS AND TIPS

You can use an interactive nomogram to quickly and easily estimate the post-test probability by entering in an individual's pre-test probability and the likelihood ratio. An interactive nomogram is accessible from the 'Centre for Evidence-Based Medicine' website: http://www.cebm.net

A library of likelihood ratios can be found on the Bandolier website: http://www.medicine.ox.ac.uk/bandolier

- A diagnostic test is most important and informative when the pre-test probability of the individual having the disease is between 40 and 60%. At this level of pre-test probability, a positive test result essentially confirms the disease diagnosis, while a negative test result essentially rules it out (unless the values of the likelihood ratios are close to 1). Therefore a test is more useful if it changes the pre-test probability of the disease by a relatively large extent.
- It is important to realise that a test may increase or decrease the probability (or likelihood) that the disease is present (Fig. 14.7). For example, a positive sputum culture for *Mycobacterium tuberculosis* has a likelihood ratio of 31, which is associated with a marked increase in the probability of a patient having tuberculosis. However, a negative sputum culture is only associated with a likelihood ratio of 0.79. Referring to Fig. 14.7, this only causes a very small reduction in the likelihood of the patient having tuberculosis. This is because *Mycobacterium tuberculosis* often fails to grow in culture; thus there are many false negatives.
- If the post-test probability is equivocal and you still have your clinical suspicion that the patient has the disease in question, the post-test probability can, in turn, be used as a pre-test probability for additional tests.

Fig. 14.7 The likelihood ratio.

Likelihood ratio (LR)		Likelihood of test to change the pre-test probability
Negative LR	Positive LR	
< 0.1	>10	Causes a very large change
0.1–0.2	5–10	Causes a moderate change
0.2–0.5	2–5	Causes a small change
> 0.5	< 2	Causes very little change
LR = 1	LR = 1	Causes no change

Should I order a test if the pre-test probability is low?

In some situations it is necessary to request a test despite starting with a low pre-test probability. For example, if:

- the test is relatively inexpensive and has a reasonable likelihood ratio.
- the test does not cause any distress or any harmful side-effects.
- you are screening for a disease in a population.
- the disease is associated with atypical or variable clinical presentations.
- delaying the diagnosis of the disease will worsen its prognosis.
- the disease prognosis can be easily improved by early treatment initiation.

(For the latter two points, you must have enough clinical suspicion that the individual has the disease.)

EXAMPLE OF A DIAGNOSTIC TEST USING PREDICTIVE VALUES

Graded exercise stress testing (EST) is an inexpensive, well-validated, readily available and easy-to-perform test. A 12 000-patient meta-analysis on the overall diagnostic accuracy of EST for coronary artery disease (>50% coronary artery stenosis) diagnosis showed that the test had 68% sensitivity and 77% specificity, using coronary angiography as the gold standard. That means that 68% of people with coronary artery disease (CAD) will test positive, but for every 100 people without CAD, 23 of them will also test positive (i.e. false-positive rate = 100% – 77% = 23%). Figures 14.8–14.10 show the results of using EST in three different populations. As we shall demonstrate, despite the test having the same sensitivity and specificity in all three populations, the positive predictive value varies.

Let's look at three different presentations of chest pain. The pre-test probability for each case is the same as the prevalence in each respective reference (gold standard) group used to establish the positive predictive value (i.e. the post-test probability) of the test.

Case 1: Low pre-test probability/ low prevalence

A 31-year-old woman presents with a 3-week history of intermittent central chest pain unrelated to activity, unrelieved by rest (sometimes relieved by nitroglycerine), and is non-radiating. The onset of the pain is

		Coronary artery disease (according to gold standard test)		
		Disease (positive)	*Disease (negative)*	*Total*
Exercise stress test	*Positive*	68	207	275
	Negative	32	693	725
	Total	100	900	1000

Sensitivity	68/100 = 68%	PPV	68/275 = 25%
Specificity	693/900 = 77%	NPV	693/725 = 96%
Prevalence	100/1000 = 10%		

Fig. 14.8 The effect of low prevalence on the predictive value.

		Coronary artery disease (according to gold standard test)		
		Disease (positive)	*Disease (negative)*	*Total*
Exercise stress test	*Positive*	340	115	455
	Negative	160	385	545
	Total	500	500	1000

Sensitivity	340/500 = 68%	PPV	340/455 = 75%
Specificity	385/500 = 77%	NPV	385/545 = 71%
Prevalence	500/1000 = 50%		

Fig. 14.9 The effect of moderate prevalence on the predictive value.

		Coronary artery disease (according to gold standard test)		
		Disease (positive)	*Disease (negative)*	*Total*
Exercise stress test	*Positive*	612	23	635
	Negative	288	77	365
	Total	900	100	1000

Sensitivity	612/900 = 68%	PPV	612/635 = 96%
Specificity	77/100 = 77%	NPV	77/365 = 21%
Prevalence	900/1000 = 90%		

Fig. 14.10 The effect of high prevalence on the predictive value.

usually associated with food intake. She has no cardiovascular risk factors.

Referring to Fig. 14.8:

- Her pre-test probability of CAD is approximately 10%.
- With a low prevalence and relatively high specificity, the negative predictive value is high. Therefore, with an NPV of 96%, if the test is negative, the individual is likely to be a true negative.
- With a PPV of only 25%, if the test is positive, this won't help the clinician in making a clinical decision about whether the patient has CAD. A total of 75% of individuals who test positive will not have CAD. Based on these findings, it is unlikely that the patient would need an angiogram if the EST result is positive.

Case 2: Equivocal pre-test probability/high prevalence

A 41-year-old female who has a background of hypertension and smoking presents with a 2-week history of central, stabbing chest pain. It is sometimes precipitated by moderate exertion and there is some costochondral tenderness.

Referring to Fig. 14.9:

- Her pre-test probability of CAD is approximately 50%.
- With a moderate prevalence of 50%, and a relatively high sensitivity and specificity, both the PPV and the NPV are high. Therefore, the results are likely to be correct, whether positive or negative.
- Based on these findings:
  - it is likely that the patient would need an angiogram if the EST result is positive.
  - it is unlikely that the patient would need an angiogram if the EST result is negative; however, as the patient still has a 29% probability (100% − NPV%) of having CAD, an angiogram may be warranted if resources are available and there is enough clinical suspicion.

Case 3: High pre-test probability/high prevalence

A 65-year-old male with a background of hypertension presents with a 6-week history of intermittent central, crushing chest pain that radiates to his jaw. It is usually precipitated by mild exertion and relieved by nitroglycerine or rest.

Referring to Fig. 14.10:

- His pre-test probability of CAD is approximately 90%.
- With a high prevalence of 90% and relatively high sensitivity and specificity, the PPV is high. Therefore, with a PPV of 96%, only 4% of individuals who test positive will not have CAD.
- The NPV is only 21%. Therefore, 79% of individuals who test negative will actually have CAD!
- Overall, if the pre-test probability is high, EST doesn't help with clinical decision-making; i.e. with a very high initial pre-test probability of 90%, you would perform an angiogram in this patient anyway!

BIAS IN DIAGNOSTIC STUDIES

When assessing the validity of a diagnostic study it is important to consider whether the study design may have been affected by potential biases. For an introduction to study error and bias, please refer to the Chapter 7 section 'Bias'.

Spectrum bias

- Spectrum bias is a type of selection bias which depends on the type of patients recruited for the diagnostic study.
- It may occur when only cases with a limited range of disease spectrum are recruited for the study.
- The performance of a diagnostic test may be artificially overestimated if a case–control study design is used in which healthy volunteers ('fittest of the fit') are compared to a population with advanced disease ('sickest of the sick') (Fig. 14.11A). As demonstrated using the example in the previous section, this diagnostic test will have limited value as these cases have already been diagnosed; i.e. the pre-test probability is already very low or very high and the test will make little difference!
- On the other hand, if the diagnostic study is based on a cohort study design, during which a representative population is evaluated, (Fig. 14.11B), there will be less spectrum bias.
- The likelihood ratio is not affected by spectrum bias and can be used in case-control studies that separately recruit people with and without the disease.

Verification bias

- Verification bias:
  - generally only occurs when patients are tested with the study test before the reference (gold standard) test.
  - is a type of non-random misclassification measurement bias (discussed in Chapter 7).
  - can be divided into:
    - Partial verification bias, or
    - Differential verification bias.

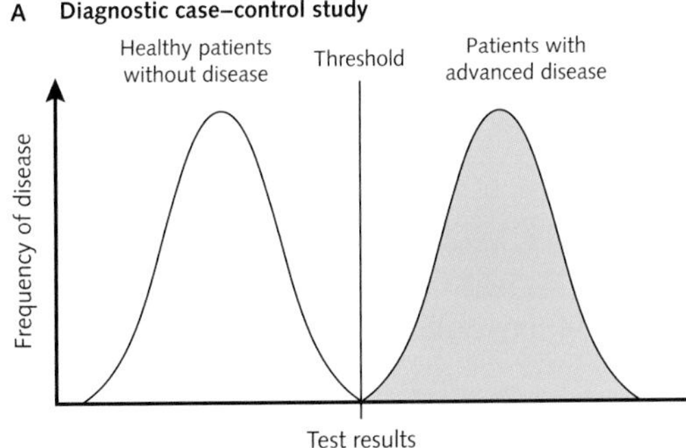

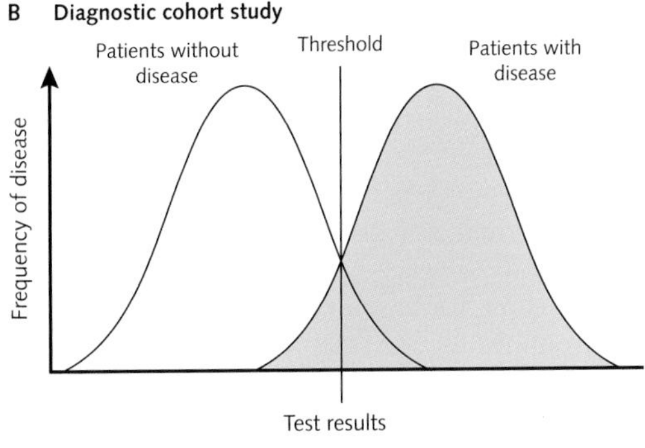

Fig. 14.11 Spectrum bias: more likely in case–control than in cohort studies. (A) Diagnostic case–control study. (B) Diagnostic cohort study.

Partial verification bias

- Partial verification bias (also known as work-up bias):
    - occurs when the decision to perform the reference (gold standard) test on an individual is based on the results of the diagnostic study test. For example, the gold standard test may only be performed on those patients who have a positive study test result. Consequently, more unwell individuals (than healthy ones) undergo gold standard testing. This will lead to an underestimation of the false-negative rate and an overestimation of both the negative predictive value and the sensitivity of the study test. Therefore, if individuals who have negative study test results do not undergo gold standard testing, the diagnostic test would be perceived to be better as the number of positive cases detected would be higher. However, the degree of partial verification bias would also be higher in this situation.
    - Is usually an issue if the gold standard test is:
        1. invasive, such as surgery or biopsy, and therefore unethical for use in individuals in whom there is very minimal clinical suspicion of disease.
        2. expensive.
    - may be an issue if those individuals with a positive study test result undergo a more extended period of follow-up than those individuals with a negative study test result.
    - may be avoided if the reference test is always performed prior to the study test. However, this is not always possible; for example, you wouldn't perform surgery prior to imaging!
    - may be minimised in some study designs by blinding the investigator between the study test and reference test results.

Differential verification bias

- Differential verification bias occurs when different reference tests are used to verify the results of the study test.
- It may be an issue if patients testing positive on the study test receive a more accurate, often more invasive, reference test than those with negative test results.
- Therefore, using a less invasive, often less accurate, reference test on those individuals with a negative study test result may lead to an increase in the specificity of the study test.

Loss-to-follow-up bias

- Loss-to-follow-up bias is a type of selection bias.
- All patients that meet the eligibility criteria and have consented to participate in the study should have both the diagnostic study test and the gold standard test.
- Loss-to-follow-up bias occurs when individuals who are lost to follow-up differ systematically from those who remain in the study.
- If the proportion of subjects lost is substantial (e.g. 20% lost to follow-up), this will affect the validity of the study, can lead to data misinterpretation, and limit the generalisability of the study results.
- It is useful to have a 'flow diagram of study participants' so it is clear what happened to all the patients who entered the study. For example, did individuals drop out because they were too unwell to re-attend?

HINTS AND TIPS

While both verification bias and loss-to-follow-up bias involve study participants not having both the study test and the reference test, the key difference between the two is that verification bias is influenced by the investigator while loss-to-follow-up bias is influenced by the study participant.

Reporting bias

- Reporting bias (also known as review bias) is a type of non-random misclassification measurement bias (discussed in Chapter 7).
- The concept behind reporting bias is similar to blinding in interventional studies (discussed in Chapter 6).
- Interpreting the results of the study test may be influenced by knowledge of the results of the reference standard test, and vice versa. This is especially an issue if there is a degree of subjectivity in interpreting the results.
- If possible, the test results (of either the study test or reference test) should be interpreted blind to the results of the other test.

SCREENING TESTS

Diagnostic tests versus screening tests

- Figure 14.12 summarises the key differences between screening tests and diagnostic tests.

HINTS AND TIPS

Screening tests are not diagnostic tests!

Screening programmes

- Screening involves investigating 'apparently' healthy individuals with an aim to identify disease early, thus enabling earlier intervention and management in the hope of reducing morbidity and mortality from the disease.
- Screening may involve:
  - the whole population (mass screening).
  - selected groups, which have been shown to have an increased risk or prevalence of a certain condition or disease (targeted screening).
- There may be:
  - a systematic screening programme, where people are invited. For example, women aged between 50 and 70 years are invited for mammography screening for breast cancer every 3 years.
  - an opportunistic screening programme, where a screening test is offered to someone who presents for a different reason; for example, *Chlamydia* screening in a university student presenting with depression!

Fig. 14.12 Diagnostic tests versus screening tests.

	Diagnostic test	Screening test
Primary objective	To establish a definitive diagnosis of a disease which will inform subsequent management.	• To detect unrecognised disease early. • To detect those individuals at high risk of developing a disease (due to having risk factors).
Target population	• Symptomatic individuals. • Asymptomatic individuals with a positive screening test result.	Healthy, asymptomatic but potentially at-risk individuals.
Description of test	May be expensive, invasive and complex but justifiable to make the diagnosis.	Relatively cheap, simple and acceptable to patients and staff (non-invasive). The costs of screening should be justified by the benefits from screening.
Validity of test	The ability of the test to distinguish between people with the disease and those without it is defined by the sensitivity and specificity of the test.	
Threshold level	• High sensitivity and specificity is usually achieved through carrying out multiple tests. • In reality, a high specificity (at the expense of a lower sensitivity) diagnostic test is preferred to ensure that healthy cases are not mistakenly diagnosed with a disease.	Ideally, a screening test should have: • High sensitivity to ensure the false-negative rate is kept low, thus reducing the number of individuals who are falsely reassured. • High specificity to ensure the false-positive rate is kept low, thus reducing the number of unnecessary follow-up tests and investigations. In reality, a high sensitivity (at the expense of a lower specificity) screening test is preferred to ensure no potential disease cases are missed.
Meaning of a positive result	A definitive diagnosis of the disease.	There is suspicion that the individual has the disease being screened for, which warrants further investigation.

Fig. 14.13 Advantages and disadvantages of screening.

Advantages	Disadvantages
• Detects unrecognised disease early, where the prognosis can be improved. For example, survival is increased in women with breast cancer who were diagnosed and treated early. • Detects those individuals at high risk of developing a certain disease, where the individual or clinician can take measures to delay (or even prevent) the development of the disease by reducing the risk; e.g. screening for high blood pressure and offering lifestyle advice and/or drug intervention. • Identifies people with infectious disease, where an intervention can treat the infection and prevent transmission of the disease to others; e.g. *Chlamydia* screening in sexually active people under 25 years.	• A false sense of security if cases are missed (i.e. a false-negative screening result), which may delay the final diagnosis. • Those tested negative may feel they have avoided the disease and therefore continue with their risk behaviour; e.g. an individual who eats more than his recommended daily allowance of saturated fat may continue to do so if his cholesterol is within the normal range when tested by his GP. Looking at the bigger picture, this may undermine primary prevention programmes, e.g. to prevent coronary artery disease by promoting healthy eating. • For cases that are true positives, treatment of early disease may be associated with potential side effects, even though the disease may not have actually progressed. • Involves using medical resources and substantial amounts of money which could be used elsewhere, especially as the majority of people screened do not need treatment. • Stress and anxiety caused by false alarms (i.e. a false-positive screening result). The stress may be related to unnecessary investigations, especially if it involves an invasive procedure.

- Figure 14.13 highlights the key advantages and disadvantages of screening.

Screening programme evaluation

- The gold standard study design used to evaluate screening programmes is a randomised controlled trial, where screening is compared with no screening in a population.
- In addition to considering the cost, feasibility and ethics involved in implementing a screening programme, it is important to measure the extent to which the programme affects the relevant outcomes, i.e. the prognosis of a disease.
- There are various types of bias which influence the outcomes recorded in a study evaluating the effectiveness of a particular screening programme, including:
    - Selection bias
    - Length time bias
    - Lead-time bias.

Selection bias

- People who participate in screening programmes often have different characteristics from those who do not. For example, when screening women aged between 50 and 70 years for breast cancer, those women with a family history of breast cancer are more likely than other women to join the mammography screening programme. Consequently, there would be higher rates of morbidity/mortality amongst this select population than in the general population. The screening test would therefore be associated with a worse prognosis and will look worse than it actually is.
- On the other hand, if the screening programme is more accessible to young and healthy individuals, there would be lower rates of morbidity/mortality amongst this select population than in the general population. The screening test would therefore be associated with a better prognosis and will look better than it actually is.

Length time bias

- Length time bias occurs when screening tests selectively detect slowly developing cases, which have a long pre-symptomatic (or pre-clinical) phase, e.g. less aggressive cancers associated with a better prognosis. The data are therefore skewed.
- For example, referring to Fig. 14.14, let's look at length time bias in the context of cancer screening. In general, fast-growing tumours have a shorter pre-clinical phase than slow-growing tumours. Therefore, there is a shorter phase during which the tumour is asymptomatic in the body (and therefore a shorter phase during which the tumour may be detected via screening). These aggressive tumours may become symptomatic in-between screening events, during which the patient may seek medical

Fig. 14.14 Length time bias.

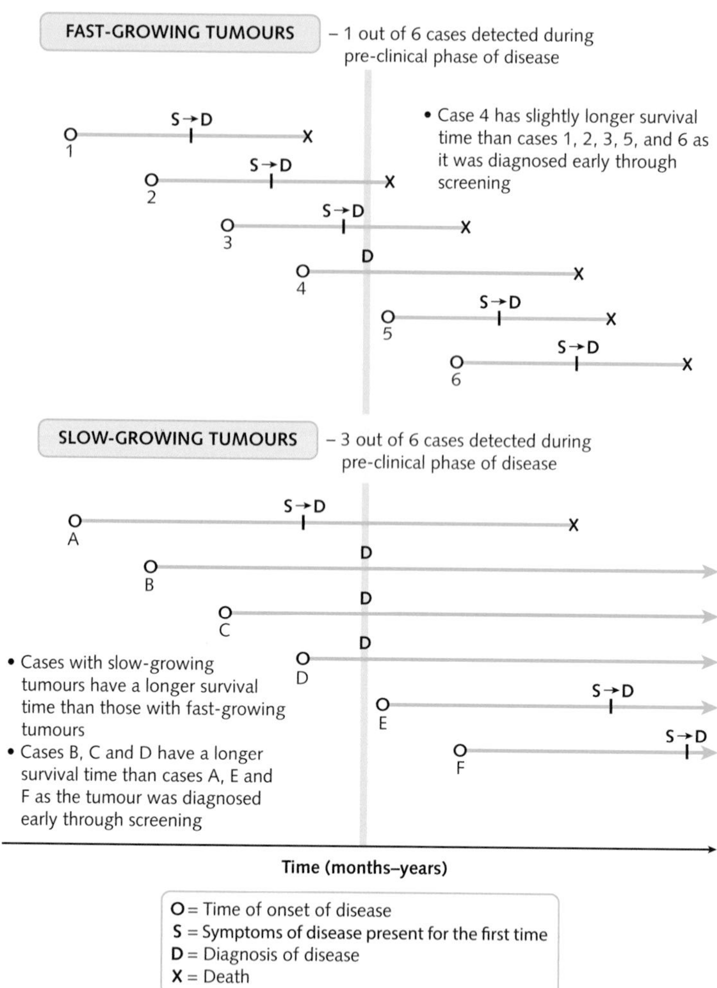
FAST-GROWING TUMOURS
– 1 out of 6 cases detected during pre-clinical phase of disease
• Case 4 has slightly longer survival time than cases 1, 2, 3, 5, and 6 as it was diagnosed early through screening
SLOW-GROWING TUMOURS
– 3 out of 6 cases detected during pre-clinical phase of disease
• Cases with slow-growing tumours have a longer survival time than those with fast-growing tumours
• Cases B, C and D have a longer survival time than cases A, E and F as the tumour was diagnosed early through screening
Time (months–years)
O = Time of onset of disease
S = Symptoms of disease present for the first time
D = Diagnosis of disease
X = Death

care and be diagnosed without screening. Putting this all together, if there are equal numbers of slow- and fast-growing tumours in a year, the screening test will detect more slow-growing cases (demonstrated in Fig. 14.14). Assuming that the slow-growing tumours are less likely to be fatal than the fast-growing tumours, the tumour cases detected through screening will have a better prognosis, on average, than those individuals who are diagnosed when the tumour becomes symptomatic. Screening is therefore unfairly favoured.

Lead-time bias

- The intention of screening is to diagnose a disease during its pre-clinical phase. Without screening, the disease may only be discovered later, when the disease becomes symptomatic. Consequently, through screening, survival time (the time from diagnosis to death) appears to increase due to earlier diagnosis, even if there is no change in the disease prognosis.
- By analysing the raw statistics, screening will appear to increase the survival time. As shown in Fig. 14.15, this gain is called lead time.
- Referring to Fig. 14.15:
  - Suppose the biological onset of a particular disease is at the same time in both Case 1 and Case 2.
  - Case 1 is diagnosed through screening in the pre-clinical phase of the disease and survives for 6 years from diagnosis.
  - Case 2 is diagnosed only when the subject becomes symptomatic, 4 years after Case 1 was diagnosed, and survives for 2 years from diagnosis.
  - Therefore, it seems as if Case 1 survives for 3 times as long as Case 2 (6 versus 2 years).
  - However, the life span has not been prolonged, as both cases survive for the same amount of time since the *biological onset* of the disease.

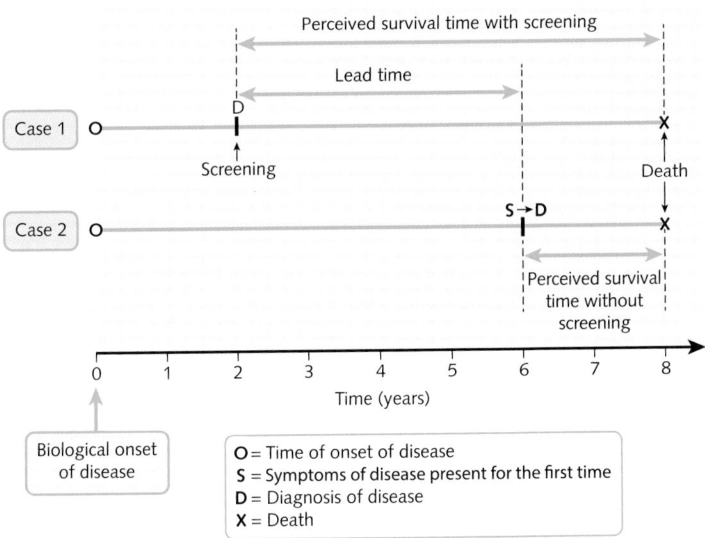

Fig. 14.15 Lead-time bias.

- Therefore, if early diagnosis of a disease has no effect on its biological course, lead-time bias can affect the interpretation of survival rates, e.g. the 5-year survival rate.

EXAMPLE OF A SCREENING TEST USING LIKELIHOOD RATIOS

Suppose a 60-year-old woman has a positive mammogram and asks you, her clinician, whether she has breast cancer. You explain that further testing is required; however, your patient wants to know the actual probability of her having breast cancer. Fortunately, you read this book and carry out the following calculations:

Regardless of the mammogram result, the clinician knows that the prevalence of breast cancer in the population is approximately 0.8%. A recent study has shown that the sensitivity and specificity of mammography testing in being able to detect breast cancer is 95% and 88.8%, respectively.

The pre-test probability is 0.008 or 0.8%

$$\text{Pre-test odds} = \frac{\text{Pre-test probability}}{1 - \text{Pre-test probability}} = \frac{0.008}{1 - 0.008} = 0.00806$$

The likelihood ratio of breast cancer if the mammogram test is positive is:

$$\frac{\text{Sensitivity}}{1 - \text{Specificity}} = \frac{0.95}{1 - 0.888} = 8.50$$

The post-test odds in a person with a positive result are:

$$\text{Post-test odds} = \text{Pre-test odds} \times \text{Positive likelihood ratio} = 0.00806 \times 8.50 = 0.0684$$

The post-test odds can be converted back into a probability:

$$\text{Post-test probability} = \frac{\text{Post-test odds}}{\text{Post-test odds} + 1} = \frac{0.0684}{0.0684 + 1} = 0.064 = 6.4\%$$

An alternative approach would be to use the Fagan nomogram to work out the post-test probability (Fig. 14.16).

You can explain to your patient that, based on this positive mammogram, she has a 6.4% probability of having breast cancer. Therefore, a positive mammogram screening test is in itself poor at confirming breast cancer and further investigations must be undertaken.

With a sensitivity of 95%, the screening test has correctly identified 95% of all breast cancers. Furthermore, with a specificity of 88.8%, 11.2% of positive test results will be false positives (100% – 88.8%).

PROGNOSTIC TESTS

- Prognosis:
  - is a prediction of the natural history (or course) of a disease, with or without treatment.
  - consists of defining the possible disease outcomes (i.e. recovery, disability or death) and also how often they are expected to occur.

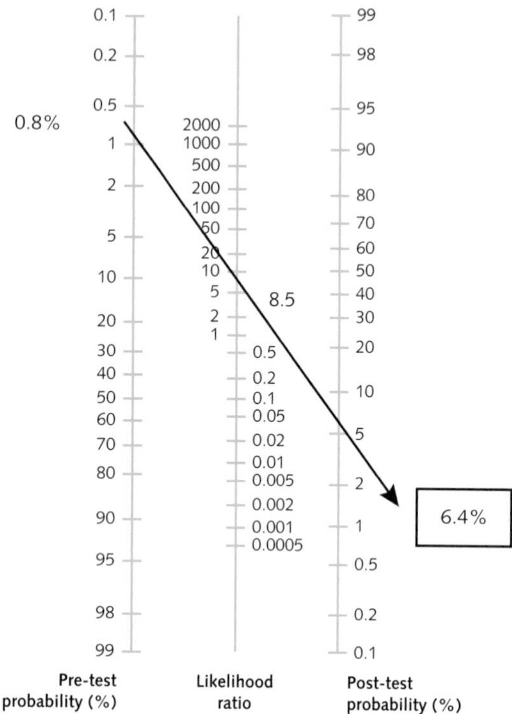

Fig. 14.16 Using the Fagan nomogram.

- It is sometimes possible to refine the prediction of the patient's likely outcome based on the characteristics of the particular patient. These characteristics are known as prognostic factors, which are not necessarily causing the outcome but are associated with its development (including the speed of progression to an outcome). However, it's never possible to predict the *actual* outcome, except by chance.
- It is important to not get confused between risk factors and prognostic factors. They are not the same! Figure 14.17 summarises the key differences between risk factors and prognostic factors. For example, sharing used needles and unprotected sexual intercourse are both risk factors for HIV infection, while the prognostic factors associated with the disease prognosis include age, viral load, CD4 count and the specific treatment used.

Fig. 14.17 Risk factors vs prognostic factors.

	Risk factors	Prognostic factors
Stage of disease spectrum	Influence the onset of disease.	Influence the outcome of disease once diagnosed.
Description of outcome(s)	Particular disease.	Range of disease consequences, e.g. morbidity or mortality.
Factors	Factors associated with the disease *onset* are not necessarily the same as those associated with the disease *outcome*.	Factors associated with the disease *outcome* are not necessarily the same as those associated with the disease *onset*.

Prognostic studies

The best design for a prognostic study is a cohort study (discussed in Chapter 7) as it usually impossible, as well as unethical, to randomise patients to different prognostic factors. The following five key features of a prognostic study should be considered when reading/appraising a prognostic study:

1. Study participants
   - Prognostic studies should begin by identifying patients with the disease.
   - The study population should be clearly defined as measures of prognosis can vary depending on the clinical or demographic features of a population.
   - The eligibility criteria should include a description of the participants at the start of the follow-up period; i.e. all participants should be at the same stage of disease, e.g. when symptoms begin or when the disease is diagnosed.
   - If patients were enrolled when the disease was diagnosed, it is important to specify how the diagnosis was made.
2. Follow-up
   - The study participants should be followed up for an adequate length of time to allow any important outcomes to occur.
   - All participants should be followed up for the same period of time.
   - It is important to document the response rate and document why patients were lost to follow-up, in an attempt to minimise loss-to-follow-up bias (discussed in Chapter 7).
3. Prognostic factors
   - As there is usually more than one way of assessing whether *prognostic factors* are present (or absent), these should be defined and measured appropriately.
   - Validated and reliable methods for measurement should be used.
4. Prognostic outcomes
   - The prognostic outcomes measured should include all aspects of the disease that are important to the patient, including recovery, death and symptoms such as pain.

- The prognostic outcome should be adequately defined.

5. Confounding factors
   - Important confounding factors should be clearly defined and measured (discussed in Chapter 13).
   - Confounders can be controlled for at the design or analysis stage of the study.

Measuring prognosis

Morbidity

Some of the measurements used to assess disease progression, in terms of patient morbidity, include:

- *Non-fatal incidents*, e.g. hospitalisations, asthma attacks, recurrence of a cardiac event, etc.
- *Symptoms*, e.g. pain duration and pain severity using validated scales.
- *Quality of life*, e.g. activities of daily living, EQ-5D (discussed in Chapter 18).
- *Disease-free survival*. Having been diagnosed with a disease in the past, the length of time during which the patient subsequently remains *disease-free* (usually after treatment) is recorded. This measure is important for conditions that relapse and recur over the course of the disease, e.g. multiple sclerosis.
- *Progression-free survival*. As the name describes, this is the period of time during which a disease does not progressively worsen, e.g. due to treatment.

Mortality

Some of the measurements used to assess disease progression, in terms of patient mortality, include:

- *Case fatality rate*: This refers to the proportion of people with a disease who actually die from that disease. It is suited for acute, short-term conditions, such as myocardial infarctions, acute infections, etc. The case fatality rate usually takes time into account, e.g. the 28-day case fatality rate after an acute myocardial infarction is 11% in men and 15% in women. The 5-year survival is used for longer-term conditions such as cancer.
- *Five-year survival*: This is the proportion of people with a disease expected to die from that disease within 5 years of diagnosis. There is nothing special about 5 years! It has traditionally been used as it is the length of time after diagnosis during which most cancer deaths occur; however, other time periods may be used. The 5-year survival can be described for different stages of a disease.
- *Median survival*: This is the length of time by which 50% of cases with the disease have died.
- *Survival curves*: These plot survival over time, with '% still alive' on the vertical axis and 'time since diagnosis' on the horizontal axis. They usually start at 100% survival at the time of diagnosis (e.g. 100% still alive at 0 months since diagnosis) and then each death is plotted as it occurs. They are useful when describing the impact of treatment over time.

HINTS AND TIPS

The case fatality rate, 5-year survival and median survival all describe survival at a single point in time. However, these measures don't describe the pattern of mortality. For example, a median survival of 6 years may involve 50% of deaths occurring over the first year since diagnosis and 10% of deaths occurring every year over the next 5 years. Survival curves are better at describing survival patterns.

Statistical techniques

Objectives

By the end of this chapter you should:

- Understand the steps involved in selecting the most appropriate statistical test when analysing data.
- Know when it is necessary to choose a non-parametric test over a parametric test.
- Know the implications of sample size when interpreting the results of parametric, non-parametric and normality tests.
- Be able to follow the flowcharts provided to assist you when choosing the correct statistical test for a data set.

CHOOSING APPROPRIATE STATISTICAL TESTS

- In previous chapters we discussed how to calculate and interpret the different measures of association, including the risk ratio (Chapter 7) and odds ratio (Chapter 8). On some occasions we compare two competing variables by calculating the difference between the group means (or group proportions) (Chapter 3).
- We can also calculate the 95% confidence interval for these measures of association to determine how precisely we have determined the differences of interest. It combines the variability (standard deviation) and sample size to generate a confidence interval for the population measure (Chapter 3).
- We use the measure of association and the confidence interval to put the result in a scientific context.
- However, we must also determine whether the results obtained are statistically significant by calculating the *P*-value (please refer to Chapter 3 for a discussion on how to interpret the *P*-value).
- Having defined the null and alternative hypotheses for your comparison, an appropriate statistical test is used to compute the *P*-value from the sample data. The *P*-value provides a measure of evidence for or against the null hypothesis. If the *P*-value shows evidence against the null hypothesis being tested, then the alternative hypothesis must be true.
- In some undergraduate curriculums you are expected to know which statistical tests to use (to calculate the *P*-value) when analysing different data sets.
- Selecting the most appropriate statistical test depends on three key pieces of information:
  1. The goal of the data analysis
  2. The type of variable you are analysing
  3. The distribution of the data.

Data analysis goal

- What is the aim of your analysis? Are you:
  - comparing one group to a hypothetical value?
  - comparing two unpaired groups?
  - comparing two paired groups?
  - comparing three or more unmatched groups?
  - comparing three or more matched groups?
  - quantifying the association between two variables?

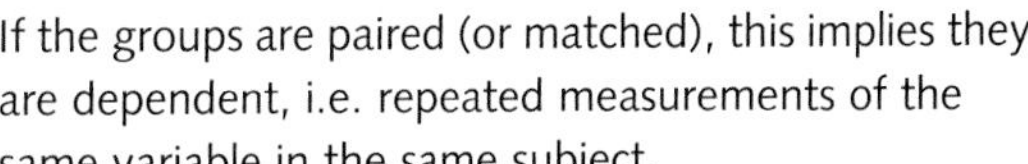

HINTS AND TIPS

If the groups are paired (or matched), this implies they are dependent, i.e. repeated measurements of the same variable in the same subject.

If the groups are unpaired (or unmatched), this implies they are independent; i.e. the same variable is measured in two different groups of subjects.

Type of variable

- It is important to define the type of variable you are analysing.
- Research data usually fall into one of the four types of variables:

- Nominal
- Ordinal } Categorical variable
- Interval
- Ratio } Numerical variable

- Please refer to Chapter 2 for a discussion on these different types of variables.

HINTS AND TIPS

It can sometimes be difficult to distinguish between an interval and ratio variable. For the purpose of choosing an appropriate statistical test for your data, it is important to only identify whether your data is numerical or not.

Data distribution

Gaussian versus non-Gaussian distributions

- Choosing the right statistical test to compare measurements also depends on the distribution of the data.
- There is no need to check the distribution of the data when dealing with nominal or ordinal variables.
- The distribution of the data should only be checked for interval or ratio variables.
- Statistical tests based upon the assumption that the data are sampled from a Gaussian (or normal) distribution are referred to as parametric tests. Some parametric tests also assume that the variance (or standard deviation) is equal in all groups being compared.
- Statistical tests that do not assume that the data follow a Gaussian distribution are referred to as non-parametric tests.
- Commonly used non-parametric tests involve ranking the outcome variable values from low to high and then analysing the distribution of the ranks.

When to choose a non-parametric test

- Formal statistical tests, such as the D'Agostino–Pearson test or the Kolmogorov–Smirnov test, are frequently used to check the distribution of the data.
- The null hypothesis of these tests (known as normality tests) state that the data are taken from a population that follows a Gaussian (normal) distribution.
- If the *P*-value is low, demonstrating that the data do not follow a Gaussian distribution, a non-parametric test is usually chosen.
- However, normality tests should not be used to automatically decide whether to use a non-parametric test or not.
- While the normality test can assist you in making your decision, the following considerations should also be made:
  - If your data do not follow a Gaussian distribution (i.e. the distribution is skewed), consider transforming the data, perhaps using reciprocals or logarithms, to convert non-Gaussian data to a Gaussian distribution (discussed in Chapter 2). The data can subsequently be analysed using a parametric statistical test.
  - The results from a single normality test should be interpreted in context. This is usually an issue if additional data from another experiment need to be analysed in the same way. Consequently, you cannot rely on the results from a single normality test.
  - Whether or not to choose a non-parametric test matters the most when the samples are small.
- On some occasions, you may decide to use a non-parametric test if, in addition to the data not having a Gaussian distribution, the variances are not equal between the groups being compared. Considering skewness and differences in variances often coexist, correcting for one (e.g. by transforming the data) may also correct the other! However, some parametric tests can still be used if they are adjusted to take account of these unequal variances.

Sample size matters

- When the sample size is small (i.e. $n < 15$):
  - parametric tests are not very robust when analysing data that do not follow a Gaussian distribution.
  - non-parametric tests have little power to detect a significant difference when analysing data that follow a Gaussian distribution.
  - you are likely to get a high *P*-value when using a non-parametric test to analyse data that follow a Gaussian distribution.
  - normality tests have little power to detect whether a sample comes from a Gaussian distribution.
- When the sample size is large (i.e. $n > 100$):
  - parametric tests are robust when analysing data that do not follow a Gaussian distribution.
  - non-parametric tests almost have as much power as parametric tests when analysing data that follow a Gaussian distribution.
  - normality tests have high power to detect whether or not a sample comes from a Gaussian distribution.
- Figure 15.1 summarises the implications of sample size when interpreting the results of parametric, non-parametric and normality tests.

Fig. 15.1 The effect of sample size on statistical testing.

	Small sample size	Large sample size
Using parametric tests on data with a non-Gaussian distribution	Not very robust – may produce misleading results	Robust
Using non-parametric tests on data with a Gaussian distribution	Little powern – may produce misleading results	Almost have as much power as parametric tests
Normality test (e.g. D'Agostino–Pearson test)	Low power for detecting whether or not a sample comes from a Gaussian distribution	High power for detecting whether or not a sample comes from a Gaussian distribution

HINTS AND TIPS

When dealing with large sample sizes, the decision to choose a parametric or non-parametric test matters less.

Data analysis

You can access online calculators, which will assist you in calculating a number of the statistical tests outlined in this chapter. GraphPad have an online version of their statistical package that can be accessed at http://www.graphpad.com/quickcalcs/

COMPARISON OF ONE GROUP TO A HYPOTHETICAL VALUE

When the primary aim of your analysis is to compare one group to a hypothetical value, the flowchart in Fig. 15.2 should be followed to identify the most suitable statistical test for your data.

COMPARISON OF TWO GROUPS

When the primary aim of your analysis is to compare two groups, the flowchart in Fig. 15.3 should be followed to identify the most suitable statistical test for your data.

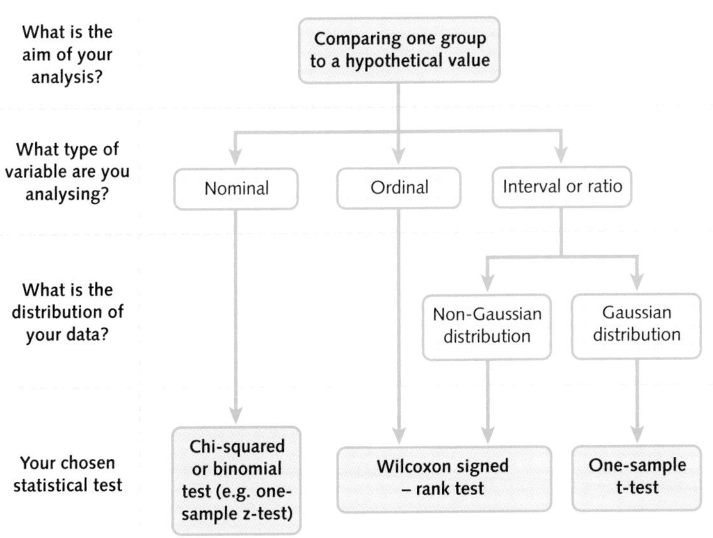

Fig. 15.2 Flowchart for selection of statistical tests comparing one group to a hypothetical value.

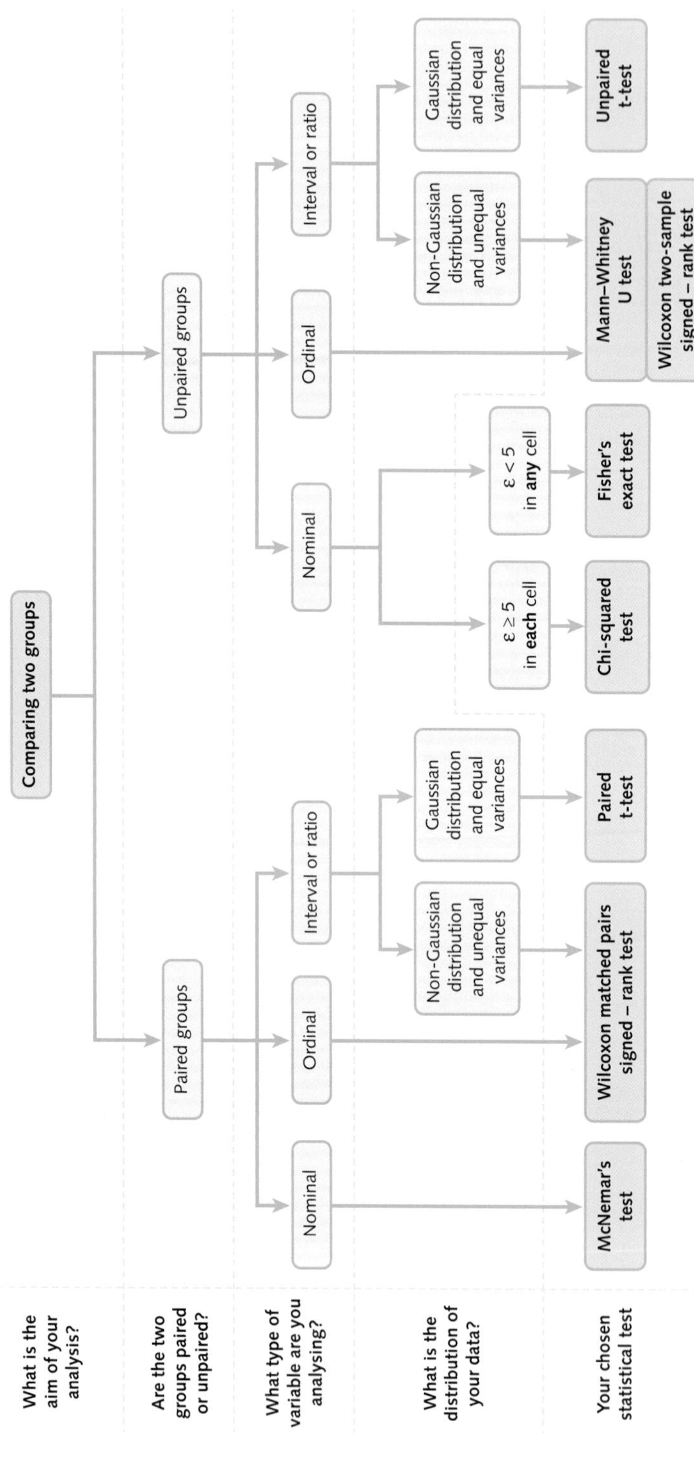

Fig. 15.3 Flowchart for selection of statistical tests comparing two groups.

Chi-squared test and Fisher's exact test

- The chi-squared test and Fisher's exact test compare the proportions of outcomes in different groups. In other words, they test for an association between two categorical variables.
- The data are obtained, initially, as 'observed' frequencies; i.e. the numbers with and without the outcome in each of the two groups (exposed and unexposed) being compared.
- These frequencies can be entered into a contingency table. If the table has two rows and two columns, it is known as a 2×2 contingency table (Fig. 15.4).
- For an example of a contingency table used as part of a study, please refer to Fig. 8.9.
- We can subsequently calculate the frequency that we would expect in each of the four cells of the contingency table if the null hypothesis were true. These are known as the 'expected' ('E') frequencies (Fig. 15.5).

COMPARISON OF THREE OR MORE GROUPS

When the primary aim of your analysis is to compare three or more groups, the flowchart in Fig. 15.6 should be followed to identify the most suitable statistical test for your data.

MEASURES OF ASSOCIATION

When the primary aim of your analysis is to quantify the association between two variables, the flowchart in Fig. 15.7 should be followed to identify the most suitable statistical test for your data.

		Characteristic (Outcome)		
		Yes	*No*	*Total*
Groups	*1*	a	b	a + b
	2	c	d	c + d
	Total	a + c	b + d	a + b + c + d

Fig. 15.4 Observed frequencies in a contingency table.

		Characteristic (Outcome)	
		Yes	*No*
Groups	*1*	$\frac{(a+c) \times (a+b)}{(a+b+c+d)}$	$\frac{(b+d) \times (a+b)}{(a+b+c+d)}$
	2	$\frac{(a+c) \times (c+d)}{(a+b+c+d)}$	$\frac{(b+d) \times (c+d)}{(a+b+c+d)}$

Fig. 15.5 Expected frequencies in a contingency table.

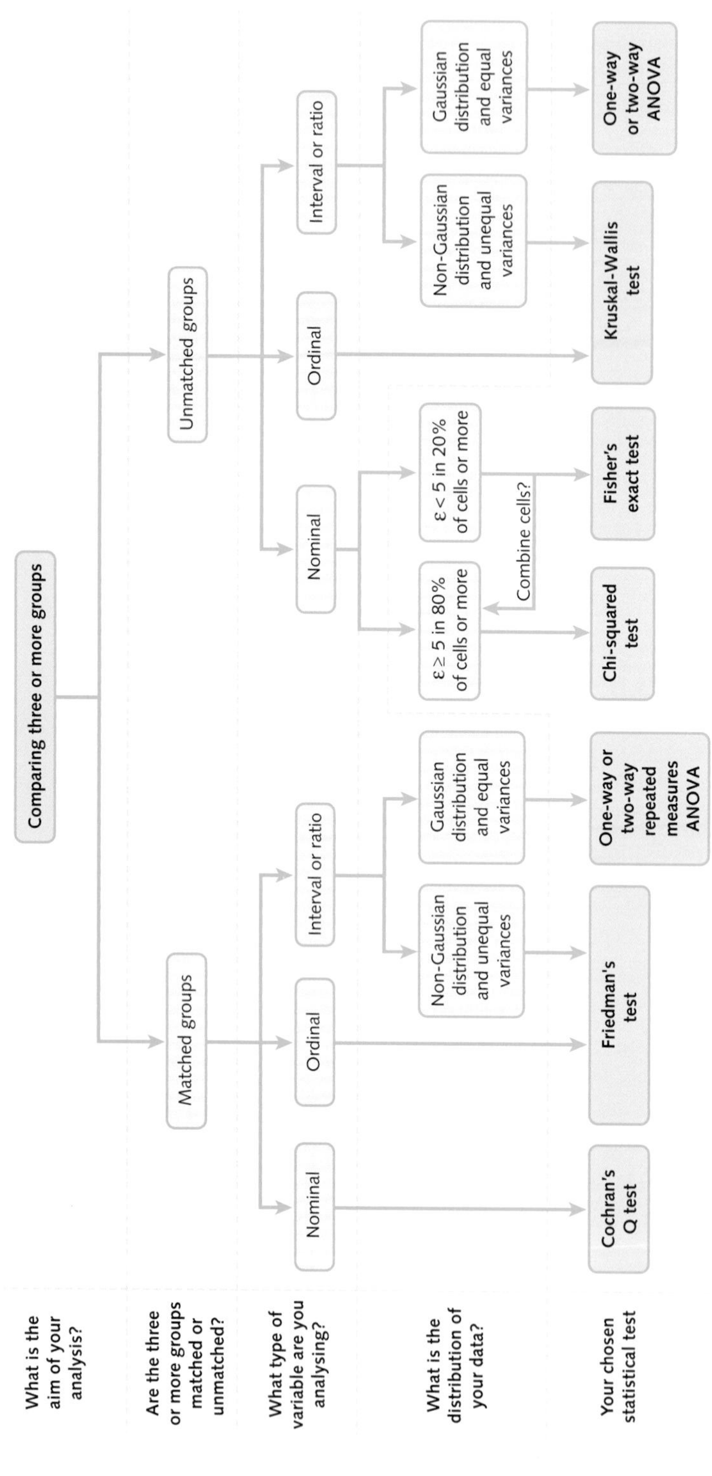

Fig. 15.6 Flowchart for selection of statistical tests comparing three or more groups.

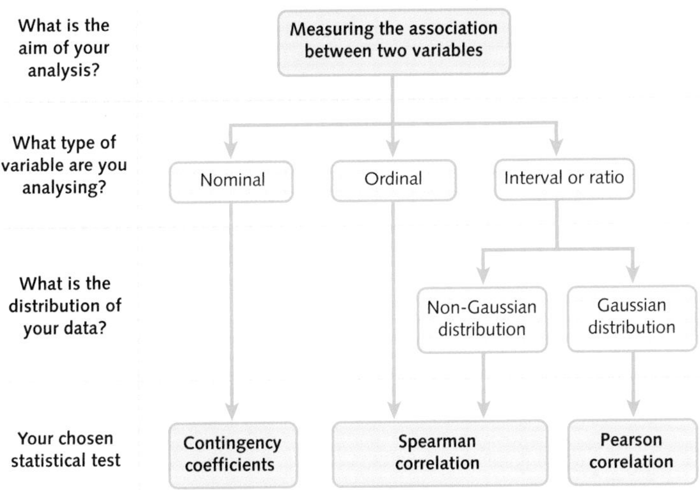

Fig. 15.7 Flowchart for selection of statistical tests measuring the association between two variables.

Clinical audit 16

Objectives

By the end of this chapter you should:
- Understand the importance of clinical governance.
- Know what steps are involved in conducting a clinical audit cycle.
- Be able to list the differences and similarities between audit and research.
- Be able to formulate an audit question and know how standards are chosen.
- Know how the sample frame is defined and the differences between prospective and retrospective sampling.
- Understand the steps involved in collecting and analysing audit data.
- Be able to list the differences between 'implicit' and 'explicit' audit criteria.
- Understand what steps are involved in implementing change after evaluating the results of an audit.

INTRODUCTION TO CLINICAL AUDIT

Clinical governance

- There is public and professional belief in the provision of high-quality care that is not only effective but also safe.
- Clinical governance is the systematic approach used to maintain and improve the quality of patient care within a health system.
- Key areas of clinical governance include:
  - Research
  - Education and training
  - Clinical audit
  - Clinical effectiveness.

What is clinical audit?

- Clinical audit is at the heart of clinical governance, reviewing the quality of care against explicit criteria of expected healthcare standards.
- The audit process is usually represented by a cycle, which emphasises its ongoing nature (Fig. 16.1).
- Audits use a systematic approach to confirm the quality of clinical services, highlighting the need for quality improvement (at an individual, team or service level) where necessary.
- However, how do we define high-quality care? How do we determine what best practice is? The answer to both these questions, in addition to life's many mysteries, is research!

Clinical audit versus clinical research

- The key difference between audit and research is in the aim of the study.
- While clinical research aims to establish what is the best or most effective practice, clinical audit evaluates how closely local practice resembles this.
- Audits may generate new research questions, which may subsequently be investigated using a research protocol. Audit and research may therefore follow each other in a cycle (Fig. 16.2).
- There may be a number of audit cycles prior to identifying an important or relevant question, if any.

Similarities between audit and research

With fundamental goals of improving healthcare, a number of similarities exist between audit and research. They both:

- address an important question related to clinical practice.
- involve writing protocols, specifying the appropriate type and size of sample.
- collect necessary information required to answer the question.
- involve analysing the data collected and interpreting the results.
- involve sharing the results in order to promote healthcare change.

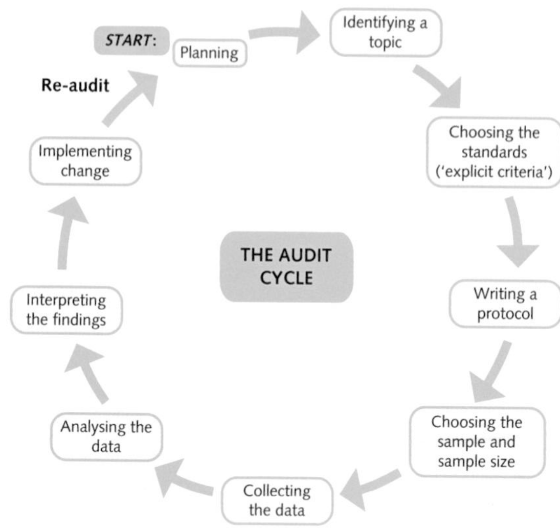
START:
Planning
Identifying a topic
Choosing the standards ('explicit criteria')
Writing a protocol
Choosing the sample and sample size
Collecting the data
Analysing the data
Interpreting the findings
Implementing change
Re-audit
THE AUDIT CYCLE

Fig. 16.1 The audit cycle.

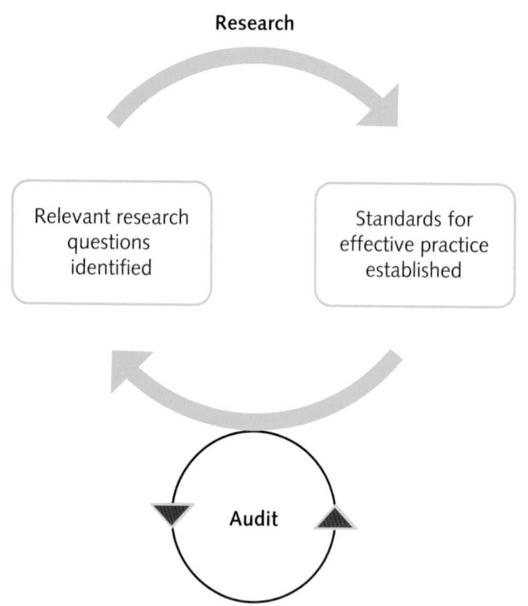

Fig. 16.2 Research–audit cycle.

Fig. 16.3 Audit versus research.

	Research	Audit
Aims	To establish what best practice is.	To determine whether current local practice resembles best practice.
Results	The results are compared with the hypothesis stated at the start of the study.	The results are compared with standards that define best practice.
Project motivation	Theory-driven.	Practice-based.
Ethical approval	Formal ethical review and approval is required.	Not always required (project should be reviewed by the audit department).
Treatment administration	May involve administration of a placebo or a completely novel treatment.	Never involves administering a placebo or a novel treatment.
Random allocation	Patient groups may be randomly allocated to different interventions.	Never involves randomly allocating patients to different interventions.
Generalisability of findings	Yes – the results can be generalised to other similar group or populations.	No – the results are only specific to the local patient group audited.
After completing the project?	An ongoing process involving investigation of *new* research questions with every project.	An ongoing process involving a number of audit cycles evaluating the *same* clinical standards.

Differences between audit and research

- It is sometimes difficult to distinguish between audit and research, or decide whether an audit or research study is required to answer your question.
- Figure 16.3 summarises the key differences between clinical audit and clinical research.

HINTS AND TIPS

As healthcare professionals, it is important that we not only understand the principles and methodology of the audit process, but that we undertake our own audit projects under appropriate guidance and supervision. Participating in clinical audit forms a routine part of clinical training and practice.

PLANNING THE AUDIT

Prior to starting the audit project, it is important to:

- ensure you have enough time to plan and complete the audit cycle prior to starting.
- identify a supervisor or relevant clinical lead in whom you can rely upon for advice and support.
- make yourself known to the local audit department who will advise you on data protection and confidentiality issues.
- consider whether you will need support in collecting data.

Identifying a topic

Sources of inspiration

- Even if you decide to carry out your audit project independently, it is important to involve stakeholders who have an involvement in the health service, when deciding on potential topics. Stakeholders may include:
  - Patients
  - Clinicians
  - Medical records personnel
  - Audit department staff.
- The audit question may be based on your clinical experience. For example:
  - when new clinical guidelines have been implemented into practice (based on research evidence) and you want to audit how well they have been introduced.
  - when you feel there is variation in healthcare practice between different wards at the same hospital.
  - in areas where there is a high risk to the patients, staff or the organisation.
  - in areas involving high-cost interventions.
- It is important to perform a literature search and consider the findings of recently published reviews to identify those areas where clinical practice could be improved.
- Other *simpler* ways of identifying an appropriate audit question may include:
  - looking at already prepared tools, e.g. using templates provided by the National Institute for Clinical Excellence that audit the implementation of their clinical guidelines.
  - asking the audit department whether they have any audits scheduled to be repeated or whether they have already identified a list of relevant audit questions (sometimes based on local priorities).
  - looking for protocols used in the department that performance could be audited against.

Formulating the audit question

- Having decided which area of healthcare you wish to audit, is important to formulate a specific question that may address one of the following:
  - An outcome, such as cost-effectiveness, patient satisfaction, quality of life, survival, infection or re-admission rates.
  - A process, which refers to protocols, such as involving follow-up, team handovers or whether, for example, the troponin level was measured in patients presenting with central chest pain.
  - A structure, which refers to the resources available, including the number of patient beds on a ward and the current knowledge, skills and attitudes of the staff.
- It is important to define the overall purpose of the project at its start, stating why the audit is being carried out and what it intends to achieve.
- You are unlikely to deliver full impact without a clear audit question or objective.

CHOOSING THE STANDARDS

- Current clinical practice should be compared to a defined set of 'explicit *criteria*' that:
  - reflect best practice.
  - are evidence-based.
  - focus on key parts of the care pathway.
  - cover the different aspects of service, including the structure, process and outcome of care.
  - must be measureable.
- The *standards* define the threshold of the expected performance for each criterion.
- They are usually expressed as a percentage, for example:
  - you expect criterion one to be achieved by 100% of the cases audited. This may represent the performance level of the top 5% in the region.
  - you expect criterion one to be achieved by 90% of the cases audited. This may represent an average performance level.
- Choosing the appropriate level of performance that you are trying to achieve is known as 'benchmarking'.

HINTS AND TIPS

If the level of care is measured without comparing the performance to a defined standard, this is known as a service evaluation.

AUDIT PROTOCOL

- Having already identified a topic of interest, defined the audit criteria and chosen the benchmark for your standards, a protocol that provides enough detail to allow someone to repeat the audit at a later date needs to be prepared.
- It should describe the various steps of the audit cycle from start to finish.
- In addition to helping to ensure that the project is on track, it will allow potential problems to be identified and addressed before they occur.
- The following points should be outlined in your protocol:
  - Title of audit project.
  - Background information, describing the clinical setting and the importance of the topic selected.
  - The audit question.
  - A definition of the explicit criteria.
  - A definition of the sample type and how sample size will be determined.
  - A description of what information will be required and how will it be collected.
    - Will administrative staff need to pull patient notes?
    - Are the data available electronically?
  - A design for the data collection form.
  - How will the data be analysed?
  - A plan to draw conclusions and make appropriate recommendations.
    - Will the results need to be compared to previous audit results?
  - How will the findings be disseminated?
  - A plan to repeat the audit cycle to ensure any changes have been made.
  - What is your timeline for all steps of the audit cycle?
- Your supervisor or clinical lead should review a draft copy of the audit protocol.
- The feedback received should be considered and amendments made to the protocol, if necessary.

DEFINING THE SAMPLE

A detailed account outlining which patients are eligible for your audit should be discussed. The sampling frame should be described in terms of:

- Sampling method
  - *Random sampling*: For example, each patient in the chosen setting has an equal probability of selection; eligible patients are allocated a number and a random number generator is used to identify your sample.
  - *Consecutive sampling*: For example, the first patient is randomly selected then patients consecutively admitted are selected until the required sample size is achieved.
- Sample size
  - This will depend on:
    - resource constraints, such as costs and the number of hours you can afford to invest for data collection prior to your deadline.
    - the degree of confidence you want in your findings.
  - There is often a compromise between the statistical validity of the results and the practical issues associated with data collection.
- Person
  - Demographic profile, i.e. age range or sex?
  - A particular group of patients, i.e. those with a particular diagnosis or who are having a particular intervention?
- Place
  - Primary care?
  - Hospital ward?
  - In-patient or out-patient clinic?
  - Health authority?
- Time
  - Depending on the resources available and the admission rate, what are the starting and predicted finishing dates for data collection?
  - Are samples going to be chosen prospectively or retrospectively (Fig. 16.4)?

Fig. 16.4 Retrospective versus prospective sampling.

Retrospective	Prospective
Involves reviewing previously collected information about the patient.	Data are collected from new admissions.
Routinely documented patient information is used. Adequate sources of retrospective data may not exist.	Within the remit of the audit criteria, additional information can be collected to what is routinely documented for the patient.
Less resources (cost, time, manpower) are required to collect the data.	More resources are usually required to collect the data.
Less prone to measurement bias: • As information has already been collected, the data reviewed are a snapshot of the level of performance at that time.	More prone to measurement bias: • Normal practice may change if people are aware that their performance is being audited.

DATA COLLECTION

- The data may be collected from various sources, including:
  - paper medical records
  - electronic medical records
  - disease registries.
- The data collected should:
  - be valid by ensuring that it relates directly to the agreed objectives and audit criteria.
  - be reliable by ensuring that the same (or almost the same) judgements about performance are made at different times and by different people.
  - comply with the accepted ethical principles.
  - be consistent with the accepted confidentiality principles by ensuring patient and staff identities are not revealed (identifiable information should not be used).
- A paper data collection form or template should be designed that includes very precise definitions of the variables that need to be filled out for each subject.
- The data collection form should be piloted to ensure that the information collected is:
  - informed by the audit criteria.
  - consistent.
  - comparable between cases.
  - kept at a minimum.
- It is advisable to collect additional information that may come into use when analysing the data (discussed below). This may include information on:
  - patient demographics, such as age, ethnicity and gender.
  - service provision, such as the healthcare professional involved and the healthcare setting.

HINTS AND TIPS

To ensure patient confidentiality, the data collected should:

- only be stored for the duration of the audit project and up until the audit cycle is repeated.
- be locked in a secure office on-site if paper data collection forms are being used.
- be safely stored on the organisation's computer server, with restricted access and password protection if electronic data collection forms are being used.

ANALYSING THE DATA

- Appropriate methods should be used to group, analyse and evaluate the data collected.
- The data collected, which represents the performance of your service, should be compared against every audit criterion and the pre-specified standards.
- The extent to which actual practice represents best practice can be calculated using the formula:

$$\textbf{Performance}\,(\%) = \text{Percentage of cases matching audit criterion} = \frac{\text{Number of cases that satisfy the explicit criterion}}{\text{Total number of cases audited}} \times 100$$

- Depending on your sample size, you may wish to perform a subgroup analysis to see whether the performance percentage varies according to different groups that share similar characteristics, such as:
  - age
  - sex
  - health professional providing care
  - healthcare setting.
- The aim of a subgroup analysis is to assist you in identifying the reasons as to why some standards are not being met (and also why the performance in some areas is above standard).
- The following should be included in your audit report when presenting and analysing your audit data:
  - The data displayed in a tabular format (Chapter 2).
  - The data displayed in a graphical format (Chapter 2).
  - The central tendency of the data (Chapter 2).
  - The variability of the data (Chapter 2).
  - A statistical test calculating the relationship (degree of association) between two or more variables (Chapter 15).
  - A statistical test calculating the difference between two or more groups (Chapter 15).
- The methods used to display and statistically analyse your data will depend on the type of data (nominal, ordinal, interval or ratio) collected for each criterion.

EVALUATING THE FINDINGS

Standards achieved

- Your service may have achieved the standards specified. Excellent! The service providers should stand up and take a bow! However, this doesn't necessarily mean there is no room for improvement.
- During your project, you may have identified certain areas of service delivery (not related to the standards) that could potentially be improved.
- The audit should be repeated at a suitable interval to ensure the high standards achieved are maintained.

Standards not achieved

- If there is substandard performance in achieving certain 'explicit' criteria, the audit group should identify as to whether there is any clinical justification for this variation.
- More experienced members of the audit group can apply 'implicit' measures about what constitutes good practice.
- Implicit measures allow senior healthcare professionals to use their experience, knowledge and judgement to make a decision regarding good practice for those cases where standards were not met.
- The differences between explicit and implicit criteria are summarised in Fig. 16.5.
- The performance percentage calculated on the previous page should therefore be adjusted to take account of those situations which did not satisfy the explicit criteria but were judged to be clinically acceptable:

$$\textbf{Adjusted performance (\%)} = \text{Percentage of cases matching audit criterion} = \frac{\text{Number of cases that satisfy the 'explicit' criterion} + \text{Number of cases that satisfy the 'implicit' criterion}}{\text{Total number of cases audited}} \times 100$$

- If cases fail to satisfy both the explicit and implicit criteria, potential causes for this substandard service provision should be identified.
- The issues raised should be listed, in order of priority, and recommendations for improvements made (discussed below).

Fig. 16.5 Explicit measures versus implicit measures.

Explicit measures	Implicit measures
Usually objective in nature.	Can be subjective in nature.
Developed in the design stage, prior to data collection.	Developed following data collection for those cases not meeting service standards.
Describes in detail the evidence required to confirm good practice.	Judgement, experience and knowledge is used to confirm good practice.
Can be used by audit staff with relatively little supervision.	Usually applied by senior health professionals.

IMPLEMENTING CHANGE

- Identifying what changes need to made can be a difficult process and may involve:
  - discussing the project with members of the multidisciplinary team (doctors, nurses, pharmacists, porters, etc.).
  - carrying out a literature search to discover how similar examples of substandard healthcare practice were addressed.
- Once appropriate changes have been identified, an action plan should be designed, which may answer the following questions:
  - What must be done?
  - Who will implement the change?
  - How will the change be monitored?
  - By when will the change be implemented?
  - When should the re-audit be planned?
- After an agreed period of time, the audit cycle should be repeated, using the same strategies for identifying the sample, data collection and data analysis.
- The aim of the re-audit is to ensure that changes have been implemented and that improvements have been made.
- The findings of your audit should be disseminated both locally (team meetings, grand rounds, regional conferences) and nationally (national conferences) where possible.
- Some professional journals also publish high-quality audits, especially if the methodology is generalisable.

EXAMPLE OF A CLINICAL AUDIT

- Non-valvular atrial fibrillation is a powerful risk factor for cardio-embolic stroke.
- Warfarin is an oral anticoagulant that reduces this risk, however, it requires regular monitoring to ensure that the target INR (international normalised ratio; measure of the clotting tendency of blood) is achieved.
- Dabigatran may be a useful alternative for patients who are not managing the monitoring requirements for warfarin, or have poor INR control.
- Current NICE guidelines recommends 'Dabigatran etexilate for the prevention of stroke and systemic embolism in atrial fibrillation'.

Audit question

- A simple audit question may be: 'How good is your practice at safe prescribing of dabigatran?'

The standards

- The standards are based on the NICE technology appraisal guidance on dabigatran etexilate for the prevention of stroke and systemic embolism in atrial fibrillation.

- The appraisal guidance defines two main criteria, but the one you choose to focus on is looking at the counselling patients receive prior to being started on dabigatran:
  - Before starting treatment of patients (with non-valvular atrial fibrillation) with dabigatran, was there a discussion with the person about the risks and benefits of the drug compared with warfarin?
- This particular criterion has defined:
  - The treatment received: dabigatran.
  - A process: counselling patients on starting dabigatran.

The sample

- *Sampling method*: consecutive sampling until the sample size has been reached.
- *Sample size*: 80 patients.
- *Person*: patients with non-valvular atrial fibrillation who were started on dabigatran during their current admission.
- *Place*: hospital.
- *Time*: prospective.

Data collection

- The information required for this audit was collected from:
  - the patent's medical notes
  - the patient.
- The following additional information was also collected to help interpret the findings:
  - The language spoken by the patient
  - The capacity of the patient to make an informed decision about the treatment
  - The consultant who prescribed the dabigatran

Analysing data

- The audit found that only 38% of patients received some form of counselling about the risks and benefits of dabigatran prior to being started on the drug. (Fig. 16.6).
- As the 100% standard expected was not achieved, potential causes for this substandard service provision should be identified.

Evaluating performance

- Prior to developing an action plan, additional information was reviewed and implicit measures applied by a senior clinician.
- As 10 of the 80 patients audited did not have the capacity to make an informed decision about the treatment, they did not receive any detailed counselling.
- The results therefore show that:
  - 51.4% (36/70) of eligible patients were counselled.
  - 48.6% (34/70) of eligible patients were not counselled.
- Looking at the subgroup analysis (Fig. 16.7), 61.8% (21/34) of the patients who were not counselled were non-English speaking nationals.

Fig. 16.6 Practice performance.

Criterion	Standard (%)	Sample size	Satisfied criteria?	Performance (%)
Before starting treatment of patients (with non-valvular atrial fibrillation) with dabigatran, was there a discussion with the person about the risks and benefits of the drug compared with warfarin?	100%	80	36	38%

Fig. 16.7 Subgroup information.

Subgroup	Counselling provided	No counselling provided	Total
Language			
English speaking	26	13	39
Non-English speaking	10	21	31
Total	36	34	70
Prescribed by:			
Dr A (F2)	3	19	22
Dr B (ST1)	8	15	23
Dr C (Consultant)	25	0	25
Total	36	34	70

- As we are looking at nominal data, a chi-squared test could be performed to assess the association between language and counselling (discussed in Chapter 15).
- Furthermore, despite doctors of all grades prescribing similar amounts of dabigatran over the audit period, a clear trend emerged:
  - The more senior the doctor, the better they were at ensuring that counselling was provided prior to starting the treatment.

Implementing change

- Following discussions with the multidisciplinary team, the suggested action plan was:
  - to improve the amount of training on safe prescribing of dabigatran (especially for the junior doctors).
  - to ensure that systems are in place to employ the services of a translator when communicating with non-English speaking patients.
  - to ensure there is a patient leaflet on dabigatran available in a number of languages.
  - to repeat the audit at 4 months, to allow enough time for the staff to participate in further training and for the patient leaflets to be designed.

Quality improvement

Objectives

By the end of this chapter you should:

- Be able to state the three fundamental questions that inform the model for quality improvement.
- Know the steps involved in developing an effective aim statement.
- Know that there are three kinds of measures: process, outcome and balancing measures.
- Understand the importance of benchmarking when identifying areas for improvement in healthcare practice.
- Be able to explain the steps involved in a Plan-Do-Study-Act (PDSA) cycle.

QUALITY IMPROVEMENT VERSUS AUDIT

- Quality improvement should *not* be seen as a separate entity from clinical audit. In fact, the ultimate goal of both a clinical audit and a quality improvement project is quality improvement!
- When examining a clinical service, with an aim to improve it, indeed there are circumstances where a clinical audit is appropriate.
- In some cases, using a less rigid quality improvement project is the best model for service improvement. With this in mind, you should acquire the skills involved in implementing both types of service improvement.
- Figure 17.1 summarises the key differences between a clinical audit and a quality improvement project.

THE MODEL FOR QUALITY IMPROVEMENT

- As highlighted in the Institute of Medicine report, 'To Err Is Human', the majority of the medical errors in healthcare practice are due to faulty systems or processes, not because of individual errors or mistakes.
- There is an unquestionable need for quality and safety improvement initiatives in healthcare.
- The Institute for Healthcare Improvement (IHI) uses a simple mantra to describe the key elements for improvement:
    - *Will*: You must have the 'will' to want to improve.
    - *Ideas*: You must have 'ideas' about which areas of service need improvement.
    - *Execution*: You must 'execute' your ideas!
- The Associates in Process Improvement group developed a model for improvement which begins with three fundamental questions:
    1. *Aim*: What are you trying to accomplish?
    2. *Measures*: How will you know whether a change in practice has led to an improvement?
    3. *Changes*: What change can be made that will result in an improvement?
- Having answered these three questions, the next stage is to carry out a Plan-Do-Study-Act (PDSA) cycle (Fig. 17.2). This four-phase *cycle* allows us to test the effectiveness of any changes in service on a small scale, prior to implementing anything on a larger scale.
- The remainder of this chapter will discuss this model for quality improvement in further detail.
- An example of a quality improvement project is discussed at the end of the chapter.

THE AIM STATEMENT

Writing the statement

- The first step is to decide which area of healthcare you are trying to improve. It is usually helpful to think of something that forms part of your regular workday.
- As highlighted by Professor Sir Bruce Keogh in 'A Junior Doctor's Guide to the NHS', '[junior doctors] have penetrating insight into how things really work – where the frustrations and inefficiencies lie, where the safety threats lurk and how quality of clinical care can be improved'.
- The aim statement should be specific about the following:
    - What degree of improvement you are expecting to achieve.

Fig. 17.1 Clinical audit versus quality improvement project.

	Clinical audit project	Quality improvement project
Emphasis of project	Data collection with a fixed endpoint.	A resource that indicates that a change in clinical practice is needed and whether an improvement has been made.
Data collection method	A single person collecting data based on nationally agreed criteria and standards.	A team approach to investigating problems, identifying solutions and raising standards.
Criteria and standards	Often derived from clinical guidelines, focusing mainly on the effectiveness of a service from a medical/clinical point of view. However, there are usually no agreed standards or criteria for areas affecting patient experience, patient safety or service improvement.	In addition to focusing on clinical problems, a wide range of issues can be addressed, including patient experience, patient safety or service improvement.
Context of project	Local practice is compared against national standards; therefore the results may lack local context.	Focuses on local practice, identifying specific local problems. The results therefore have a local context.

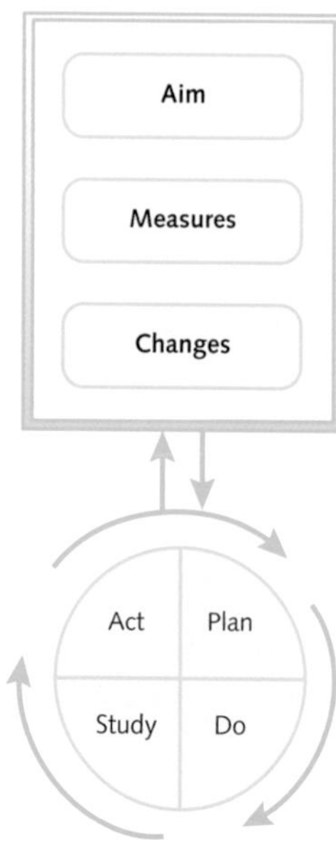

Fig. 17.2 Model for quality improvement.

- By when you wish to accomplish this.
- Who (or what system) will be affected.

Example

- You are a general practitioner. The aim of your quality improvement project is to decrease the average blood pressure of your population of patients with hypertension to less than 140/90 mmHg within 9 months.

Statement

- It is important to include the right people in your team when conducting a quality improvement project.
- Your team may include members who are familiar with the different aspects of the process or system you are trying to improve, e.g. managers, doctors, nurses, or pharmacists.
- It is important to have senior support, ideally from someone who understands the implications of the proposed change and has authority in all areas affected by the change.

Dimensions for improvement

- To assist organisations in developing an aim statement in a complex clinical setting, the Institute of Medicine put forth six dimensions for improvement in healthcare. Healthcare must be:
  1. Safe
     - Patients shouldn't be harmed by the care intended to help them.
     - *Primum non nocere*, which translates to 'first, do no harm', is one of the principal precepts of medical ethics.
  2. Effective
     - Care should be based on the best available evidence on what is likely to help a patient.
     - It is important that only effective services are provided to those likely to benefit from them, thus avoiding:
       - overuse of procedures, medications, surgeries, etc., that are not supported by the scientific literature.
       - underuse of care that has shown to be effective by the scientific literature.

3. Patient-centred
   - It is important to provide care that is respectful of the individual patient's culture, specific needs, preferences and values.
   - The patient should play an active role when guiding clinical decisions about his or her own healthcare.
4. Timely
   - Unintended waiting times are a healthcare system defect, which may be detrimental to both the patient and the caregiver.
5. Efficient
   - The healthcare provided should avoid waste (and therefore cost) of equipment, ideas, capital, supplies and time.
6. Equitable
   - The care provided should not vary in quality based on patient characteristics such as ethnicity, gender, age, socioeconomic status or geographic location.

MEASURES FOR IMPROVEMENT

Types of measures

- It is important to receive feedback to assess whether the change has led to an actual improvement. The most useful form of feedback is usually provided by taking measurements.
- The three main types of measures used in quality improvement are:
  1. Outcome measures
  2. Process measures
  3. Balancing measures.

Outcome measures

- Outcome measures inform us whether the change made has led to an improvement in the outcome we are ultimately trying to improve.

Process measures

- In order to improve your outcome measure, the processes involved need to be improved first. We therefore need to measure the results of these process changes.
- Are the steps in the system performing as originally planned?

Balancing measures

- Balancing measures inform us whether changes in one part/step of the system are causing 'new' problems in other parts of the system.
- There is usually no direct relation between this measure and the project aim.

Example

- Returning to our project on lowering the blood pressure in patients with hypertension, the following measures may be assessed:
  - *Outcome measure*: Average blood pressure in population of patients with hypertension.
  - *Process measure*: Percentage of patients with hypertension registered at your practice who had:
    - their blood pressure measured twice in the past year.
    - counselling on lifestyle changes to improve their blood pressure.
  - *Balancing measure*: The amount of extra time spent with each patient with hypertension, thus cutting into the amount of time you have to see other patients registered at your practice.

DEVELOPING THE CHANGES

- The next step is to think about the host of changes that will lead to an improvement in healthcare practice.
- Reflecting on the current system is a good starting point and may help you identify key issues.
- It is useful to draw a flowchart of the steps involved in the current process. This will help you identify any flaws in the system that aren't functioning as planned.
- It is important to compare the steps involved in your own system to 'best practice' as reported in the literature. This approach, known as benchmarking, can help you identify areas where your own system falls short.
- You should take as many perspectives into account as possible, not just from the caregivers. For example, a patient may see opportunities for improvement in the care system that weren't apparent to the caregivers.

Example

- Sticking with our scenario on lowering blood pressure in patients with hypertension, you may decide to make the following changes:
  - You use your register of patients with hypertension to set up a reminder system to automatically notify everyone with hypertension that they need their blood pressure measured at least twice a year.
  - You set up a notification on your patient management computer software, which pops up when a

patient with hypertension has a consultation with the doctor. The notification reminds the doctor to:
- measure the blood pressure.
- review the patient's anti-hypertensive medications.
- offer advice to promote a healthy lifestyle.

THE PLAN-DO-STUDY-ACT CYCLE

- The next step is to implement your ideas for change in your work setting.
- The PDSA cycle approach allows you to test this change using a systematic approach.
- An example of a quality improvement project PDSA cycle is discussed at the end of the chapter.

Plan

- A plan should be devised which states:
  - the objective for the cycle.
  - the changes necessary to achieve the improvement expected.
    - Despite having discussed a number of changes, you may decide to keep it simple and test only one change first.
  - your approach to data collection:
    - Who will measure the change?
    - What change are they measuring?
    - When will the change be measured?
    - What data will be collected?

Do

- The plan is implemented on a small scale.
- In addition to measuring the change, any issues or unexpected outcomes are documented.

Study

- The data collected are analysed and the results compared to the predictions stated as part of your project aim.
- Graphically displaying the data makes it easier to identify trends in the measurements taken over several PDSA cycles.
- Plotting the data over time is a simple and effective way of assessing whether the changes made are leading to an improvement.
- Having studied the results, the next step is to reflect on your findings.

Act

- Based on the feedback received, you start planning the next cycle:
  - If there were significant differences between the planned and actual measurements, you may decide to modify the current change for the next cycle.
  - If the change was successfully implemented, you may decide to add another new change for the next cycle.

If your changes have previously been shown to be effective elsewhere, why test them at your setting?

Testing the change will:
- allow you to evaluate the related costs and compromises at your setting.
- increase your belief as well as the belief of your colleagues, that the change will lead to an improvement in *your* setting.
- minimise the amount of resistance from the organisation when implementing the change on a larger scale, if proven to be effective.

REPEATING THE CYCLE

- Having finished one PDSA cycle, the next step is to repeat the cycle again, incorporating the changes discussed as part of the 'Act' stage of the previous cycle.
- The measurements recorded should improve with every PDSA cycle until you're ready to implement the change on a larger scale (Fig. 17.3).

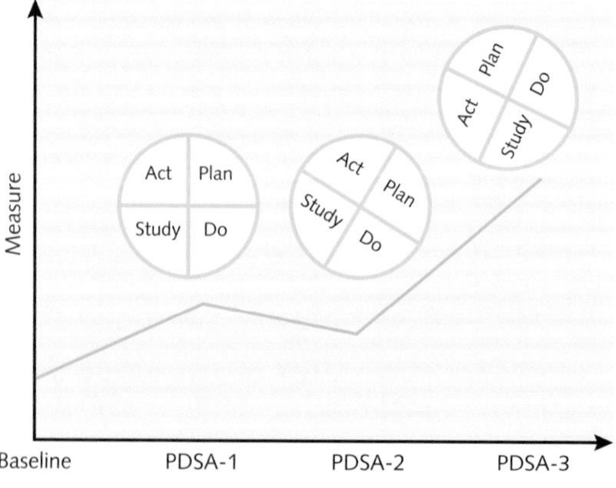

Fig. 17.3 Linking PDSA cycles.

- However, as illustrated in Fig. 17.3, some changes may not go as planned, leading to a decline in improvement.

EXAMPLE OF A QUALITY IMPROVEMENT PROJECT

Background

- Foundation Programme doctors raised concerns about the quality of information handed over to out-of-hours medical and surgical teams. At present, out-of-hours doctors received either verbal or written handover of the ward jobs required for in-patients.
- However, key patient history and management details were inconsistently handed over. Similarly, summarised key medical information about all ward patients was rarely available, though many ad hoc reviews were likely during out-of-hours service.
- This was due to the lack of a systematic or consistent method for patient handover, which was felt to be having an impact on the safety, effectiveness and efficiency of in-patient care delivered by out-of-hours medical and surgical teams.
- While all junior doctors carried a ward list, which had key summarised information about their ward patients, this was not accessible to the on-call team.
- Furthermore, there was much variation in the layout and information included in the ward lists.
- A quality improvement project was therefore developed in order to create a standardised method of handover that would allow communication of clinically significant information in a timely and effective manner.

Plan

Objective

The objective of the project was to achieve the following aims over a 3-month period:

1. Improve junior doctors access to accurate key summarised in-patient medical information whilst on-call, with an average satisfaction score of 4 out of 5.
2. Decrease the time taken for a doctor to gain an accurate impression of an in-patient by 50%.
3. Decrease the percentage of occasions whereby out-of-hours jobs were performed without reviewing any medical records to 0%.

Changes

- Doctors of all grades, from Foundation Programme doctors to consultants, were invited to focus group meetings for a discussion on methods of how to improve the handover process.
- A consensus was reached and a patient summary and handover proforma (Fig. 17.4) was created with the following headings:

Patient summary proforma (standardised ward list)

1. Bed number
2. Demographic information
3. Presenting complaint and diagnosis
4. Co-morbidities
5. Operations/procedures
6. Current issues
7. Management plan
8. Discharge plan and social issues
9. Key blood results
10. Jobs

Location:	Details	Current admission	Co-morbidities	Operation/ Radiology	Social issues	Current issues:	Management plan	Key blood results:
Bed 1	Patient name: Amit Kaura Date of birth: 08/02/1922 Hospital number: 111 1111 111	Presenting complaint: Shortness of breath Diagnosis: LRT1 Atrial flutter → T2RF → BiPAP	1) T2DM 2) MI – 09/11 3) AF – on warfarin 4) HT 5) Hypothyroid	Echo – mild LV impairment LVH Δ cor pulmonale X Rt Shoulder: loss of rotator cuff tendon, degen changes	Lives alone Carer's BD	1) Peripheral oedema 2) Pain/↓ROM right shoulder 3) Reduced mobility 4) LRT1	Medical: Physiotherapy OT Fluid management on co-trimoxazole until 19/02/12 Discharge plan:	ANA +'ve (28/02/12) CRP 52 (27/02/12)
Jobs:								

Patient name and bed	Additional relevant medical details	Out-of-hours job	HO	SHO
Amit Kaura Bed 1	Patient on co-trimoxazole for LRT1 – possible interaction with warfarin	Patient has atrial fibrillation Please prescribe warfarin	X	

Fig. 17.4 Patient summary and handover proforma.

Patient handover proforma

1. Patient name and bed number
2. Additional relevant medical details
3. Out-of-hours jobs
4. Job For completion by: HO or SHO

- All doctors would be informed of the pilot handover system via trust email.
- The initial rounds of data collection would be carried out on the Care of the Elderly ward.
- The day-based ward doctors would electronically complete the patient summary and handover proforma and subsequently print out hard copies for the out-of-hours doctors.
- Additionally, the on-call team would have access to the proforma via the trust intranet.
- The ward doctors would update the proforma on a daily basis.

Measures

- Following each out-of-hours shift, the Foundation Programme doctor would provide questionnaire feedback on the effectiveness of the proforma. The following measures would be determined:

Outcome measure

- Time taken for the out-of-hours doctor to gain an accurate impression of the patient admission.
- The satisfaction score of the handover process as perceived by the on-call doctor.
- The proportion of jobs carried out without reviewing any medical records about the patient.

Process measure

- Is there a summary proforma for each patient on the ward?
- Is the proforma being updated on a daily basis?

Balancing measure

- The amount of time spent updating the proforma on a daily basis by the ward doctors versus the amount of time saved by the on-call team by using the proforma.
- Baseline measurements would be taken from 20 Foundation Programme doctors.
- Feedback would be received from 20 Foundation Programme doctors for each PDSA cycle.

Do

- The proforma was implemented on the Care of the Elderly ward.
- Qualitative feedback from the ward doctors and the on-call team highlighted key issues with the proforma:
  - *Ward doctor*: 'There should be an empty "Notes" box on the proforma to allow different specialties to tailor the list accordingly. For example, on the Care of the Elderly ward, it would be necessary to note the Mini Mental State Examination score and the Do Not Attempt CPR status.'
  - *On-call doctor*: 'The proforma is too busy. There are too many boxes.'

Study

- Compared to baseline, all measures recorded showed signs of improvement:
  - The outcome measures all improved (Fig. 17.5).
  - The proforma was welcomed by the Care of the Elderly ward doctors and was updated on 96% of occasions.
  - It would take on average 7 minutes for the ward doctors to update the list on a daily basis. With an average review of 30 patients during an on-call service, referring to Fig. 17.5, the proforma saved the on-call doctor approximately 1 hour (30 patients × 2 minutes saved) during his or her 13-hour shift.

Act

- With an aim to further improve the outcomes measured, amendments were made to the proforma based on the feedback received from those involved in the project.
- The PDSA cycle was repeated a further two times, to ensure that all the kinks in making the change work were addressed.
- The proforma used as part of PDSA cycle 3 is illustrated in Fig. 17.6. As shown, the layout issues were addressed and a 'Notes' box was added.
- The feedback received as part of each PDSA cycle is graphically displayed in Fig. 17.7.
- By the end of PDSA cycle 3, all objectives set at the start of the project were successfully accomplished.
- While the on-call doctor would still need to review the medical records, having the proforma as an

Fig. 17.5 Measurements from PDSA Cycle 1.

	Baseline	PDSA Cycle 1
Satisfaction score	2.47	2.95
Time taken to gain accurate impression of patient admission	13 minutes	11 minutes
Percentage of jobs carried out without reviewing any medical records	68%	32%

Bed	Demographic information	Presenting complaint and diagnosis	Co-morbidities	Operations/ procedures	Current issues:	Management plan	Discharge plan and social issues	Key blood results:	Notes:	Jobs:
1	Amit Kaura 08/02/1922 90 **111 1111 111** Admitted: 12/02/12	Shortness of breath LRT1 Atrial flutter → T2RF → BiPAP	1) T2DM - drug 2) MI – 09/11 3) AF – on warfarin 4) HT 5) Hypothyroid	Echo – mild LV impairment LVH Δ cor pulmonale X Rt Shoulder: loss of rotator cuff tendon, degen changes	1) Peripheral oedema 2) Pain/↓ROM right shoulder 3) Reduced mobility 4) LRT1	Physiotherapy OT Fluid management on co-trimoxazole until 19/02/12	Lives alone, Carer's BD	ANA +'ve (28/02/12) CRP 52 (27/02/12)	MMSE: - AMT 6/6 **DNACPR** TTA: No	
2										

Fig. 17.6 Revised proforma – PDSA Cycle 3.

adjunct saved the on-call doctor approximately 3 and a half hours (30 patients × 7 minutes saved) during his or her 13-hour shift.

- Having demonstrated the effectiveness of the proforma on a small scale, the next step would be to implement this proforma on other medical and surgical wards.

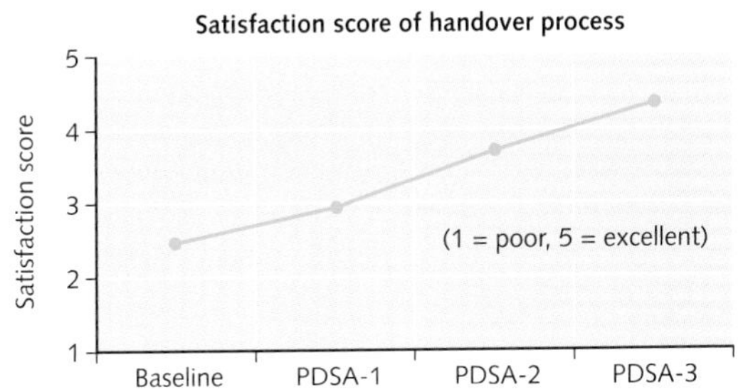

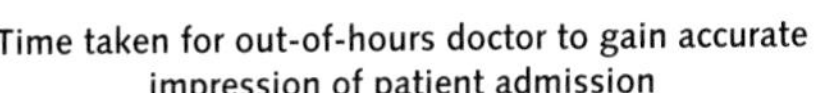

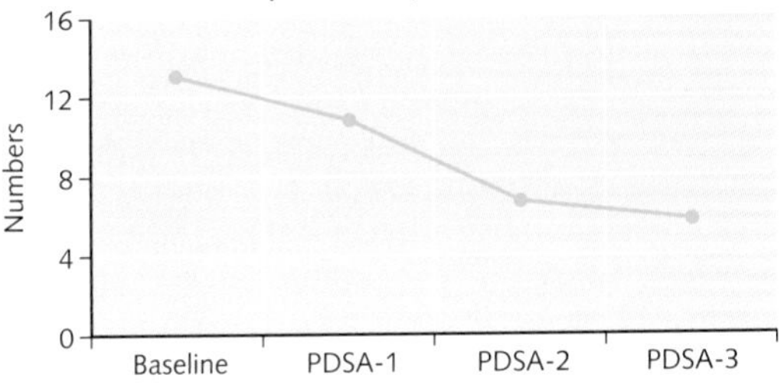

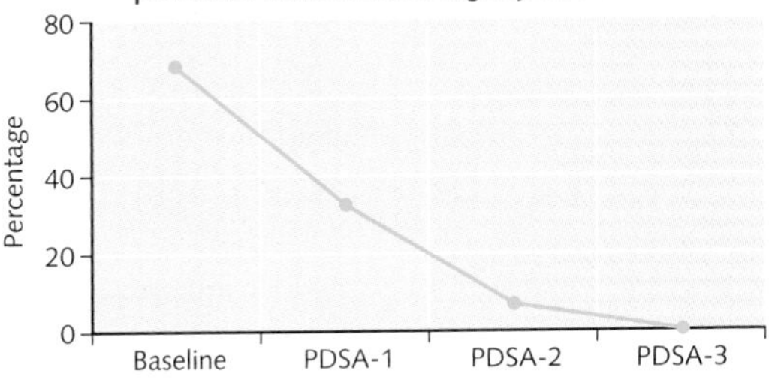

Fig. 17.7 Repeating the PDSA cycle.

Economic evaluation

Objectives

By the end of this chapter you should:

- Understand the basic concepts of economics in relation to health.
- Understand the importance of resource efficiency and opportunity costs.
- Be able to distinguish between the main types of economic evaluation.
- Know how quality-adjusted life year (QALY) measurements are calculated.
- Understand that sensitivity analysis is used to test all the assumptions used in an economic model.

WHAT IS HEALTH ECONOMICS?

Background

- Scarcity of resources (e.g. land, labour, time and money) is a fact of life.
- Health economics analyses how choices are made to obtain maximum value for money within the constraints of the resources available.
- Healthcare decision-makers must prioritise their choices through analysis of the costs and benefits of competing interventions. In other words, both the cost-effectiveness and the clinical effectiveness of healthcare provision must be considered.

Efficiency

When resources are scarce it is important to evaluate how well they are being used to achieve a desired outcome. There are three key concepts of efficiency: technical, productive and allocative efficiency.

Technical efficiency

- Technical efficiency:
  - is the effectiveness with which a given set of inputs (resources) is used to achieve a desired output (health outcome).
  - is achieved when the maximum possible improvement in a health outcome is achieved from a combination of available resources.
- An intervention is technically inefficient if the same (or greater) health outcome is achieved with less resource input. For example, if the results of a randomised controlled trial comparing the effectiveness of low- and high-dose drug preparations on disease outcome show that both dose preparations have similar outcome effects, the lower dose drug would be technically more efficient for use in clinical practice.
- Alternatively, the technical efficiency of a new intervention may come into question if shown to improve survival rates at the cost of reducing the quality of life.

Productive efficiency

- Productive efficiency involves assessing the relative value for money of different interventions, which have outcomes that are directly comparable. In other words, productive efficiency compares alternative interventions based on the relative costs of these different resources.
- The concept of productive efficiency is, therefore, to minimise the cost of resources for a given healthcare outcome or maximise the outcome for a given cost.

HINTS AND TIPS

While technical efficiency involves maximising outcome using the resources available, productive efficiency involves comparing alternative interventions to achieve the maximum health outcome benefit for a given cost.

Allocative efficiency

- Allocative efficiency involves measuring the extent to which the available resources are allocated to individuals or (a group of people) who will benefit the most.
- The allocative efficiency takes into account the productive efficiency of the resources available and the efficiency of distribution of the outcomes in society. For example, the use of statin treatment in reducing the amount of low-density lipoprotein ('bad'

cholesterol) in the body and therefore, the risk of developing cardiovascular disease, is more beneficial when prescribed to high-risk patients (such as those individuals who have had a myocardial infarction in the past) than to low-risk patients. In terms of allocative efficiency, high-risk patients are targeted as a priority as the health outcome associated with statin use will be most beneficial in these patients.

- Allocative efficiency has implications for the definition of opportunity costs, as discussed underneath.

Opportunity costs

- In order to understand the concept of 'opportunity cost', it is necessary to first distinguish between the financial and economical concepts of cost.
- Financial costs relate to the actual monetary spend on resources that someone is willing to pay for in order to develop a service (i.e. financial cost related to the resources consumed).
- Economical costs incorporate not only the financial cost of resources but also the time, energy and effort involved for which there may be no associated financial payment. For example, in the healthcare setting, when members of the public visit the accident and emergency department, the time spent waiting to be seen by a doctor represents an economic cost to the patient (i.e. the time and stress associated with waiting), despite there being no financial payment involved.
- When financial and non-financial resource costs (the economical cost) are used to develop a particular service, these resources, and the costs associated with their consumption, become unavailable to provide benefits to an alternative service.
- 'Opportunity cost' is what is lost when an alternative service is not provided because resources are directed elsewhere. For example, on receiving my first pay slip as a foundation doctor, I was faced with a huge dilemma. Do I splash out on a new car or do I travel abroad on a de-stressing holiday!? Having decided to trade in a life of stress for two weeks of sun, sea and sand, the true opportunity cost of going on holiday was the forgone benefits of purchasing a new car.

HINTS AND TIPS

The concept of opportunity cost highlights the struggle that policy-makers are faced with when deciding how resources are allocated to various competing services.

Economic evaluation

A full economic evaluation of healthcare involves systematically comparing the costs (inputs) and benefits (outcomes) of at least two alternative interventions (e.g. novel treatment versus usual treatment, disease prevention versus disease treatment measures, care provided at location A versus care provided at location B) to evaluate the best use of the scarce resources available. In addition to full economic evaluation studies, Drummond and colleagues (2005) highlighted a number of partial evaluations as outlined in Fig. 18.1.

HINTS AND TIPS

A full economic evaluation involves:

1. comparing two or more alternative interventions.
2. considering both the costs and benefits of all alternative interventions being compared.

A number of steps are followed when undertaking a full economic evaluation:

1. Frame the economic question clearly.
2. Choose the study design, e.g. randomised controlled trial-based economic evaluation.
3. Choose an appropriate economic evaluation method.
4. Perform a sensitivity analysis of the results.

Fig. 18.1 Different types of cost and outcome evaluations.

	Costs only	**Outcomes only**	**Costs and outcomes**
One intervention (no comparison to alternative interventions)	Cost *description*	Outcome *description*	Cost outcome *description*
Comparison of 2 or more alternative interventions	Cost *analysis*	Effectiveness or efficacy evaluation	**FULL ECONOMIC EVALUATION**

ECONOMIC QUESTION AND STUDY DESIGN

Economic question

As with most research questions, the PICO method can be used to formulate the economic question:

- *Patient/population*, e.g. in-patients diagnosed with hospital-acquired pneumonia.
- *Intervention*, e.g. novel antibiotic regimen.
- *Comparator/control*, e.g. current antibiotic regimen.
- *Outcome*, e.g. *benefits* and *costs* of the alternative antibiotic regimens.

In previous chapters we have shown that research studies usually identify and measure the outcome of the alternative interventions being compared by looking at their clinical *benefit*. However, for the purposes of an economic evaluation study, the research question must also incorporate methods for identifying, measuring and valuing the *costs* of the alternative interventions.

Costs

As highlighted above, economical costs imply both financial and non-financial costs and may include:

1. Costs to the service providers
   a. Running costs
      i. Managerial costs
      ii. Administrative costs
      iii. Staff costs
      iv. Drug costs
   b. Capital
      i. Equipment costs, e.g. CT scanner
      ii. Building costs
2. Costs to patients
   a. Out-of-pocket expenses
      i. Travel costs
      ii. Prescription costs
   b. Non-financial costs
      i. Stress
      ii. Pain
      iii. Side effects
3. Productivity costs
   a. Production losses
   b. Other uses of time.

The costs measured in a study will depend on whether the evaluation is from the health service perspective, the patient perspective or from an even wider perspective. The outcome measured will have an implication on which economic evaluation method is chosen for the study design.

Study design

Before considering whether an intervention is cost-effective, it is important to decide whether there is sufficient evidence showing its clinical effectiveness. Considering randomised controlled trials are at the top of the pecking order in the hierarchy of evidence, randomised controlled trial-based economic evaluations have the most robust study design. Data on both cost and benefit should ideally be measured at the same time.

The study design stage also involves choosing the most suitable economic evaluation method. There are five main types of economic evaluation:

1. Cost-minimisation analysis
2. Cost-utility analysis
3. Cost–consequence analysis
4. Cost-effectiveness analysis
5. Cost–benefit analysis

It is important to match the economic evaluation method to the economic question being asked. As discussed below, the main difference between these methods is the way in which the outcomes are measured.

COST-MINIMISATION ANALYSIS

- Cost-minimisation analysis is a tool that should only be used when there is unambiguous evidence of clinical equivalence between the alternative interventions being compared.
- The cost-minimisation analysis itself consists of measuring all costs inherent to the delivery of the therapeutic intervention.
- The least expensive intervention is preferred in a cost-minimisation analysis. For example, if a randomised controlled trial shows the treatment effects of both a generic drug and a brand-name drug to be identical, a cost-minimisation analysis would prefer the cheaper generic drug as it achieves the same outcome at a lower cost.

COMMUNICATION

When to use a cost-minimisation analysis study design?

- A cost-minimisation analysis cannot be planned in advance of knowing the results of a clinical trial.
- A cost-minimisation analysis should only be used when the health outcomes of two or more competing interventions are similar.
- Having demonstrated the above, the quality of clinical evidence dictates the appropriateness of carrying out a cost-minimisation analysis.

Clinical equivalence

What is clinical equivalence?

- Clinical equivalence implies that both the primary health outcome benefits (e.g. clinical improvement of a hospital-acquired pneumonia infection) and the secondary health outcome benefits (e.g. similar safety, efficacy and side-effect drug profiles) are the same in two or more competing interventions.
- In fact, the definition for clinical equivalence varies according to what perspective is taken, i.e. clinicians', patients' or society's view. However, regardless of whose views of clinical equivalence are assessed, the health outcome measured should be clinically important to the patient.
- If a randomised controlled trial shows there is clinical equivalence between the alternative interventions, it is important that this is demonstrated over a sustained and clinically significant period of time.

Demonstrating clinical equivalence

- Trials should be specifically designed to demonstrate that clinical equivalence exists, or does not exist, between competing interventions.
- The 'gold standard' method for demonstrating clinical equivalence is through a randomised controlled trial.
- Three different types of randomised controlled trial study designs may be used:
  1. Superiority trials
  2. Equivalence trials
  3. Non-inferiority trials.
- All three involve comparing one or more interventions against a gold standard. They differ in their initial assumptions and, therefore, also in the statistical methods used.

Superiority trials

- The most common study design performed to prove clinical equivalence between competing interventions is the superiority trial.
- Superiority trials are primarily used to determine whether a new intervention is more efficacious than the gold standard intervention.
- The null hypothesis (H_0) of a superiority trial would typically state that the new intervention has the *same* health outcome benefits as the gold standard intervention.
- The alternative hypothesis (H_1) of a superiority trial would typically state that the new intervention and gold standard intervention have significantly *different* health outcome benefits.
- The higher the P-value, the more likely the null hypothesis is not rejected and there is no difference between the health outcome benefits generated by the competing interventions.
- Alternatively, the more significant the result (i.e. the lower the P-value), the more likely it is that the null hypothesis is rejected and a difference does exist. For a discussion on how to interpret the P-value, please refer to Chapter 3.

Equivalence trials

- When a new healthcare intervention has already been introduced into clinical practice, equivalence trials are used to confirm the absence of a significant difference between the new intervention and the existing gold standard intervention.
- The objective of the study would be to evaluate whether the health outcome effect of the new intervention is not different to the effect of the gold standard intervention by a *pre-established equivalence margin*.
- As the goal of an equivalence trial is to prove that the competing interventions have equal health outcomes, the alternative hypothesis (H_1) must reflect that the interventions have the same health outcomes.
- The null hypothesis (H_0) of an equivalence trial would therefore state that a clinically significant difference in clinical outcome exists between the competing interventions.
- The alternative hypothesis of clinical equivalence is accepted when the entire confidence interval of the point estimate of the health outcome benefit falls exclusively within the equivalence margin (Fig. 18.2).
- The hypothesis of equivalence is rejected (therefore the null hypothesis is not rejected) if the confidence interval lies partially or entirely outside the equivalence margin.

Non-inferiority trials

- Non-inferiority trials are designed to ensure that the new intervention does not have an unacceptably worse clinical outcome than the gold standard intervention. In other words, is the new intervention as good as the current gold standard intervention?
- The objective of the study would be to evaluate whether the health outcome effect of the new intervention is *not worse* than the effect of the gold standard intervention by more than a pre-established clinical margin (non-inferiority margin).
- The alternative hypothesis (H_0) of a non-inferiority trial would typically state that the treatment difference is superior to the non-inferiority margin.
- The null hypothesis (H_0) of a non-inferiority trial would therefore state that the new intervention is inferior by more than the non-inferiority margin.
- The null hypothesis is not rejected when the entire confidence interval of the point estimate of the

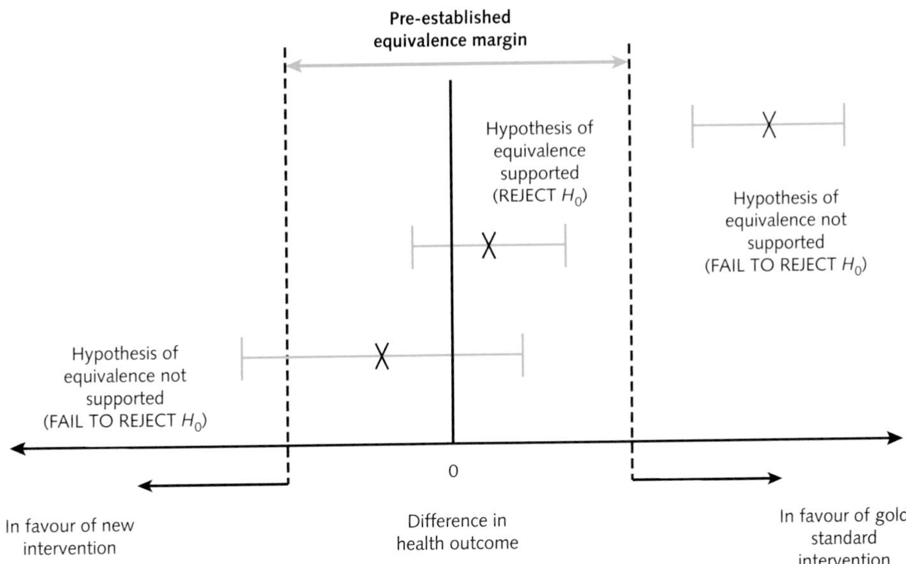

Fig. 18.2 Interpreting equivalence trials using confidence intervals.

difference in health outcome benefit between the competing interventions falls exclusively inferior to the non-inferiority margin (Fig. 18.3).

- The null hypothesis is rejected when the confidence interval lies partially or entirely superior to the non-inferiority margin.

COST-UTILITY ANALYSIS

In health economics, utility measurements are typically combined with survival estimates to generate quality-adjusted life years (QALYs), which are used when carrying out a cost-utility analysis of competing healthcare interventions.

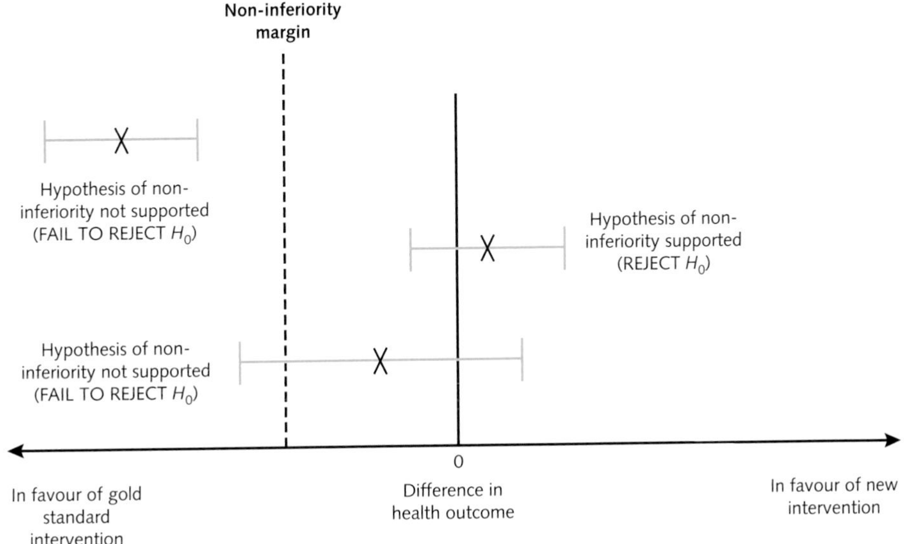

Fig. 18.3 Interpreting non-inferiority trials using confidence intervals.

Health utilities

- It is important to have a common quality of life outcome measure when comparing competing interventions. In health economics, such an outcome measure is referred to as utility measurement. In other words, utilities are values that reflect what preferences individuals have for different states of health.
- Utility measurements are made on an interval scale between 0 and 1, with:
  - 0 reflecting health states equivalent to death.
  - 1 reflecting perfect health (Fig. 18.4).
- It is necessary to identify, define and measure the health states of interest. Having measured these health states, the next step is to 'value' the health gains from any improvement in quality of life.
- Utilities can be measured either directly or indirectly, as discussed below.

COMMUNICATION

When to use a cost-utility analysis study design?

Cost-utility studies are usually employed when:
- The quality and/or the quantity of life is the main outcome of the intervention.
- A range of different outcomes arising from different interventions are measured.

Direct measurement of utilities

- Direct utility measurement methods are usually used for condition-specific health states.
- It is crucial that all relevant health attributes (health-related quality of life components) of the condition or disease are assessed.
- Key health attributes include:
  - Cognitive function
  - Physical function
  - Emotional/psychological well-being
  - Social function
  - Symptoms
  - Occupational status.
- Details of these key health attributes should be included when describing the health state (clinical vignette) for the particular condition or disease of interest.
- The clinical vignette will enable individuals to undertake an informed utility valuation of the condition or disease.
- Utility valuation methods commonly used in direct measurement studies include the visual analogue scale, time trade-off and standard gamble.

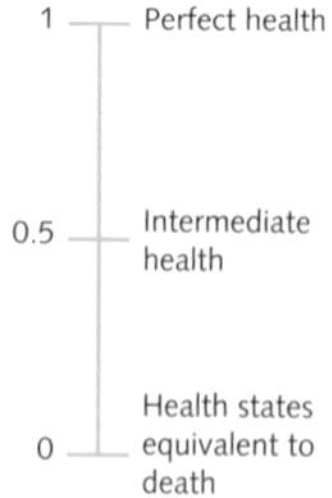

Fig. 18.4 Utility measurement interval scale.

Visual analogue scale

- The visual analogue scale is a rating scale with a very simple approach.
- Volunteers are given a clinical vignette and must try to imagine what it would be like to have the health attributes associated with the condition or disease.
- Respondents must indicate on a scale of 0 to 1 (Fig. 18.4) how good or bad the perceived health state is for the condition or disease described.
- The visual analogue scale generates values that can be compared between different clinical vignettes for different conditions/diseases.

Time trade-off

- The time trade-off approach involves asking volunteers to consider the relative amount of time (e.g. number of life years) they would be prepared to sacrifice in order to avoid living with a certain poorer health state. For example, imagine you are told that you can remain in your current health state (with the health attributes associated with the condition or disease) for 20 years before dying! On the other hand, you could choose to give up some life years to live for a shorter period of time, but in full health! How many years in full health would you think is of equal value to 20 years with the health attributes associated with the condition or disease?
- The time trade-off utility score can be calculated with the equation

$$\text{Utility score} = \frac{\text{Number of years alive at full health}}{\text{Number of years alive at poorer health state}}$$

- For example, using the same scenario as discussed above, if you had been indifferent at 12 years (i.e. 12 years in full health is equivalent to 20 years in the relevant degree of poor health) the time trade-off utility score would be 12/20 = 0.6.

Method of response	Question frame	
	Uncertainty	*Certainty*
Choice	Standard gamble	Time trade-off
Scaling		Visa analogue scale

Fig. 18.5 Comparison of direct utility measurement methods.

Standard gamble

- So you call yourself a gambler? Would you gamble with your life?
- The standard gamble approach involves presenting volunteers with a choice between two different health states:
  1. A health state that is *certain*, e.g. chronic unremitting abdominal pain for 20 years.
  2. A health state that is *uncertain*: You have $X\%$ chance of an improved heath state (e.g. perfect health) and $(100 - X)\%$ chance of a worse health state (e.g. immediate death).
- Volunteers must determine what probability ($X\%$) of having the better health state would make them indifferent between gambling for the current certain health state or going for the risky health state option.
- For example, using the same scenario as discussed above, if you are indifferent between the chronic abdominal pain health state and a gamble with a probability of 0.75 (75% chance) of having a better outcome (and, therefore, a 25% chance of a worse outcome), the standard gamble utility measurement of the chronic abdominal pain health state would be 0.75.

Which valuation method is best?

- While the visual analogue scale is the simplest method of the three valuation methods (a scaling exercise), with only limited demands on the mathematical capability of the respondents, it is the least favoured in the world of health economics for placing value on health-related quality of life.
- The visual analogue scale does not require volunteers to make a choice, or to make decisions when the outcome is uncertain (Fig. 18.5). It therefore informs us of the ordinal preferences that individuals may have for various health states.
- Although the standard gamble method is similar to the time trade-off method for utility measurement (there are two alternative options for volunteers to choose between, with one option varied until there is indifference between the two options), the former approach offers a degree of uncertainty in the question due to the element of risk in one arm of the choice (Fig. 18.5).
- Considering the prospect of mortality is incorporated as an option for the standard gamble and time trade-off methods, these approaches are considered more valid for estimating health-related quality of life values.
- While the aim of each valuation method is to obtain a representative utility measurement, there are in fact consistent differences in the results produced from all three of the methods discussed above.
- A systematic review on utility measurements across 995 acute and chronic health states found a tendency for the standard gamble method to yield the highest, the visual analogue scale to yield the lowest and the time trade-off method to yield an intermediate utility value for the same health states.

Public versus patients

- The valuation can be performed by different groups of individuals, including:
  - Patients
  - Clinicians
  - Carers
  - Government
  - General population.
- In practice, the main debate centres on whether the utility valuation is performed by patients or the general population (Fig. 18.6).

Fig. 18.6 Comparison between patients versus general population for utility measurements.

General population	Patients
As the National Health Service is publically funded, society's resources are being allocated, so the views of the general population are important.	They have first-hand experience of the impact of the condition or disease and its treatment on their health; therefore their preferences are important.
Members of the general public may unintentionally bring in stereotypes or prejudice when asked to value a specific health state.	It may be challenging to find patient volunteers with the specific health state of interest (however, hypothetical health states can also be used).
Compared to identifying patients with specific health states, it is relatively easier to survey the general public about a range of health states.	If patients have a chronic disease, they may become accustomed to their health state, therefore unintentionally undervaluing their utility measurement scores.

- Utility scores may differ depending on whose preferences are measured.
- There is evidence to suggest that utility scores are higher than those from the general population if patients with a condition/disease are asked to value a hypothetical health state that is likely to be worse than their own health state. This may be due to patients becoming accustomed to their own condition, therefore developing coping mechanisms when in poor health.

HINTS AND TIPS

Studies have shown that clinicians are fairly poor judges of the symptoms felt by their patients! Some food for thought guys!

Indirect measurement of utilities

- Indirect methods of utility valuation are made using utility algorithms.
- Patients with any health condition/disease are asked to categorise their health status on a variety of health attributes (e.g. pain and anxiety) using specific quality of life questionnaires (e.g. EuroQol-5D (EQ-5D) and Short Form Six Dimension (SF-6D)). These health attributes have already been pre-valued by a sample of individuals from the general population (using one of the three direct valuation methods described above) and a scoring algorithm developed.
- The EQ-5D method (Fig. 18.7) is the most frequently used questionnaire for generating utility measurements in the UK.
- The EQ-5D instrument is usually valued using the time trade-off method, while the SF-6D instrument relies on the standard gamble approach.
- Based on the patient response, the appropriate utility from the scoring algorithm is measured. For example, referring to Figure 18.7, if the patient volunteer categorises their health state with having no problems walking about (1), no problems with washing or dressing (1), slight problems with performing usual activities (2), moderate pain or discomfort (3) and no anxiety or depression (1), the utility valuation for a 11231 health state would be 0.767.
- The maximum EQ-5D health state score is 1.0. The higher this score, the better the health state. This hybrid approach addresses some of the practical difficulties associated with the direct methods of utility valuation as highlighted above.
- A potential limitation of the indirect method of utility valuation is that it may have limited use when scoring acute health conditions (e.g. angina attack, asthma attack).

Quality-adjusted life years (QALYs)

- As discussed above, the main outcome of an intervention has two key components – the quality and quantity of life.
- The quality-adjusted life year (QALY) incorporates both outcome components.
- The quantity of life is simply expressed in terms of life expectancy or survival.
- The health-related quality of life is measured using direct or indirect methods of utility valuation, as discussed above.
- A QALY is the arithmetic product of the period of time spent in a particular health state and the utility measurement for the same health state. For example, a QALY of 1 is generated if an individual has perfect health (utility score = 1) for one year.

Example 1: QALY – intervention A versus intervention B (Fig. 18.8)

Even though both interventions generate four additional years of life, the utility scores differ between intervention A and intervention B. Intervention A generates 1 more QALY than intervention B.

Example 2: QALY – intervention C versus intervention D (Fig. 18.9)

In this example, interventions C and D both generate eight additional years of life. However, for intervention D, the utility score ranges from 0.5 for the first 4 years to 0.25 for the final 4 years. Overall, intervention C generates 1 more QALY than intervention D.

Implementing QALYs

- QALYs can be used to compare the effectiveness of competing interventions and are combined with costs associated with each intervention to generate a cost-utility ratio, which is also known as the 'incremental cost-effectiveness ratio' (ICER).
- An ICER, can be calculated using the formula

$$\text{ICER} = \frac{\text{Cost of intervention A} - \text{Cost of intervention B}}{\text{Number of QALYs for intervention A} - \text{Number of QALYs for intervention B}}$$

- The units for an ICER are cost per QALY.
- If an intervention has an ICER below a threshold ICER it is likely to be funded by the healthcare system.
- The threshold ICER is determined by the willingness to pay for health gain, which depends on the budget available to the healthcare service.

Under each heading, please tick the **ONE** box that best describes your health **TODAY**

MOBILITY

I have no problems in walking about ❑
I have slight problems in walking about ❑
I have moderate problems in walking about ❑
I have severe problems in walking about ❑
I am unable to walk about ❑

SELF-CARE

I have no problems washing or dressing myself ❑
I have slight problems washing or dressing myself ❑
I have moderate problems washing or dressing myself ❑
I have severe problems washing or dressing myself ❑
I am unable to wash or dress myself ❑

USUAL ACTIVITIES *(e.g. work, study, housework, family or leisure activities)*

I have no problems doing my usual activities ❑
I have slight problems doing my usual activities ❑
I have moderate problems doing my usual activities ❑
I have severe problems doing my usual activities ❑
I am unable to do my usual activities ❑

PAIN / DISCOMFORT

I have no pain or discomfort ❑
I have slight pain or discomfort ❑
I have moderate pain or discomfort ❑
I have severe pain or discomfort ❑
I have extreme pain or discomfort ❑

ANXIETY / DEPRESSION

I am not anxious or depressed ❑
I am slightly anxious or depressed ❑
I am moderately anxious or depressed ❑
I am severely anxious or depressed ❑
I am extremely anxious or depressed ❑

Fig. 18.7 EuroQol-5D (EQ-5D) questionnaire. *(© EuroQol Group Foundation, reproduced with permission.)*

Fig. 18.8 QALY: intervention A versus intervention B.

Intervention	Additional years in health	Utility score	QALYs
A	4	0.5	2
B	4	0.25	1

Fig. 18.9 QALY: intervention C versus intervention D.

Intervention	Additional years in health	Utility score	QALYs	
C	8	0.5	4	
D	4	0.5	2	3
	4	0.25	1	

HINTS AND TIPS

QALYs can be calculated over an extended period of time even if the health state profile changes over this time. This is possible, as the utility of a health state is *not* affected by:

- previous health states
- subsequent health states
- the amount of time spent in that health state.

The QALYs calculated over the proposed period of time can be summed up to estimate the total QALY.

The net monetary benefit statistic

- The net monetary benefit (NMB) statistic:
  - is mainly used in 'cost per QALY' (cost-utility analysis) studies.
  - provides an alternative approach in how the primary results of an economic evaluation study are reported.
  - requires us to know the amount that healthcare service providers are willing to pay per QALY.
- The NMB can be calculated using the formula

$$\text{NMB} = [(\text{Number of QALYs for intervention A} - \text{Number of QALYs for intervention B}) \times \lambda] - (\text{Cost of intervention A} - \text{Cost of intervention B})$$

where λ is the amount that society are willing to pay per QALY

- The value for λ in the NHS is roughly between £20 000 and £30 000.
- A positive NMB suggests that the intervention has good value for money, while a negative NMB is cost-ineffective.
- The intervention with the greatest NMB (and therefore the most cost-effective) is usually chosen.
- For example, suppose:
  - Intervention A, which is associated with a QALY of 1.1, costs £23 000 per patient
  - Intervention B, which is associated with a QALY of 0.65, costs £7000 per patient
  - Healthcare providers are willing to pay £30 000 per QALY.

  Therefore, the NMB is:

$$= [(1.1 - 0.65) \times 30\,000] - (23\,000 - 7000)$$
$$= 13\,500 - 16\,000$$
$$= -£2500$$

This means intervention B has a NMB statistic that is £2500 greater than intervention A. Therefore, although intervention A is associated with a greater QALY than intervention B, it is less cost-effective.

Advantages and disadvantages of a cost-utility analysis

What are the advantages and disadvantages of a cost-utility analysis (Fig. 18.10)?

While a cost-utility analysis values health-related benefits of competing interventions for different health conditions or diseases (one of the limitations of a cost-effectiveness analysis, see below), QALYs do not capture the non-health-related impacts of the interventions. This limitation in using a cost-utility analysis prompted

Fig. 18.10 Advantages and disadvantages of cost-utility analysis.

Advantages	Disadvantages
Allows valuation of specific health states.	Which group of individuals should provide health-related quality of life utility measurements? Patients? General population?
Takes into account not only the quantity of life gained from a particular intervention, but also the quality of this life.	Concerns over lack of sensitivity of utility measurements for particular diseases, e.g. milder conditions.
Allows comparisons of the effectiveness of two competing interventions for the same condition or disease.	The utility of a health state is independent of the time spent in that health state. This poses an issue for chronic conditions.
Guides priority setting.	The utility of a health state is not affected by previous or subsequent health states. This again poses a problem for chronic conditions where disability may worsen over time.
Standardised indirect utility instruments, such as the EQ-5D questionnaire, have been developed.	There is evidence to suggest that the improvement in the quality of life associated with an intervention is valued higher for the more severe health states.

health economists to measure not only health benefits but also a profile of all the non-health impacts of the competing interventions. This type of analysis is referred to as a *cost–consequence analysis*. The subjective weighting of costs and benefits is left to the policy-makers.

COST-EFFECTIVENESS ANALYSIS

- Cost-effectiveness analysis forms the majority of the economic evaluations in the health economics literature.
- It compares the costs and health effects of competing interventions.
- The intervention effect is measured using a single 'natural' health unit (e.g. life years gained, new cases detected, deaths avoided).
- Competing interventions are compared in terms of cost per unit of effectiveness.
- Interventions can be completely independent (one intervention has no effect on the costs and effects of another intervention) or mutually exclusive (one intervention results in changes to the costs and effects of another intervention).

HINTS AND TIPS

While a cost-utility analysis measures the outcome for as long as the intervention effects last, a cost-effectiveness analysis measures the outcome at a particular point in time, e.g. 6 months after the intervention ends.

COMMUNICATION

When to use a cost-effectiveness analysis study design?

Cost-effectiveness studies are usually employed to compare the financial costs of competing interventions whose outcomes are *only* measured in terms of health effect (e.g. life years gained, infections treated).

Independent interventions

- For independent interventions, average cost-effectiveness ratios (CERs) are calculated for each intervention:

$$\text{Cost-effectiveness ratio} = \frac{\text{Cost of intervention}}{\text{Health effect outcome}}$$

- For example, if there are three independent interventions for *different patient groups/conditions*, we must first calculate the CER for each intervention programme (Fig. 18.11).
- The CERs calculated for the interventions being compared are placed in rank order to decide which programme to implement.
- Referring to Fig. 18.11, intervention A should be given priority over interventions B and C since it has the lowest CER. However, this doesn't necessarily mean intervention A is fully implemented. The extent of the resources (budget) available needs to be reviewed first (Fig. 18.12).

Mutually exclusive interventions

- When there are competing interventions for treatment of the *same patient group/condition*, incremental cost-effectiveness ratios (ICERs) are calculated:

$$\text{ICER} = \frac{\text{Cost of intervention A} - \text{Cost of intervention B}}{\text{Health effects of intervention A} - \text{Health effects of intervention B}}$$

- The competing interventions are ranked in order of ascending health effectiveness and ICERs calculated working down the list (Fig. 18.13).
- As demonstrated in Fig. 18.13, the least effective intervention is compared with the alternative intervention of 'nothing'. The negative ICER calculated for intervention B implies that not only does this intervention have a better health effect than intervention A but also it is associated with a cheaper cost. The ICER for intervention C of 118 means that it costs £118 to generate each additional life-year gained compared with intervention B.

Fig. 18.11 Cost-effectiveness ratios of independent interventions.

Intervention	Cost (£) [C]	Health effect (life years gained) [E]	Cost-effectiveness ratio (£/life years gained) [C/E]
A	300 000	2350	127.66
B	220 000	1700	129.41
C	250 000	1850	135.14

Fig. 18.12 Which interventions are implemented?

Available budget (£)	Intervention(s) implemented		
	A	B	C
< 300 000	As much as budget allows		
300 000	Fully implemented		
300 000 < Budget < 520 000	Fully implemented	Implemented as much as budget allows	
520 000	Fully implemented	Fully implemented	
520 000 < Budget < 770 000	Fully implemented	Fully implemented	Implemented as much as budget allows
770 000	Fully implemented	Fully implemented	Fully implemented

Fig. 18.13 Incremental cost-effectiveness ratios for mutually exclusive interventions.

Intervention	Cost (£) [C]	Health effect (life years gained) [E]	Incremental cost [ΔC]	Incremental effect [ΔE]	ICER [ΔC/ΔE]
A	160 000	1100	160 000	1100	145.45
B	130 000	1250	–30 000	150	–200
C	195 000	1800	65 000	550	118
D	170 000	2100	–25 000	300	–83.33
E	200 000	2300	30 000	200	150

- It is important to exclude those interventions that are more expensive and less effective. As interventions B and D are more effective and less expensive (have negative ICERs) than interventions A and C, respectively, interventions A and C are excluded. With exclusion of interventions A and C, ICERs are subsequently recalculated for the remaining interventions (Fig. 18.14).
- Referring to Fig. 18.14, intervention D is 'dominant' over intervention B, as the former is more effective and less expensive for each additional unit of health effect. In other words, the ICER is lower for intervention D than for intervention B.
- Having excluded intervention B, the ICERs are recalculated for the remaining two interventions (Fig. 18.15).
- Whether to implement interventions D or E will depend on the available budget.
- If the available budget is:
    - £170 000, all patients should be treated with intervention D.

Fig. 18.14 Incremental cost-effectiveness ratios for mutually exclusive interventions with exclusion of more costly and less expensive interventions.

Intervention	Cost (£) [C]	Health effect (life years gained) [E]	Incremental cost [ΔC]	Incremental effect [ΔE]	ICER [ΔC/ΔE]
B	130 000	1250	130 000	1250	200
D	170 000	2100	40 000	300	83.33
E	200 000	2300	30 000	200	150

Fig. 18.15 Incremental cost-effectiveness ratios for mutually exclusive interventions with 'further' exclusion of more costly and less expensive interventions.

Intervention	Cost (£) [C]	Health effect (life years gained) [E]	Incremental cost [ΔC]	Incremental effect [ΔE]	ICER [ΔC/ΔE]
D	170 000	2100	170 000	2100	80.95
E	200 000	2300	30 000	200	150

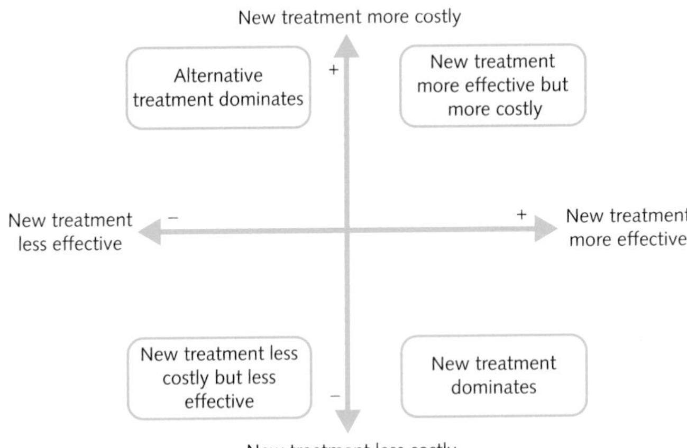

Fig. 18.16 Cost-effectiveness plane.

- £200 000, all patients should be treated with the more effective intervention E.
- £190 000, two-thirds of patients can be treated with the more effective intervention E and the remaining one-third of patients treated with intervention D. This is because the cost difference between intervention D and intervention E is £30 000 and the budget surplus is £20 000.

The cost-effectiveness plane

- The cost-effectiveness plane illustrates the process used for deciding which intervention to finance when carrying out a cost-effectiveness analysis.
- There are four possible scenarios as highlighted by the four quadrants of the cost-effectiveness plane (Fig. 18.16).
- Using the example above, intervention D would lie in the south-west quadrant (relative to intervention E) and intervention E would lie in the north-east quadrant (relative to intervention D).

Advantages and disadvantages of a cost-effectiveness analysis

What are the advantages and disadvantages of a cost-effectiveness analysis (Fig. 18.17)?

COST–BENEFIT ANALYSIS

- If information is required on which interventions lead to overall resource savings, a cost–benefit analysis is performed.

Fig. 18.17 Advantages versus disadvantages of cost-effectiveness analysis.

Advantages	Disadvantages
Useful for interpreting which interventions provide the best value for money.	Problematic when comparing across different patient groups/conditions with different outcome measures.
Allows comparisons of the effectiveness of competing interventions for the same condition or disease.	Doesn't take quality of life measurements into account.
Guides priority setting.	Dependent on the quality of the data on health effectiveness used, thus requiring a detailed sensitivity analysis (see below).

- In a cost–benefit analysis, all individual benefits are measured in monetary terms, meaning all costs and consequences are measured in the same units.
- We are trying to determine whether the monetary value of benefits outweighs the costs. However, measuring all health gains in monetary terms is sometimes challenging.
- In a cost–benefit analysis, the monetary value placed on a health benefit is usually estimated using a willingness-to-pay valuation method.
- The willingness-to-pay is the maximum amount an individual would be willing to pay, exchange or sacrifice in order to receive a service or avoid an undesired event/condition.
- If only one intervention can be funded, the one with the highest excess financial benefit over costs is chosen.

COMMUNICATION

When to use a cost–benefit analysis study design?

Cost–benefit studies are useful when there are a number of diverse outcomes associated with the interventions being compared. It enables comparisons between interventions in different areas of healthcare.

SENSITIVITY ANALYSIS

- Economic models are useful tools for determining the value for money of an intervention, aiding decision-makers in healthcare. However, the interpretation of the results of an economic evaluation will depend upon the level of uncertainty associated with a number of factors.
- Uncertainty may be due to:
  - issues associated with the model structure used.
  - potential variation in the values used for the economic evaluation.
  - issues regarding the validity of the values taken from different groups of individuals.
- A sensitivity analysis is used to test all the assumptions made in the economic model. For example, using a cost-effectiveness economic model:
  - what would happen if the 'true' cost of a particular intervention was lower than the estimate used in the evaluation?
  - what would happen if the 'true' measure for life years gained for a particular intervention was higher than the estimate used in the evaluation?
- There are three types of sensitivity analysis:
  1. One-way sensitivity analysis
  2. Multi-way sensitivity analysis
  3. Probabilistic sensitivity analysis.

One-way sensitivity analysis

- Estimates for each uncertain parameter in the economic model are varied by a given amount, one at a time, in order to investigate their impact on the model's results. For example, if the value for the quality of life of patients with a particular disease is increased by 20%, the ICER for the intervention may increase by 30%.
- By using this approach, it is therefore possible to identify which parameters have the greatest influence on the model's output.
- There are several ways in which an investigator may attempt to vary the parameters. For instance:
  - by using the upper and lower limit of the confidence intervals of the data, if known.
  - by using the range of values found in the literature for the parameter.
- Finally, it is possible to assess the impact of a full range of values of a particular parameter on the model's results. Using this approach, the main model outcome (e.g. ICER) can be plotted against each of the parameter values (e.g. the values for the quality of life of patients with a particular disease). Having plotted such a graph, a line of best fit can be drawn to demonstrate the relationship between the parameter values and the main model outcome. A threshold analysis on this data can be applied to determine the parameter value at which a pre-specified outcome threshold is met. For example, referring to Fig. 18.18, the ICER of an intervention will remain below £8000 (the pre-specified outcome threshold) provided that the cost of the intervention stays below £37.

Multi-way sensitivity analysis

If two or more different parameters are changed simultaneously, this is known as a multi-way sensitivity analysis. One approach is to perform a scenario analysis where all the parameters in a model are varied to represent the 'best' possible case (e.g. the intervention is cheaper than the study case and its effects continue to magnify after the follow-up period) and the 'worst' possible case (e.g. the intervention is more expensive than the study case and its effects diminish after the follow-up period). In other words the best- and worst-case values for all parameters are chosen and the model's results reviewed accordingly.

Probabilistic sensitivity analysis

- In a probabilistic sensitivity analysis, a distribution of potential values is assigned to all the parameters,

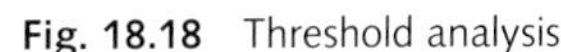

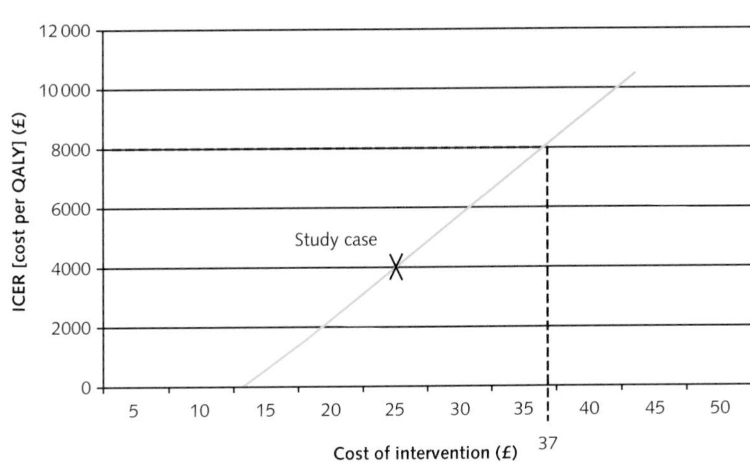

Fig. 18.18 Threshold analysis.

rather than a point estimate. Computer software will calculate this distribution by using:

- the standard deviation (discussed in Chapter 2).
- the mean value.
- the 'shape' of the spread of the data (e.g. positive skewness – discussed in Chapter 2).

- The software will run a number of iterations by randomly selecting one value for each parameter from the distribution and recording the model output. The model results for all the iterations are then plotted on a cost-effectiveness scatter plane. If there is a wide distribution of parameter values, the spread of results will be large. On the other hand, if the values were associated with a higher level of confidence (i.e. there is a narrow distribution of parameter values), there would be a tighter spread of results.
- The data can be used to indicate the percentage of iterations that have results below a pre-specified cost-effectiveness threshold value.
- As the threshold (and therefore the willingness to pay per QALY) increases, the percentage/proportion of iterations with results below that threshold also increases. This can be demonstrated using a cost-effectiveness acceptability curve (CEAC) (Fig. 18.19).
- The CEAC shows 'the probability that the intervention is cost-effective' on the *y*-axis. This value depends on the amount the NHS is willing to pay per QALY (the *x*-axis).
- Referring to Model A in Fig. 18.19, if the NHS is willing to pay £30 000 per QALY, there is a greater than 95% chance that the new intervention is cost effective. In Model A, the CEAC rises steeply to >0.90,

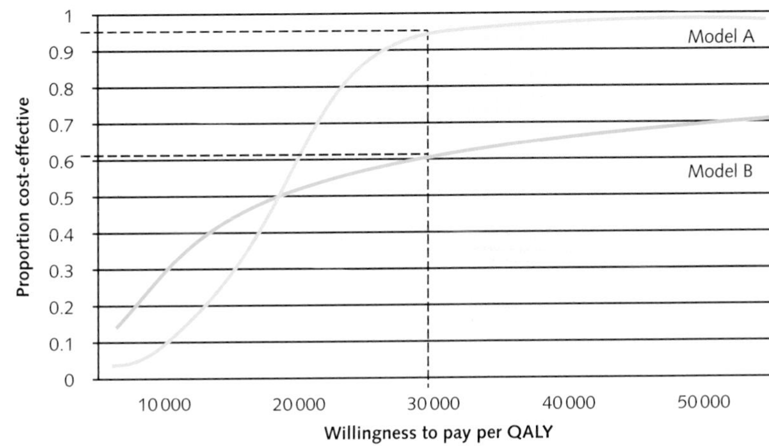

Fig. 18.19 Cost-effectiveness acceptability curve.

indicating that the economic trial has a good statistical power to assist us in reaching a valid conclusion about the cost-effectiveness of the intervention. In contrast, referring to Model B in Fig. 18.19, the CEAC is flatter, suggesting the economic trial is less conclusive. Again, if the NHS is willing to pay £30 000 per QALY, there is only a 60% chance that the intervention is cost-effective this time. Overall, decision-makers will have far more confidence in the results of Model A.

HINTS AND TIPS

In poorer countries, where the willingness to pay per QALY is less than that in the UK (e.g. only £15 000 per QALY), policy-makers may find it more difficult to identify interventions that are deemed cost-effective (i.e. the interventions will tend to have a lower probability of being cost-effective).

Critical appraisal checklists

Objectives

By the end of this chapter you should:

- Know the key factors to look out for when appraising research articles, regardless of the study design employed.
- Know the key questions to ask when appraising systematic reviews (and meta-analyses), randomised controlled trials, diagnostic studies and qualitative studies.
- Know the different types of selection bias and measurement bias that may operate in different study designs.

CRITICAL APPRAISAL

- Critical appraisal is the process of systematically examining the available evidence to judge its *validity*, *results* and *relevance* in a particular context.
- The appraiser should make an objective assessment of the study quality and potential for bias.
- It is important to determine both the internal validity and external validity of the study:
  - *External validity*: the extent to which the study findings are generalisable beyond the limits of the study to the study's target population.
  - *Internal validity*: ensuring that the study was run carefully (research design, how variables were measured, etc.) and the extent to which the observed effect(s) were produced solely by the intervention being assessed (and not by another factor).
- Studies such as cohort, case–control or cross-sectional studies vary in design; however, there are a number of key points that should be reviewed when appraising all research papers, regardless of the study design employed.

Clinical question

- Was there a clear clinical question stated at the start of the study?
- Have the study investigators formulated a focused and clinically relevant research question based on evidence from previously published studies?
- Is the research question novel (i.e. the question has not been addressed in a previous study)?
- Have the investigators stated a well thought out and complete study hypothesis?

Study design

- Is there a clear study design and where does it fall on the hierarchy of evidence?
- Has the best study design been chosen to investigate the specific research question?

Methodological checklists for critically appraising the different types of study designs discussed in this book will be covered in subsequent sections of this chapter.

Ethical issues

- Was the study approved by an independent Ethics Committee?
- Was 'informed' consent obtained from all the subjects who participated in the study?

Study population

- Is there a clear description of what target population was studied?
- Were sample size calculations conducted prior to starting the study? If yes, were these numbers satisfied to ensure that the study had adequate power to detect the proposed study effect?
- When recruiting the study subjects,
  - were there eligibility criteria, including clear inclusion and exclusion criteria? If the eligibility criteria are very strict, this may restrict the generalisability of the results to other populations.
  - were cases and controls clearly defined? Are the study controls representative of people without the disease?

  - were people invited to participate (with reference to a target population), or did random volunteers participate? If the latter, people with a particular 'interest' in the research question may have been motivated to take part in the study, thus introducing bias.
  - was a random sample selected from the target population, or were all people in the target population invited to participate?
  - did the study investigators keep a record of response rates?
  - were the characteristics of those participating (and those not-participating) documented to assess whether non-response may have introduced bias?
- Having recruited the study subjects, were they studied in the 'real-life' setting? If yes, the results are more likely to apply to those working in that setting than if the setting was experimental.

Study methods

- Is there a clear description of both the intervention and its comparator? Is an exposure-outcome association being investigated?
- Is there a clear description of what exposure was measured? How was the exposure status measured? Was the exposure measured using the same approach in all study groups? Is the exposure objective or subjective?
- Is there a clear description of what outcome was measured? To whom is the outcome measure important, i.e. the patient, investigator, carer, etc.? How was the outcome measured? Was the outcome measured using the same approach in all study groups? Is the outcome objective or subjective?
- Were the researchers/subjects blinded to the treatment/exposure allocation? Is there potential for measurement bias?
- For longitudinal studies, was the study follow-up sufficiently long for cases of disease to occur? Have study subjects been lost to follow-up? If yes, there is potential for bias.

Data analysis

- Did the investigators define the primary and secondary outcomes (or end-points) in advance of collecting the data?
- What are the results and how were they expressed? How strong is the association between the exposure and outcome? Has the correct method been used to display the particular type of data collected?
- Was the plan for data analysis established in advance of collecting the data? Is the data analysis appropriate to answer the research question? Were any subgroup analyses predefined or did the investigators subsequently search for an association? Remember, the nature of statistical significance dictates that if you look at 20 subgroups (when $P \leq 0.05$), one will appear to show a significant result purely by chance.
- To determine the probability of a chance finding were *P*-values calculated?
- Are confidence intervals reported? If yes, are the results precise?

Confounding and bias

- Were confounding factors controlled for in the design and/or analysis stage of the study? Were confounding factors missed, e.g. socioeconomic or environmental factors?
- Were potential sources of selection bias considered in the study design (Fig. 19.1)?
- Were potential sources of measurement bias considered in the study design (Fig. 19.2)?
- Were the study investigators and/or subjects blinded?

Discussion

- Have the study investigators reached a sound conclusion based on the results obtained? Have the study limitations been taken into account?
- Have the data been misinterpreted? Have alternative interpretations been overlooked?
- Have any causal inferences been made? Have the Bradford-Hill criteria of causality been considered?
- Are the study findings logical? That is, do the results fit alongside other research findings?
- Can the study findings have an impact on healthcare practice? Was cost information provided?

It is rare for one observational study alone to provide sufficient evidence for recommendations to be made for changes in clinical practice. However, for certain clinical questions, the only evidence available is from observational studies. Furthermore, a study should *not* be automatically dismissed if it has one or more methodological limitations. It is important to make an overall assessment on how serious these limitations are compared to the methodological strengths of the study.

The general principles for critical appraisal reviewed in this section sufficiently cover the key questions that should be asked when appraising observational studies such as cohort, case–control or cross-sectional studies.

The following sections cover specific checklists for a number of more complex study designs, including:

- Systematic reviews and meta-analyses
- Randomised controlled trials
- Diagnostic studies
- Qualitative studies.

Fig. 19.1 Potential sources of selection bias.

Type of selection bias	Study design affected
Eligible population inappropriately defined	
Hospital admission rate bias (Berkson's bias)	Hospital-based case–control study
Exclusion bias	Case–control study
Inclusion bias	Hospital-based case–control study
Overmatching bias	Case–control study
Healthy worker effect bias	Cohort study
Detection bias	
Diagnostic suspicion bias	Case–control study
Unmasking-detection signal bias	Case–control study
Participation bias	
Non-response bias	Cross-sectional study Case–control study Cohort study
Ascertainment bias	
Incidence–prevalence bias (survival bias or Neyman bias)	Cross-sectional study Case–control study (with prevalent cases)
Healthcare access bias	Cross-sectional study Case–control study Cohort study
Migration bias	Cross-sectional study Case–control study (with prevalent cases)
Bias during study implementation	
Loss-to-follow-up bias (or attrition bias)	Cohort study Randomised controlled trial
Contamination bias	Randomised controlled trial
Bias associated with randomisation	
Random sequence generation bias	Randomised controlled trial
Allocation of intervention bias	Randomised controlled trial
Reporting bias	
Citation bias	Systematic review/meta-analysis
Language bias	Systematic review/meta-analysis
Publication bias	Systematic review/meta-analysis
Multiple publication bias	Systematic review/meta-analysis
Time lag bias	Systematic review/meta-analysis

Fig. 19.2 Potential sources of measurement bias.

Type of measurement bias		Study design affected
Random misclassification bias (non-differential misclassification bias)		All studies (interventional and observational)
Non-random misclassification bias (differential misclassification bias)	Detection bias	
	Diagnostic suspicion bias	Cohort study Randomised controlled trial
	Performance bias	
	Follow-up bias	Prospective cohort Randomised controlled trial
	Recall bias	
	Participant expectation bias	Randomised controlled trial
	Rumination bias	Cross-sectional study Case–control study Retrospective cohort study
	Exposure suspicion bias	Cross-sectional study Case–control study Retrospective cohort study
	Interviewer bias	
	Observer expectation bias	All studies (interventional and observational)
	Apprehension bias	All studies (interventional and observational)

HINTS AND TIPS

Critically appraising a research paper is fine and dandy! The key question you then need to ask yourself is whether the study results can be generalised (or extrapolated) to your own practice. Are the study setting and your setting comparable?

SYSTEMATIC REVIEWS AND META-ANALYSES

- Does the systematic review address a clearly defined, well-focused and clinically important question?
- Did the review focus on the study type (e.g. randomised controlled trials or cohort studies) most relevant to address the review's question?
- Was the literature search rigorous enough to identify all the relevant studies?
- Was the methodological quality of the included studies assessed and reported?
- If a meta-analysis was performed, was it appropriate to combine the results of the studies included? Have tests for evidence of heterogeneity been performed?
- What are the results and how were they expressed (e.g. risk ratio, odds ratio, etc.)?
- Were all important outcomes (e.g. from the point of view of the patient, carers, policy-makers, etc.) considered?
- Has a scientifically rational subgroup analysis been conducted?
- Has a sensitivity analysis been conducted to determine whether the findings of the meta-analysis are robust to the methodology used to obtain them?
- Was the possibility of publication bias, language bias, time lag bias, multiple publication bias or citation bias assessed?
- Do the benefits reported outweigh the associated harms and/or costs? Should there be changes in clinical practice based on the review findings?

RANDOMISED CONTROLLED TRIALS

- Does the randomised controlled trial (RCT) ask a clearly defined, well-focused and clinically important question?

- Was it appropriate to answer this question using a RCT study design? Was there clinical equipoise?
- To avoid selection bias (systematic differences between the treatment groups being compared) study participants should be appropriately allocated to the intervention and control groups:
  - Was an appropriate method of randomisation used to allocate study participants to the treatment groups?
    - Was the allocation sequence adequately generated?
    - Was the allocation adequately concealed?
  - Have major confounding and prognostic factors been measured to ensure the treatment groups are comparable at baseline? Were there systematic differences between the intervention and control groups being compared?
- Is there any risk of contamination between subjects in the intervention and control arm?
- To avoid loss to follow-up bias (attrition bias), there should be no systematic differences between the treatment groups in terms of the number of subjects lost, or differences between those not adhering to the study protocol and those who remain in the study.
  - Were all groups followed up for an equal length of time? If not, did the results analysis take this into account?
  - If all study participants were followed up in each treatment group, was there loss to follow-up, i.e. participants who did not complete treatment?
  - Were there differences in loss to follow-up in each group?
  - Were all participants' outcomes analysed by the groups to which they were originally allocated (intention to treat analysis)?
  - Were incomplete outcome data adequately addressed? In order to avoid attrition bias, the treatment groups should be comparable in terms of outcome data availability.
  - Was a sensitivity analysis conducted to assess the impact that loss to follow-up had on the data?
- To avoid follow-up bias, which is a type of performance bias, the treatment groups being compared should receive the same care, apart from the intervention being investigated:
  - Were study investigators 'blind' to treatment allocation?
- To avoid recall bias, were the study subjects kept 'blind' to treatment allocation?
- To avoid detection bias:
  - were the investigators 'blind' to treatment allocation? This may also prevent interviewer bias.
  - were the investigators 'blind' to the baseline measurements, i.e. the confounding and prognostic factors? This may also prevent interviewer bias.
  - was the length of follow-up appropriate to detect the effect of the intervention?
  - was the outcome measure precisely defined?
  - was a valid and reliable tool used to measure the outcome? This may also prevent interviewer bias.
  - were data collected in the same way in all treatment groups? For example, were participants in both groups reviewed at the same time intervals? This may also prevent interviewer bias.
- Interviewer bias can also be prevented if the investigators conducting the interview are trained to collect data using a standardised approach. Is there any documentation of this?
- What are the results and how were they expressed (e.g. number needed to treat for benefit or harm)?
- Has a scientifically rational subgroup analysis been conducted?
- How do the results fit in locally? Does your local setting differ much from that of the study?

DIAGNOSTIC STUDIES

- Does the diagnostic study ask a clearly defined, well-focused and clinically important question? Is the aim of the study to estimate the diagnostic accuracy of a test or to compare the diagnostic accuracy between tests (or across different target populations)?
- Was there a comparison with an appropriate reference test or gold standard test?
- Was the diagnostic test evaluated in a representative spectrum of patients (i.e. similar to those in whom the test would normally be used in clinical practice)?
- Did all the patients in the study get the reference gold standard test regardless of the diagnostic study test result? In other words, was the disease status of the tested patients clearly established?
- Were individuals lost to follow-up? If yes, did individuals lost to follow-up differ systematically from those who remained in the study?
- Is the disease status of the tested population clearly defined? If only cases with a limited range of diease spectrum are recruited for the study there is potential for spectrum bias.
- Was there an independent, blind comparison between the diagnostic test and the reference gold standard test? Partial verification bias (also known as work-up bias) may occur when the decision to perform the reference gold standard test on an individual is based on the results of the diagnostic test.
- Were the methods used for performing the test described in sufficient detail? A protocol should be followed. Differential verification bias may occur when different reference tests are used to verify the results of the study diagnostic test.

- Are all the test characteristics presented? The accuracy (sensitivity and specificity) and performance (positive and negative predictive values) of the test should be reported. Confidence intervals should be provided for these measures.
- Could interpretation of the results of the diagnostic test have been influenced by knowledge of the results of the reference standard test, and vice versa? Reporting bias may be an issue if there is a degree of subjectivity in interpreting the results.
- Were the methods for performing the test described in sufficient detail to permit replication?
- Have the study findings regarding the accuracy and performance of the diagnostic test been placed in the wider context of other (potential) tests in the diagnostic process?
- How do the results fit in locally? Does your local setting differ much from that of the study?
- Can the diagnostic test be applied to your patient (or population) of interest? The following should be considered:
  - Opportunity costs.
  - Level of expertise required to perform the test and interpret the results.
  - Number of resources available.
  - Availability of services.
- What impact would the test have if used in your local setting? This may include implications for patient management or healthcare costs.

QUALITATIVE STUDIES

- Does the qualitative study ask a clearly defined, well-focused and clinically important question?
- Was it appropriate to answer this question using a qualitative study design?
- Do the study investigators explain how potential participants were selected? Why were these participants chosen in particular?
- What sampling strategy was used to address the study aims, i.e. purposive sampling, quota sampling, snowball sampling, etc.? Was this the most appropriate sampling strategy to address the study aims? Are there any major limitations to the sampling strategy?
- What methods were used for data collection, i.e. participant observation, in-depth interviews or focus groups? Was this the most suitable method of data collection? Was the data collected at the most appropriate setting, e.g. the participant's own home, at a clinic, etc.?
- What was the investigator's perspective and how did this influence (or bias) data collection, i.e. reflexivity?
- Is there any evidence of triangulation?
- Were the study findings well 'grounded' in the data? Was the constant comparison approach used to clarify emerging themes?
- Is there any evidence of iteration between data collection and analysis?
- Did the investigators continue until they reached data saturation?
- Were all data collected taken into account? For example, did the investigators include data on negative cases, i.e. those against the emerging theme?
- Was sufficient raw data included in the final report to enable the reader to draw the same conclusions as the study investigators?
- Would another researcher be able to reproduce the same data and interpret it in the same way? To assess for inter-rater reliability, did a second investigator independently code the data?
- What was the main study finding? Are the conclusions drawn justified by the findings?
- Are the findings applicable (or transferrable) to other patients and/or settings? There should be a detailed description of the context and setting in which the study was undertaken.
- Are the findings of this study likely to have any relevance for clinical practice?

Crash course in statistical formulae

20

Objectives

By the end of this chapter you should:

- Have memorised the statistical formulae listed.
- Understand the meaning of the terms used in the formulae listed, referring to the relevant chapters, if necessary.
- Be able to recall the statistical formulae from memory and use them when provided with relevant data.

The application of the formulae listed in this chapter will be expected in most evidence-based medicine undergraduate and postgraduate exams. Furthermore, some medical schools and exam bodies expect you to memorise these formulae as they may not be provided in the exam!

DESCRIBING THE FREQUENCY DISTRIBUTION

We can summarise the data (or frequency distribution) of a variables using the formulae listed in Fig. 20.1. The formulae listed in Fig. 20.1 are covered in Chapter 2 of this book.

EXTRAPOLATING FROM 'SAMPLE' TO 'POPULATION'

Having chosen an appropriate study sample, the rules of probability are applied to make inferences about the overall population from which the sample was drawn (Fig. 20.2). The formulae used to make this inference depends on whether you are dealing with:

- A single group mean
- A single group proportion
- Two independent means
- Paired means
- Two independent proportions.

The formulae listed in Fig. 20.2 are covered in Chapter 3 of this book.

STUDY ANALYSIS

Different formulae are used when analysing the results from different study designs (Fig. 20.3), including:

- Randomised controlled trials
- Cohort studies
- Case–control studies
- Cross-sectional studies.

Please refer to the relevant study design chapter for an in-depth discussion on how to apply each formula to sample data.

TEST PERFORMANCE

As clinicians, we rely on diagnostic tests to make decisions on how we treat our patients. Therefore, the performance (or validity) of a new test must be properly assessed before implementing its use in the clinical setting (Fig. 20.4). The formulae listed in Fig. 20.4 are covered in Chapter 14 of this book.

ECONOMIC EVALUATION

A full economic evaluation of healthcare involves systematically comparing the costs (inputs) and benefits (outcomes) of at least two alternative interventions to evaluate the best use of the scarce resources available. Some of the key formulae used to evaluate the cost-effectiveness of competing interventions are covered in Fig. 20.5. The formulae listed in Fig. 20.5 are covered in Chapter 18 of this book.

Fig. 20.1 Formulae used to describe the frequency distribution.

	Formula	Key
Arithmetic mean $\bar{x}$ (x-bar)	$\bar{x} = \frac{x_1 + x_2 + x_3 + \cdots + x_n}{n}$ $\bar{x} = \frac{\sum_{i=1}^{n} x_i}{n}$	• x = variable • n = number of observations of the variable • Σ (sigma) = the sum of (the observations of the variable) • Sub- and superscripts on the Σ = sum of the observations from $i = 1$ to n NOTE: The arithmetic mean of a population is denoted using the symbol μ.
Population variance σ^2	$\sigma^2 = \frac{\sum (x_i - \bar{x})^2}{n}$	• x = variable • $\bar{x}$ (x-bar) = mean of the variable x • x_i = individual observation • n = number of observations of the variable • Σ (sigma) = the sum of (the squared differences of the individual observations from the mean)
Population standard deviation σ	$\sigma = \sqrt{\sigma^2}$	• σ^2 = population variance
Sample variance s^2	$s^2 = \frac{\sum (x_i - \bar{x})^2}{n - 1}$	The symbols are identical to those used for the population variance.
Sample standard deviation s	$s = \sqrt{s^2}$	• s^2 = sample variance
95% reference range	mean – [1.96 × SD(mean)] to mean + [1.96 × SD(mean)]	• SD(mean) = standard deviation of the mean NOTE: The equation is the same whether you are calculating the 95% reference range for sample or population data.

Fig. 20.2 Formulae used when extrapolating data from sample to population.

	Formula	Key
Standard error of a single mean (SEM)	$\text{SEM} = \frac{\text{SD}}{\sqrt{n}}$	• SD = standard deviation • n = number of observations
95% Confidence interval for a single mean	mean – [1.96 × SE(mean)] to mean + [1.96 × SE(mean)]	• SE(mean) = standard error of the mean NOTE: This equation only applies for large samples.
Standard error of a single proportion SE(p)	$\text{SE}(p) = \sqrt{\frac{p \times (1 - p)}{n}}$	• p = proportion • n = number of observations
95% Confidence interval for a single proportion	proportion – [1.96 × SE(p)] to proportion + [1.96 × SE(p)]	• SE(p) = standard error of the proportion NOTE: This equation only applies for large samples.
Standard error of the difference between two independent means $\text{SE}(\bar{x}_1 - \bar{x}_0)$	$\text{SE}(\bar{x}_1 - \bar{x}_0) = \sqrt{[\text{SE}(\bar{x}_1)]^2 + [\text{SE}(\bar{x}_0)]^2}$	• $\text{SE}(\bar{x}_1)$ = standard error of mean of group 1 • $\text{SE}(\bar{x}_0)$ = standard error of mean of group 0
95% Confidence interval for the difference between two independent means	95% CI for $(\bar{x}_1 - \bar{x}_0)$ = $(\bar{x}_1 - \bar{x}_0)$ – [1.96 × $\text{SE}(\bar{x}_1 - \bar{x}_0)$] to $(\bar{x}_1 - \bar{x}_0)$ + [1.96 × $\text{SE}(\bar{x}_1 - \bar{x}_0)$]	• $(\bar{x}_1 - \bar{x}_0)$ = difference in means between two independent groups, group 0 and group 1 • $\text{SE}(\bar{x}_1 - \bar{x}_0)$ = standard error of the difference in means between group 0 and group 1
Standard error of the difference between paired means SE($\bar{d}$)	$\text{SE}(\bar{d}) = \frac{\text{SD}(d)}{\sqrt{n}}$	• SD(d) = standard deviation of the difference between all paired observations • n = number of paired observations

Fig. 20.2 Formulae used when extrapolating data from sample to population—cont'd.

	Formula	Key
95% Confidence interval for the difference between paired means	95% CI $(\bar{d}) = \bar{d} - [1.96 \times SE(\bar{d})]$ to $\bar{d} + [1.96 \times SE(\bar{d})]$	• $\bar{d}$ = mean of paired differences • $SE(\bar{d})$ = standard error of mean of paired differences
Standard error of the difference between two independent proportions $SE(p_1 - p_0)$	$SE(p_1 - p_0) = \sqrt{SE(p_1)^2 + SE(p_0)^2}$	• $SE(p_1)$ = standard error of proportion of group 1 • $SE(p_0)$ = standard error of proportion of group 0
95% Confidence interval for the difference between two independent proportions	95% CI for $(p_1 - p_0) =$ $(p_1 - p_0) - [1.96 \times SE(p_1 - p_0)]$ to $(p_1 - p_0) + [1.96 \times SE(p_1 - p_0)]$	• $(p_1 - p_0)$ = difference in proportions between group 1 and group 0 • $SE(p_1 - p_0)$ = standard error of difference in proportions between group 1 and group 0

Fig. 20.3 Analysing study data.

Study	Formula
Randomised controlled trial	
Number needed to treat to benefit (NNTB) or number needed to treat to harm (NNTH)	$\text{NNTB or NNTH} = \dfrac{1}{\lvert\text{Risk difference between two treatment groups}\rvert}$
Cohort study	
Incidence of disease	$\text{Incidence risk} = \dfrac{\text{Number of new cases of the disease in a given time period}}{\text{Total number of subjects initially disease-free}}$ $\text{Incidence rate} = \dfrac{\text{Number of new cases of the disease in a given time period}}{\text{Total number of subjects initially disease-free} \times \text{Time interval}}$
Risk ratio (RR)	$\text{RR} = \dfrac{\text{Risk in exposed group}}{\text{Risk in unexposed group}}$
Risk difference (RD)	RD = Risk in exposed group – Risk in unexposed group
Case–control study	
Odds of exposure	$\text{Odds of exposure} = \dfrac{\text{Probability of being exposed}}{\text{Probability of being unexposed}}$
Exposure odds ratio (OR)	$\text{Exposure OR} = \dfrac{\text{Odds of exposure in cases}}{\text{Odds of exposure in controls}}$
Odds of disease	$\text{Odds of disease} = \dfrac{\text{Probability of having disease}}{\text{Probability of not having disease}}$
Disease odds ratio (OR)	$\text{Disease OR} = \dfrac{\text{Odds of disease amongst exposed subjects}}{\text{Odds of disease amongst unexposed subjects}}$
Cross-sectional study	
Prevalence	$\text{Prevalence} = \dfrac{\text{Number of new and old cases of the disease at a single point in time}}{\text{Total number of people in the population at the same point in time}}$
Prevalence odds ratio (OR)	$\text{Prevalence OR} = \dfrac{\text{Odds of the disease amongst the exposed subjects at a single point in time}}{\text{Odds of the disease amongst the unexposed subjects at the same point in time}}$
Prevalence ratio	$\text{Prevalence ratio} = \dfrac{\text{Probability of the disease amongst the exposed subjects at a single point in time}}{\text{Probability of the disease amongst the unexposed subjects at the same point in time}}$

Fig. 20.4 Analysing the performance of a test.

Measure of test performance	Formula
False positive (FP) rate	FP(%) = 100% – Specificity (%)
False negative (FN) rate	FN(%) = 100% – Sensitivity (%)
Sensitivity	$\text{Sensitivity} = \frac{\text{True positive}}{\text{True positive} + \text{False negative}}$
Specificity	$\text{Specificity} = \frac{\text{True negative}}{\text{True negative} + \text{False positive}}$
Positive predictive value (PPV)	$\text{PPV} = \frac{\text{True positive}}{\text{True positive} + \text{False positive}}$
Negative predictive value (NPV)	$\text{NPV} = \frac{\text{True negative}}{\text{True negative} + \text{False negative}}$
Positive likelihood ratio (LR+)	$\text{LR+} = \frac{\text{Sensitivity}}{1 - \text{Specificity}}$
Negative likelihood ratio (LR–)	$\text{LR}- = \frac{1 - \text{Sensitivity}}{\text{Specificity}}$

Fig. 20.5 Economic evaluation.

Economic measure		Formula
Cost-utility analysis	Utility score	$\text{Utility score} = \frac{\text{Number of years alive at full health}}{\text{Number of years alive at poorer health state}}$
	Quality adjusted life year (QALY)	QALY = Period of time spent in a health state × Utility score for that health state
	Incremental cost-effectiveness ratio (ICER)	$\text{ICER} = \frac{\text{Cost of intervention A} - \text{Cost of intervention B}}{\text{Number of QALYs for intervention A} - \text{Number of QALYs for intervention B}}$
	Net monetary benefit (NMB)	NMB = [(Number of QALYs for intervention A – Number of QALYs for intervention B) × λ] – (Cost of intervention A – Cost of intervention B) where λ is the amount that society is willing to pay per QALY
Cost-effectiveness analysis	Cost-effectiveness ratio (CER)	$\text{Cost effectiveness ratio} = \frac{\text{Cost of intervention}}{\text{Health effect outcome}}$
	Incremental cost-effectiveness ratio (ICER)	$\text{ICER} = \frac{\text{Cost of intervention A} - \text{Cost of intervention B}}{\text{Health effects of intervention A} - \text{Health effects of intervention B}}$

Careers in academic medicine 21

Objectives

By the end of this chapter you should:

- Understand the significance of the Walport report in shaping the career pathway for training clinical academics.
- Understand the various stages of the integrated academic training pathway.
- Know that there are various opportunities to gain experience in academic medicine whilst at medical school.
- Understand the pros and cons of a career in academia.

CAREER PATHWAY

- A career in academic medicine involves a combination of research, teaching and patient care.
- Clinical academics make up 5 to 10% of the medical workforce.
- Until recently, there has not been a transparent career structure in academic medicine.
- In 2005, the Modernising Medical Careers (MMC) and the Joint Academic Careers Subcommittee of the UK Clinical Research Collaboration (UKCRC) produced the Walport report, named after the chair of the Academic Careers Subcommittee, Mark Walport.
- The committee identified three major issues faced by academic trainees:
    1. Lack of flexibility in the balance of clinical and academic training and in geographical mobility.
    2. Lack of both a clear route of entry and a transparent career structure.
    3. Shortage of structured and supported posts on completion of training.
- The committee sought to resolve these three major issues and recommended the development of a clear and integrated training and career pathway for medically qualified staff to embark on a career in academic medicine.
- Figure 21.1 illustrates the Integrated Academic Training Path from medical school to completion of training and beyond.
- Despite offering academic clinical fellowships in only England and Northern Ireland, the other components of the pathway are available throughout the UK.
- A key aspect of the training pathway is the flexibility involved in transferring between the clinical and academic training programme.

Academic Foundation Programme (AFP)

- On completion of medical school, the first opportunity for research on the training pathway arises in foundation year 2.
- The academic attachment usually lasts for 4 months in year 2, with some ongoing academic activity during the 20 months on clinical rotation.
- The aim is to allow academic foundation trainees to prepare for core/speciality training or apply for an academic clinical fellowship post.

Academic clinical fellowship (ACF)

- The academic clinical fellowship is intended for those who are at the start of their specialty training.
- The trainees are usually pre-doctoral clinical academics, but some appointed trainees might already have a PhD or MD.
- As part of the training post, which usually lasts for up to 3 years, 25% of the time is protected and devoted entirely for academic research.
- The aim is to allow academic clinical fellowship trainees the opportunity to identify a research interest and secure funding for a PhD or MD (training fellowship) by writing a competitive research proposal.

Academic clinical lectureship (ACL)

- The academic clinical lectureship is intended for those who are post-doctoral clinical academics.
- As part of the training post, which usually lasts for up to 4 years, 50% of the time is dedicated entirely for post-doctoral research.

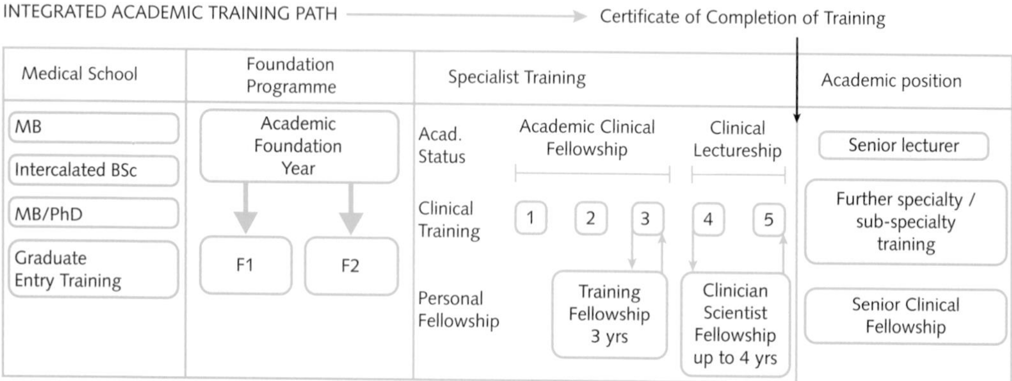

Fig. 21.1 The Integrated Academic Training Path. (Source: UK Clinical Research Collaboration, 2012. Clinical Academic Careers: England and Wales. Reproduced with permission.)

- The aim is to allow academic clinical lectureship trainees to progress into a senior academic role afterwards, such as a clinical scientist fellowship or a clinical senior lectureship.

GETTING INVOLVED

- Despite being relatively junior in my academic career, I was recently commended in the British Medical Association (BMA) Medical Academic Staff Committee (MASC), 'The Role of the Medical Academic Doctor', as a next generation medical academic role model.
- We need to value academic medicine and I hope my story inspires you to consider a career in academia.

What is my career path to date?

I graduated with a degree in medicine from the University of Bristol, in 2011. As a medical student I knew at an early stage that I wanted to pursue a career in cardiology. In 2008, I undertook an intercalated BSc degree in Physiological Sciences with selected modules in 'The Heart in Health and Disease' and the 'Cardiovascular System in Health and Disease'. I am currently on the Academic Foundation Programme at North Bristol NHS Trust/University of Bristol.

During my final year at medical school, I spent five weeks on a clinical cardiology rotation at Brigham and Women's Hospital, a teaching affiliate of Harvard Medical School. In addition to developing my clinical skills, I attended numerous seminars held by the editors of the scientific journal *Circulation*, alongside the 'TIMI' trial study group. This inspired me to co-author a peer-reviewed article in collaboration with a leading cardiologist at Harvard, on the interpretation of troponin levels in patients with renal impairment, an area of cardiology that still causes much debate on a daily basis.

Over the past four years I have actively pursued my research interests at the Microvascular Research Laboratories and the Bristol Heart Institute in my spare time. Building on from this work, my Academic Foundation research post has enabled me to formulate a relevant and incisive research question in an area of cardiology research that has fascinated me throughout my medical training: the role of angiogenesis (and anti-angiogenesis) in ischaemic heart disease.

I also have an unquestionable passion for teaching students/fellow colleagues. For this reason, in 2009, I founded the University of Bristol Cardiology Society, with an aim to teach students struggling with the fundamental or clinical aspects of cardiology.

HINTS AND TIPS

There are various opportunities to gain experience in academic medicine whilst at medical school, such as:

- by doing an intercalated degree
- during your elective period
- during student selected modules or components
- by getting involved in teaching.

What inspired me to embark upon an academic career?

During my intercalation year, I carried out a laboratory project supervised by Dr Andy Salmon, an MRC Clinical Senior Lecturer/Consultant in Renal Medicine. I investigated the role of anti-angiogenic growth factors on the water permeability of intact mice glomeruli. Mastering the experimental assay proved to be a steep learning curve. Consequently, sample size requirements for each test group were not satisfied by the end of the research period due to time constraints. I subsequently returned to my medical training with a burning desire to complete my project, with the aim of making a novel discovery that may be linked to improvements in patient care. I was successfully granted funding through a Physiological Society Studentship Award, which enabled me to continue my research and generate sufficient data in my spare time. My results were published in a leading medical journal and presented at an international conference. This triggered the realisation that academic medicine was the career path for me, providing lifelong intellectual stimulation, autonomy and variety.

HINTS AND TIPS

You need to be persistent, patient, determined and passionate to get the most out of your research project. In the process, you will encounter a number of intellectual challenges; however, it is important that you see your project through to the end. This involves publishing your innovations in a journal and presenting your results at a local, national or international level. It is necessary to teach innovation to colleagues; otherwise, it will remain a curiosity.

What do I like about being a clinical academic?

Research allows me to progress, use my imagination and face new challenges every day. My academic post provides the opportunity to work alongside highly motivated and talented individuals, to teach and hopefully inspire medical students and doctors to become involved in academia themselves. Having the opportunity to contribute to research, which may one day be translated from bench to bedside, is incredibly gratifying. The rewards are enormous. Furthermore, I have opportunities to travel and work with colleagues internationally. I can't think of anything else I would rather be doing.

What challenges have I faced?

Research is not always easy and I have encountered many challenges as a medical academic. One example is when experiments do not go according to plan. I have learnt to address this by being patient and persevering. Overcoming such difficulties forms part of the experience of a career in academic medicine and it is important to reflect on what could be done differently if faced with a similar situation in the future. During these times I would turn to my supervisor for some experienced advice.

Advice for someone considering a career in academic medicine

1. Find a role model whom you admire, someone who is supportive, understanding and encourages you to pursue your dreams.
2. Do not rush into the first project that comes your way. It is essential that you use your clinical experience to inform your research interests and look for the right supervisor to support you in achieving your goals. Visit the department before applying for a post.
3. Whether you are making career decisions or carrying out an academic project, do not be afraid to ask for advice.
4. Having established your long-term goals, set short-term objectives to assist you in achieving them. Review your goals regularly. Try and resist taking on too many things at one time.
5. Relish the intellectual challenge and enjoy all steps of the academic process; formulate a clinically relevant question, secure funding and see the project through to the end. Don't let things go!
6. Establish strong collaborations with experts in your field of research – collaboration teamwork garners recognition, greater resources and rewards.
7. While a National Institute for Health Research (NIHR) pathway for training clinical academics exists, don't be afraid to go outside of medicine to do some additional training in research methods, e.g. BSc, MSc, MD or PhD. It is important to be flexible about the path your career may take.
8. Most importantly, believe in yourself. Nothing is impossible!

HINTS AND TIPS

Having a role model is crucial. Good role models possess a number of positive characteristics, including:

- leading by example and conduct
- maintaining a broad perspective on life
- having a commitment to excellence and growth
- inspiring others to fulfil their academic potential.

PROS AND CONS

What are the pros and cons of a career in academic medicine (Fig. 21.2)?

Fig. 21.2 Pros and cons of a career in academic medicine.

Pros	Cons
• Great opportunities to carry out, publish and present cutting-edge research. • Opportunities to travel and lecture abroad. • Can balance research and clinical medicine. • Involves teaching new and old innovations to fellow clinicians and the public. • Associated with great respect in the community.	• Job security is questionable. • Less flexibility in managing your academic or clinical duties than in private practice. • Less clinically skilled than pure clinical doctors as there is less incentive to see more patients. • Pressure for securing grants can be very high as you must satisfy your employer. • Meeting deadlines for grant applications or submitting articles can be a huge burden.

References

Chapter 3

Heart Protection Study Collaborative Group, 2002. MRC/BHF Heart Protection Study of cholesterol lowering with simvastatin in 20 536 high-risk individuals: a randomised placebo-controlled trial. Lancet 360, 7–22.

Steering Committee of the Physicians' Health Study Research Group, 1988. Preliminary report: findings from the aspirin component of the ongoing Physicians' Health Study. N. Engl. J. Med. 318, 262–264.

Chapter 4

Antman, E.M., Lau, J., Kupelnick, B., Mosteller, F., Chalmers, T.C., 1992. A comparison of results of meta-analyses of randomized control trials and recommendations of clinical experts. Treatments for myocardial infarction. JAMA 268, 240–248.

Lau, J., Antman, E.M., Jimenez-Silva, J., Kupelnick, B., Mosteller, F., Chalmers, T.C., 1992. Cumulative meta-analysis of therapeutic trials for myocardial infarction. N. Engl. J. Med. 327, 248–254.

Lau, J., Schmid, C.H., Chalmers, T.C., 1995. Cumulative meta-analysis of clinical trials: builds evidence for exemplary medical care. J. Clin. Epidemiol. 48, 45–57.

Chapter 6

Gilron, I., Bailey, J.M., Tu, D., Holden, R.R., Weaver, D.F., Houlden, R.L., 2005. Morphine, gabapentin, or their combination for neuropathic pain. N. Engl. J. Med. 352 (13), 1324–1334.

Scandinavian Simvastatin Survival Study Group, 1994. Randomized trial of cholesterol lowering in 4444 patients with coronary heart disease: the Scandinavian Simvastatin Survival Study (4S). Lancet 344, 1383–1389.

van Linschoten, R., van Middelkoop, M., Berger, M.Y., Heintjes, E.M., Verhaar, J.A., Willemsen, S.P., et al., 2009. Supervised exercise therapy versus usual care for patellofemoral pain syndrome: an open label randomised controlled trial. BMJ 339, b4074.

Chapter 7

Doll, R., Peto, R., Wheatley, K., Gray, R., Sutherland, I., 1994. Mortality in relation to smoking: 40 years' observations on male British doctors. BMJ 309, 901–911.

Chapter 8

Doll, R., Hill, A.B., 1950. Smoking and carcinoma of the lung. BMJ 2 (4682), 739–748.

Imazio, M., Brucato, A., Maestroni, S., Cumetti, D., Belli, R., Trinchero, R., et al., 2011. Risk of constrictive pericarditis after acute pericarditis. Circulation 124, 1270–1275.

Chapter 9

Walsh, J.P., Bremner, A.P., Bulsara, M.K., O'Leary, P., Leedman, P.J., Feddema, P., et al., 2005. Subclinical thyroid dysfunction as a risk factor for cardiovascular disease. Arch. Intern. Med. 165, 2467–2472.

Chapter 10

Alter, D.A., Naylor, C.D., Austin, P., Tu, J.V., 1999. Effects of socioeconomic status on access to invasive cardiac procedures and on mortality after acute myocardial infarction. N. Engl. J. Med. 341, 1359–1367.

Alter, D.A., Chong, A., Austin, P.C., Mustard, C., Iron, K., Williams, J.I., et al., 2006. Socioeconomic status and mortality after acute myocardial infarction. Ann. Intern. Med. 144, 82–93.

Chapter 11

Barnard, C.L., 1967. A human cardiac transplant: an interim report of a human successful operation performed at Groote Schuur Hospital, Cape Town. SAMJ 41, 1271–1274.

Jones, H.B., 1847. Chemical pathology. Lancet 2, 88–92.

Jones, H.B., 1848. On a new substance occurring in the urine of a patient with mollities ossium. Philos. Trans. R. Soc. London 138, 55–62.

Macintyre, W., 1850. Cases of mollities and fragilitas ossium, accompanied with urine strongly charged with animal matter. Medical and Chirurgical Transactions of London 33, 211–232.

McBride, W.G., 1961. Thalidomide and congenital abnormalities. Lancet 2, 1358.

Chapter 12

Wright, E.B., Holcombe, C., Salmon, P., 2004. Doctors' communication of trust, care and respect in breast cancer: qualitative study. BMJ 328, 864.

Chapter 13

Driver, J.A., Beiser, A., Au, R., Kreger, B.E., Splansky, G.L., Kurth, T., et al., 2012. Inverse association between cancer and Alzheimer's disease: results from the Framingham Heart Study. BMJ 344, e1442.

Chapter 14

Detrano, R., Gianrossi, R., Froelicher, V., 1989. The diagnostic accuracy of the exercise electrocardiogram: a meta-analysis of 22 years of research. Prog. Cardiovasc. Dis. 32 (3), 173–206.

Gibbons, R.J., Balady, G.J., Beasley, J.W., Bricker, J.T., Duvernoy, W.F., Froelicher, V.F., et al., 1997. ACC/AHA Guidelines for Exercise Testing. A report of the American College of Cardiology/American Heart Association Task Force on Practice Guidelines (Committee on Exercise Testing). Circulation 96, 345–354.

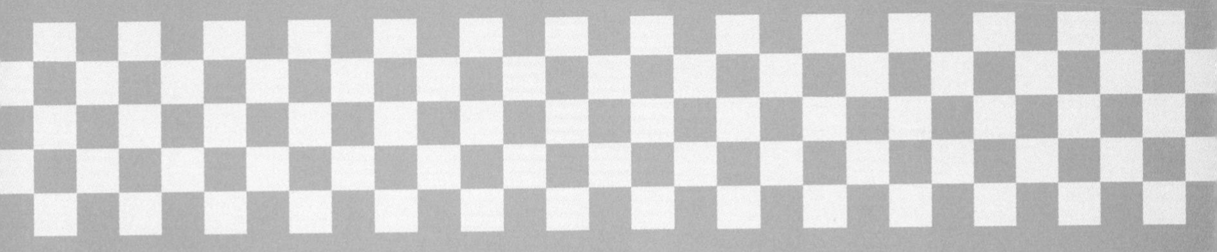

SELF-ASSESSMENT

Single best answer (SBA) questions

1. Which one of the following types of studies is considered the gold standard to assess the benefits and harms of a therapy?
   A) Case–control study
   B) Cohort study
   C) Randomised controlled trial
   D) Case report
   E) Ecological study.

2. A total of 1234 patients known to have a disease were tested using a new diagnostic test and 567 patients test positive. Furthermore, 1234 patients without the disease were tested and 1145 return a negative result. Which of the following statements is true regarding the outcome of this analysis?
   A) The sensitivity of the new diagnostic test is 54.1%.
   B) The specificity of the new diagnostic test is 7.2%.
   C) The positive predictive value of the new diagnostic test is 13.6%.
   D) The negative predictive value of the new diagnostic test is 63.2%.
   E) The sensitivity of the new diagnostic test is 41.9%.

3. Case reports are most useful when:
   A) The sample size of your study is large.
   B) Determining a cause–effect relationship between an intervention and outcome.
   C) Developing new practice guidelines.
   D) Unknown manifestations of a known disease are identified.
   E) The sample size of your study is small.

4. A case series:
   A) Is a type of observational study useful for identifying similar or differing characteristics between selected cases.
   B) Can be prospective or retrospective and usually involves only a small number of individuals.
   C) Is a descriptive study that reports on data from a group of individuals who have a similar disease or condition.
   D) A and C only.
   E) A, B and C.

5. You review the long-term complications of a new anti-diabetic treatment for patients with type 2 diabetes mellitus. A study of 5000 patients (2500 treatment, 2500 control) showed there were 114 myocardial infarctions in the treatment group and 61 myocardial infarctions in the control group over the 3-year study period. Which of the following statements is true?
   A) 47 patients would need to be treated for 1 year with the new anti-diabetic drug to cause 1 extra myocardial infarction.
   B) 53 patients would need to be treated for 3 years with the new anti-diabetic drug to prevent 1 extra myocardial infarction.
   C) 47 patients would need to be treated for 3 years with the new anti-diabetic drug to cause 1 extra myocardial infarction.
   D) 53 patients would need to be treated for 1 year with the new anti-diabetic drug to cause 1 extra myocardial infarction.
   E) 47 patients would need to be treated for 3 years with the new anti-diabetic drug to prevent 1 extra myocardial infarction.

6. In a cardiovascular disease prevention trial, patients were randomised to receive either aspirin or a matching placebo and then to either beta-carotene or a different matching placebo. What type of study design has been employed?
   A) Cross-over trial
   B) Superiority trial
   C) Factorial trial
   D) Cluster trial
   E) Equivalence trial.

7. A new blood test for diagnosing patients with syphilis infection was trialled in a high prevalence syphilis population. The specificity and sensitivity of the test were found to be 97 and 88%, respectively. The health authorities are thinking about trialling the new test in a population with a low prevalence of syphilis. How will this affect the performance of the diagnostic test?
   A) The sensitivity of the test will be lower in the low prevalence population.
   B) The negative predictive value is higher in the low prevalence population.
   C) The specificity of the test will be higher in the low prevalence population.
   D) The positive predictive value is higher in the low prevalence population.
   E) There is no change to the sensitivity, specificity, negative predictive value or positive predictive value.

8. Researchers have recently discovered a new neurological disorder that typically presents in healthcare professionals aged over 50 years. However, it is rare with a prevalence of 1 in 60 000 individuals. Little is known about the aetiology of the disease; however, it has been postulated to be due to long-term exposure to excessive amounts of caffeine. In order to test this hypothesis, which of the following study designs would be most useful?
   A) Randomised controlled trial
   B) Prospective cohort study

C) Case–control study
D) Case report
E) Retrospective cohort study.

9. Amitopril, a new angiotensin converting enzyme inhibitor (ACEi) drug has recently been licenced, marketed and made available for all patients with hypertension in the UK. The next step is to gather information on whether the drug can be used in combination with other anti-hypertensive treatments. Which clinical trial phase is warranted?
A) Phase I trial
B) Phase II trial
C) Phase III trial
D) Phase IV trial
E) Pre-clinical trial.

10. In a study investigating the clinical effectiveness of amitopril, a new angiotensin converting enzyme inhibitor (ACEi) drug, blood pressure measurements were taken prior to administering amitopril and repeated in the same subjects 1 month later. What statistical test should be used to test the hypothesis that amitopril lowers blood pressure?
A) Unpaired *t*-test
B) Chi-squared test
C) Mann–Whitney U test
D) Fisher's exact test
E) Paired *t*-test.

11. In a randomised controlled trial investigating the clinical effectiveness of amitopril, a new angiotensin converting enzyme inhibitor (ACEi), patients with hypertension were randomised to either amitopril or ramipril (the gold standard ACEi). Blood pressure measurements were taken in both treatment groups 1 year following the start of the study. A statistical test comparing blood pressure measurements in both treatment groups showed there was no statistically significant difference between the two groups. The study investigators failed to carry out sample size calculations at the start of the study. It is therefore possible that the study did not have enough power to detect a difference in blood pressure between the two treatment groups (if there truly is a difference to detect). The power refers:
A) To the sample size of the study.
B) To the probability of a type 2 error.
C) To the probability of not making a type 1 error.
D) To the probability of a type 1 error.
E) To the probability of not making a type 2 error.

12. Which of the following is not an example of a ratio variable?
A) Speed (in m/s)
B) Weight (in kg)
C) Age (in years)
D) Height (in cm)
E) Pain scale (0–5).

13. Which of the following is not true about the probability density function of the normal distribution?
A) Symmetrical about the mean
B) Defined by the variance of the population
C) Defined by the mean of the population
D) Bell-shaped
E) Becomes less peaked as the variance decreases.

14. Which of the following is not true about positively skewed distributions?
A) The mass of the distribution is concentrated on the left.
B) The median of the distribution is lower than the mode.
C) There is a long tail to the right.
D) The mean of the distribution is greater than the median.
E) The F-distribution has a positively skewed distribution.

15. The following data are on the length of stay (in days) following admission for an acute myocardial infarction in a sample of 10 patients:

6 12 6 2 17 11 6 3 21 5

Which of the following measures is correct?
A) Mean = 9.8 days
B) Mode = 21 days
C) Range = 23 days
D) Standard deviation = 2.6 days
E) Variance = 38.8 days^2.

16. A total of 4000 women attended their local breast cancer screening service and were found to not have breast cancer. Over the following 3 years, 39 of these women were diagnosed with breast cancer. The incidence rate of breast cancer among the 4000 women is:
A) 975 cases
B) 975 cases per 100 000 person-years
C) 39 cases per 4000 person-years
D) 325 cases per 100 000 person-years
E) 325 cases.

17. We measure the body weight of a sample of 100 patients admitted to hospital with a myocardial infarction. Below is a table of summary statistics of this sample:

Mean (kg)	Median (kg)	Range (kg)	Standard deviation (kg)
71.4	70.4	60.4–81.4	9.4

We expect 95% of patients in the population to have a body weight between:
A) 50.5 and 70.4 kg
B) 44.5 and 88.5 kg
C) 55.5 and 85.4 kg
D) 53.0 and 89.8 kg
E) 60.4 and 81.4 kg.

18. The I^2 statistic:
A) Is commonly used in case–control studies.
B) Is larger if there is more heterogeneity between studies.
C) Provides an estimate of the proportion of the total variation in effect estimates that is due to homogeneity between studies.
D) Is based on the *z* statistic.
E) Ranges from 0 to 1.

19. The fixed effects meta-analysis:
A) Is used when there is evidence of statistical heterogeneity between the studies.
B) Assumes that different studies are estimating different true population exposure effects.
C) Assumes that there is a single underlying 'true' effect that each study is estimating.
D) Gives more weight to the smaller studies.
E) Calculates the weight using the square of the variance of the exposure effect estimate.

20. A research group performed a meta-analysis of case–control and cohort studies investigating whether an association exists between cardiovascular risk factors and venous thromboembolism (VTE). Twenty-one case–control or cohort studies were included, showing the risk of VTE was 1.51 for hypertension, 1.42 for diabetes mellitus and 2.33 for obesity. The group wished to determine whether the findings of the meta-analysis are robust to the methodology used to obtain them. The analysis performed involves omitting low-quality studies. What type of analysis did the research group perform?
A) Sensitivity analysis
B) Quality analysis
C) Subgroup analysis
D) Random effects meta-analysis
E) Fixed effects meta-analysis.

21. One of the greatest limitations with systematic reviews is that not all studies carried out are published. The main graphical method used for identifying publication bias is by constructing a:
A) Dot plot
B) Funnel plot
C) Bar chart
D) Histogram
E) Forest plot.

22. In men with benign prostatic hyperplasia, is laser prostatectomy superior to transurethral resection of the prostate with regards to symptom relief? There is currently no evidence that one procedure is more effective than the other. What is the most appropriate research design to investigate this research question?
A) Case–control study
B) Case report
C) Cohort study
D) Cross-sectional study
E) Randomised controlled trial.

23. A research group investigates whether smoking causes a rare blood disorder known as bloodophilia. What is the most appropriate research design to investigate this hypothesis?
A) Case report
B) Cohort study
C) Case–control study
D) Randomised controlled trial
E) Cross-sectional study.

24. In prospective cohort studies, the biggest drawback is:
A) Loss to follow-up
B) Recruiting enough patients for the study
C) Inability to tolerate the intervention
D) Confounding
E) Expense.

25. In randomised controlled trials, the main aim of randomisation is to:
A) Reduce cost
B) Reduce confounding
C) Reduce bias
D) Increase the external validity of the results
E) Reduce the number of patients lost to follow-up.

26. You are interested in investigating whether an association exists between head circumference at birth and IQ at the age of 45 years. What is the most appropriate research design to investigate this research hypothesis?
A) Randomised controlled trial
B) Case–control study
C) Retrospective cohort study
D) Ecological study
E) Prospective cohort study.

27. A randomised controlled trial randomly allocated patients with hypertension to either a new anti-hypertensive drug or a placebo drug. Two months following the start of the trial, blood pressure measurements were significantly lower in the new treatment group than in the placebo group ($P = 0.023$). However, at the start of the study, the average body mass index (BMI) of patients in the new drug group was lower than the BMI of patients in the placebo drug group. This difference in BMI between the two groups may have contributed to the statistically significant difference observed in blood pressure measurements. When analysing the study results, which of the following is correct?
A) BMI is definitely not a confounding factor so the results must be correct.
B) BMI may be a confounding variable and should be corrected for using a stratified analysis approach.
C) All patients in both groups with a BMI greater than 30 (considered as obese) should be excluded from the study analysis.
D) BMI may be a confounding factor so the trial should be repeated ensuring that recruitment is restricted to those patients with a BMI less than 30.

E) As the trial is randomised, the results must be correct and the differences in BMI between the two treatment groups can be ignored.

28. A large multicentre randomised controlled trial was conducted on patients newly diagnosed with breast cancer to evaluate the effect of a new breast cancer drug on 6-month mortality compared with standard drug treatment. The results of the trial are presented below. What statistical test should be used to compare the outcome between the two treatments?

	Alive at 6 months		Total
	Yes	No	
New drug	412	88	500
Standard drug	354	146	500
Total	766	234	1000

A) Fisher's exact test
B) Unpaired *t*-test
C) Chi-squared test
D) Quality-adjusted life year (QALY) analysis
E) Paired *t*-test.

29. A doctor hypothesises that gas emissions from a newly opened factory are causing the recent increase in the number of patients admitted to the local hospital with a respiratory disease. Which of the following factors would most strongly implicate the causal relationship between the gas emissions and respiratory disease?
A) Temporarily closing the factory for 2 months had no impact on the incidence of respiratory disease in the local area.
B) The duration of exposure to the gas emission is related to the risk of respiratory disease.
C) There are no previous studies at other locations to investigate whether a causal relationship exists.
D) No potential biological mechanism has been identified.
E) The incidence of respiratory disease increased before the factory opened.

30. Any excess risk of exposure (associated with an occupation) is likely to be underestimated if the unexposed group includes subjects from the general population. The relative risk of the occupational exposure on the disease outcome will therefore be underestimated. This is because, in general:
A) The general population is healthier than the working population.
B) The unexposed group is healthier than the exposed group.
C) The working population is healthier than the general population.
D) There is no difference between the health of the general population and the working population.
E) There is no difference between the health of the exposed and unexposed groups.

31. A recent meta-analysis showed that dietary supplementation with omega-3 fatty acids significantly reduced the odds of cardiovascular deaths (odds ratio [OR]: 0.87, 95% confidence interval [CI]: 0.79–0.95, $P=0.002$). An odds ratio of 0.87 means:
A) Omega-3 fatty acids reduce the odds of cardiovascular deaths by 87%.
B) Omega-3 fatty acids reduce the odds of cardiovascular deaths by 87 times.
C) Omega-3 fatty acids reduce the odds of cardiovascular deaths by 13%.
D) Omega-3 fatty acids reduce the odds of cardiovascular deaths by 13 times.
E) Omega-3 fatty acids increase the odds of cardiovascular deaths by 87%.

32. In a case–control study, men aged between 50 and 60 years with lung cancer were selected as cases. How many control subjects should be selected?
A) One control should be selected for every case.
B) Two controls should be selected for every case.
C) Three controls should be selected for every case.
D) Four controls should be selected for every case.
E) Five controls should be selected for every case.

33. Which of the following statements is not true about the odds ratio and risk ratio?
A) When the disease is not rare, the odds ratio can underestimate the risk ratio.
B) Odds and odds ratio are usually calculated in case–control studies.
C) When the disease is rare, the odds ratio is approximately equal to the risk ratio.
D) Risk and risk ratio are usually calculated in cohort studies.
E) In general, the odds ratio is interpreted in the same way as the risk ratio.

34. A case–control study investigates the association between smoking and myocardial infarction (MI). If cases who were smokers die more quickly, there will be a lower frequency of smokers amongst the remaining cases. This will:
A) Underestimate the association between smoking and myocardial infarction. This will confound the study results.
B) Have no effect on the association between smoking and myocardial infarction.
C) Overestimate the association between smoking and myocardial infarction. This will bias the study results.
D) Overestimate the association between smoking and myocardial infarction. This will confound the study results.
E) Underestimate the association between smoking and myocardial infarction. This will bias the study results.

35. A population initially contains 30 000 people free of disease and 1324 people develop diabetes (300 have type 1 diabetes and 1024 people have type 2 diabetes) over 2 years of observation. The incidence risk of type 1 diabetes over the 2-year period was:
A) 1.7%
B) 1.0%
C) 4.4%
D) 0.05%
E) 0.5%.

36. To assist with health resource allocation decisions, a research group set out to determine the burden of a particular disease in the population. Which type of study should be undertaken?
A) Randomised controlled trial
B) Ecological study
C) Cohort study
D) Cross-sectional study
E) Case–control study.

37. A research group distributes a health survey to investigate the prevalence of depression in West London. Only 70% of the study population replied to the survey. Which factor is not associated with a low response rate?
A) Alcohol or drug misuse
B) More unwell
C) Male sex
D) Younger age
E) Higher socioeconomic status.

38. The graph underneath shows the mortality rate from stroke according to cholesterol level for four different countries. The scatter for each country displays the association between cholesterol level and stroke mortality rate at an individual level. Regarding the association between cholesterol level and stroke mortality rate, there is:

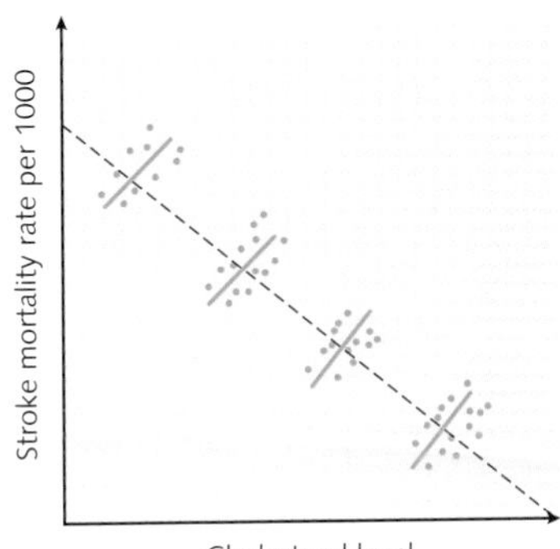

A) No association
B) No ecological fallacy
C) Ecological fallacy – negative bias
D) Ecological fallacy – positive bias
E) Ecological fallacy – reversal of association.

39. In a prospective cohort study investigating the association between drinking alcohol and liver disease amongst bartenders, the crude incidence risk ratio was 3.8. The investigators stratify the data according to smoking status. The stratum specific risk ratio of liver disease amongst bartenders who drink alcohol was 4.6 in smokers and 1.9 in non-smokers. Which of the following statements is true?
A) There is no association between drinking alcohol and liver disease.
B) Smoking status is a confounding factor.
C) Alcohol intake is an effect modifier.
D) Smoking status is an effect modifier.
E) Alcohol intake is a confounding factor.

40. In qualitative research, which of the following refers to reviewing and analysing the data in conjunction with data collection?
A) Saturation point
B) Deductive approach
C) Quota sampling
D) Iterative approach
E) Triangulation.

41. In a qualitative study of chronic heart failure patients' understanding of their symptoms and drug therapy, all but one participant described how prescribed medications had improved their symptoms. This one patient attributed his symptom improvement to a herbal remedy. When analysing the data, all cases were reviewed. What type of sampling method was used?
A) Quota sampling
B) Negative sampling
C) Snowball sampling
D) Maximum variation sampling
E) Positive sampling.

42. A qualitative study is carried out to investigate the attitudes of medical students on the feedback they receive from their medical school on exam performance. The researchers openly acknowledge (and address) that the relationship among the researchers, the research topic and subjects may have influenced the study results. This concept is known as:
A) Triangulation
B) Iteration
C) Grounding
D) Reflexivity
E) Transferability.

43. In a clinical audit, current clinical practice should be compared to a defined set of explicit criteria. Which of the following descriptions of the explicit criteria is not true?
A) Reflect worst practice
B) Evidence-based
C) Measureable
D) Cover the structure of care
E) Cover the outcome of care.

44. Which of the following is not true about clinical audits?
A) Clinical audit is an ongoing process involving a number of audit cycles evaluating the same clinical standards.
B) The results are compared with standards that define best practice.
C) The results are generalizable.
D) Clinical audits never involve randomly allocating patients to different interventions.
E) The aim of clinical audit is to determine whether current local practice resembles best practice.

45. The majority of medical errors in healthcare practice are due to:
A) Individual errors
B) Faulty systems and processes
C) Team errors
D) Poor financial resources
E) Managerial errors.

46. A foundation doctor carries out a quality improvement project on access to out-patient appointments. As part of the project, she measures the average daily clinician hours available for appointments. What type of measure is she measuring?
A) Outcome measure
B) Sample measure
C) Balancing measure
D) Process measure
E) Population measure.

47. A pharmacist carries out a quality improvement project on the number of adverse drug events on the cardiology ward over the past month. She records that there were 8 drug events per 100 doses. Following a series of tutorials on 'good prescribing practice' for the junior doctors on the ward, the pharmacist checks to see whether this education may have led to a reduction in the number of adverse drug events, again on the cardiology ward. What type of measure is the pharmacist measuring?
A) Outcome measure
B) Sample measure
C) Balancing measure
D) Process measure
E) Practice measure.

48. A medical student at East Hospital carries out a quality improvement project assessing the average HbA1c level in a population of patients with diabetes. Having carried out a number of Plan-Do-Study-Act cycles, there is a gradual improvement in the average HbA1c level compared to baseline. A registrar at West Hospital wishes to implement similar changes at his hospital setting. Which one of the following statements is correct?
A) There will be more resistance by healthcare staff to repeat the project at West Hospital as the changes have been already shown to be effective at East Hospital.
B) The registrar should repeat the quality improvement project at West Hospital, despite there being evidence that the changes were effective at East Hospital.
C) As the changes were shown to be cost-effective at East Hospital, the changes will be cost-effective at West Hospital.
D) Considering the changes led to an improvement in the average HbA1c level in the population of patients at East Hospital, there will be a similar improvement in the average HbA1c level in the population of patients at West Hospital.
E) When implementing changes 'on a large scale', it is unnecessary to first test the changes out on a smaller scale.

49. Which of the following is an agreed method of assessing the quality of reporting systematic reviews and meta-analyses?
A) NHS
B) WHO
C) PRISMA
D) CONSORT
E) NICE.

50. The most clinically useful measure that helps inform the likelihood of having a disease in a patient with a positive result from a diagnostic test is the:
A) Sensitivity
B) Confidence interval
C) Specificity
D) Positive predictive value
E) *P*-value.

51. A recent trial shows that a new asthma treatment reduces the annual rate of admissions for acute exacerbations of asthma by 25% compared to placebo. How many patients will need to be treated to prevent one admission?
A) 50
B) 4
C) 5
D) 40
E) 6.

52. A research group wishes to determine whether drug A is more cost-effective than drug B in treating depression. They gather the following information about each treatment:

Treatment	Cost	Effect (number of weeks patient has no depression)
Drug A	£7000	70 weeks
Drug B	£13 000	80 weeks

What is the cost effectiveness ratio for drug B?
A) £100/week
B) £50/week
C) £325/week
D) £35/week
E) £162.50/week.

53. Using the data presented in Question 52, what is the incremental cost-effectiveness ratio (ICER) for drug B?
A) £1000 per additional week free of depression
B) £450 per additional week free of depression
C) £30 per additional week free of depression
D) £1200 per additional week free of depression
E) £600 per additional week free of depression.

54. Based on the study discussed in Question 52, the NHS trust decides to finance drug B instead of drug A for first-line drug treatment of depression. The opportunity cost is:
A) The cost (financial and non-financial) of providing drug A as a second-line drug treatment for depression.
B) The cost (financial and non-financial) of what is lost when drug A is not provided as first-line drug treatment for depression.
C) The cost (only financial) of what is lost when drug A is not provided as first-line drug treatment for depression.
D) The cost (financial and non-financial) of providing drug B instead of drug A as first-line drug treatment for depression.
E) The cost (only financial) of providing drug A as a second-line drug treatment for depression.

55. When assessing the validity of a diagnostic study it is important to consider whether the study design may have been affected by potential biases. Partial verification bias:
A) Occurs when only cases with a limited range of disease spectrum are recruited for the study.
B) Occurs when the decision to perform the reference test on an individual is based on the results of the diagnostic study test.
C) May be avoided if the study test is always performed prior to the reference test.
D) Occurs when different reference tests are used to verify the results of the study test.
E) Can always be prevented if a diagnostic study is carefully designed.

56. A research group wishes to determine the diagnostic accuracy of the two verbally asked questions for screening for depression:
1) During the past month have you often been bothered by feeling down, depressed, or hopeless?
2) During the past month have you often been bothered by little interest or pleasure in doing things?

The group compared the performance of this study test against the International Classification of Disease (ICD) diagnostic criteria (reference test). Using the data in the following table, what is the sensitivity of the two-question screening test for depression?

		ICD depression diagnostic criteria: depression?		**Total**
		Yes	**No**	
Two-question screen: depression?	Yes	44	140	184
	No	9	307	316
	Total	53	447	500

A) 17.0%
B) 100.0%
C) 75.7%
D) 83.0%
E) 91.4%.

57. Using the data in the table presented in Question 56, what is the specificity of the two-question screening test for depression?
A) 68.7%
B) 91.3%
C) 84.0%
D) 15.0%
E) 76.9%.

58. Suppose a 44-year-old woman answers 'yes' to both the screening questions for depression, as stated in Question 56. The prevalence of depression in the population is 10%. Using the data in the table presented in Question 56, what is the probability of her actually having depression?
A) 93.4%
B) 23.9%
C) 29.6%
D) 10.0%
E) 68.4%.

59. The table below displays a contingency table with the results of a randomised controlled trial investigating the incidence of coronary artery restenosis within 3 months after angioplasty with either a bare metal stent (control group) or drug-eluting stent (intervention group). What is the expected frequency, if there is no difference between the two treatments, for the number of patients randomised to the bare metal stent who get coronary artery restenosis within 3 months after angioplasty?

		Restenosis within 3 months after angioplasty		Total
		Yes	No	
Treatment group	Drug-eluting stent	124	301	425
	Bare metal stent	155	270	425
	Total	279	571	850

A) 155
B) 139.5
C) 69.75
D) 279
E) 279.

60. Which one of the following statements about study sample size is correct when considering the most appropriate statistical test for your data?

A) When the sample size of a study is small, parametric tests are robust when analysing data that do not follow a Gaussian distribution.
B) When the sample size of a study is small, normality tests have high power to detect whether a sample comes from a Gaussian distribution.
C) When the sample size of a study is small, non-parametric tests have little power to detect a significant difference.
D) When the sample size is large, non-parametric tests have much less power than parametric tests when analysing data that follow a Gaussian distribution.
E) When dealing with large sample sizes, the decision to choose a parametric or non-parametric test matters more.

Extended matching questions (EMQs)

1. Describing the frequency distribution

A. Median
B. Range
C. Arithmetic mean
D. Reference range
E. Inter-quartile range
F. Standard deviation
G. Standard error
H. Geometric mean
I. Confidence interval
J. Mode

For each of the following definitions, select the appropriate answer from the list of options. Each option may be used once, more then once, or not at all.

1. Adding up all the values in a set of observations and dividing this by the number of values in that set.
2. The middle value when the data are arranged in order of size.
3. A measure of the spread (or scatter) of sample means around the true population mean.
4. The range of values that includes the middle 50% of values when the data are arranged in order of size.
5. A measure of the spread (or scatter) of observations about the mean.

2. Randomised controlled trials

A. Cluster trial
B. Blinding
C. Clinical equipoise
D. Randomisation
E. Allocation concealment
F. Selection bias
G. Measurement bias
H. Factorial trial
I. Cross-over trial
J. Superiority trial

For each of the following definitions/statements, select the appropriate answer from the list of options. Each option may be used once, more then once, or not at all.

1. The patients and the investigators enrolling the patients cannot foresee treatment group assignment.
2. The patients and investigators (including those involved in recruitment and assessing the outcome) have no knowledge of treatment allocation.
3. Healthcare professionals treating the patients have sufficient doubt about the relative effectiveness of the treatments being compared in the randomised controlled trial.
4. In a trial in which patients were randomised to receive the intervention ($n = 100$) or usual care ($n = 100$), 6 months of follow-up were achieved for 70 and 91 patients, respectively.
5. In a specific type of trial, groups of patients, clinics or communities are randomised to receive the intervention or a control.

3. Types of variables

A. Nominal
B. Distribution
C. Qualitative
D. Ratio
E. Discrete
F. Multinomial
G. Ordinal
H. Frequency
I. Interval
J. Dichotomous

For each of the following examples of variables, select the *best-suited* type of variable it represents from the list of options. Each option may be used once, more then once, or not at all.

1. Gender
2. Dates
3. Disease staging
4. Height
5. Marital status, i.e. single, married, divorced

4. Calculating the strength of an association

A. 0.541
B. −0.413
C. 0.133

D. 13.1
E. 0.493
F. 0.154
G. 0.184
H. 0.602
I. 11.2
J. −0.333

A hypothetical randomised controlled trial set out to examine the effect of a new cholesterol-lowering drug, statstatin, on the incidence of myocardial infarction in patients with high cholesterol. In total, 1000 patients with high cholesterol were randomised to receive either the intervention, statstatin ($n=500$) or usual treatment for high cholesterol, simvastatin ($n=500$), with 5-year follow-up data obtained for 450 and 465 patients, respectively. The primary outcome was the proportion of patients who suffered a myocardial infarction during the follow-up period. Of those who received statstatin, 60 patients had a myocardial infarction compared to 103 patients from the simvastatin group.

For each of the following questions, select the appropriate answer from the list of options. Each option may be used once, more then once, or not at all.

1. What are the odds of having a myocardial infarction in the statstatin group?
2. What is the risk of having a myocardial infarction in the statstatin group?
3. What is the odds ratio of having a myocardial infarction in the statstatin group compared to the simvastatin group?
4. What is the risk ratio of having a myocardial infarction in the statstatin group compared to the simvastatin group?
5. What is the number needed to treat with statstatin instead of simvastatin to prevent one myocardial infarction?

5. Extrapolating from sample to population – working with proportions

A. −12.4 to −4.6%
B. 18.4 to 26.0%
C. −13.8 to −4.0%
D. 16.8 to 28.4%
E. 10.2 to 16.4%
F. −8.9%
G. −4.45%
H. 34.5 to 47.5%
I. Chi-squared test
J. Unpaired *t*-test

The results of a randomised controlled trial examining the effect of a new cholesterol-lowering drug, statstatin, on the 5-year incidence of myocardial infarction in patients with high cholesterol are as follows:

	Myocardial infarction	No myocardial infarction	Total
Statstatin	60	390	450
Simvastatin	103	362	465
Total	163	752	915

For each of the following questions, select the appropriate answer from the list of options. Each option may be used once, more then once, or not at all.

1. What is the 95% confidence interval of the percentage of cases of myocardial infarction in the statstatin group?
2. What is the 95% confidence interval of the percentage of cases of myocardial infarction in the simvastatin group?
3. What is the difference between the percentage of cases of myocardial infarction in the two treatment groups?
4. What is the 95% confidence interval of the difference in the percentage of cases of myocardial infarction in the two treatment groups?
5. What statistical test should be used to compare the percentage of cases of myocardial infarction in the two treatment groups?

6. Extrapolating from sample to population – working with means

A. −0.6
B. 0.0227
C. 0.0113
D. 0.0233
E. 0.5
F. −0.65 to −0.55
G. 0.32 to 0.42
H. One-way ANOVA
I. Paired *t*-test
J. Unpaired *t*-test

A hypothetical randomised controlled trial was set out to examine the effect of a new cholesterol-lowering drug, statstatin, on the incidence of myocardial infarction in patients with high cholesterol. In total, 1000 patients with high cholesterol were randomised to receive either the intervention, statstatin ($n=500$) or usual treatment for high cholesterol, simvastatin ($n=500$), with 5-year follow-up data obtained for 450 and 465 patients, respectively. The mean cholesterol level (and standard deviation) 5 years after the start of the study was 3.6 mmol/L (0.24 mmol/L) and 4.2 mmol/L (0.49 mmol/L) in the statstatin and simvastatin groups, respectively.

For each of the following questions, select the appropriate answer from the list of options. Each option may be used once, more then once, or not at all.

1. What is the standard error of the mean cholesterol level in the statstatin group?
2. What is the standard error of the mean cholesterol level in the simvastatin group?
3. What is the difference between the mean cholesterol level in the two treatment groups?
4. What is the 95% confidence interval of the difference in mean cholesterol level in the two treatment groups?
5. Assuming the data follow a normal distribution, what statistical test should be used to compare the mean cholesterol level in the two treatment groups?

7. Meta-analyses

A. Subgroup analysis
B. Forest plot
C. −15, 95% CI −20 to −10
D. 0, 95% CI −30 to 20
E. Fixed effects
F. Funnel plot
G. Statistical heterogeneity
H. −25, 95% CI −30 to −20
I. Random effects
J. Sensitivity analysis

A research group performs a meta-analysis of clinical trials investigating the effect of group exercise versus a single workout routine on systolic systemic blood pressure. The figure underneath presents the results of the meta-analysis.

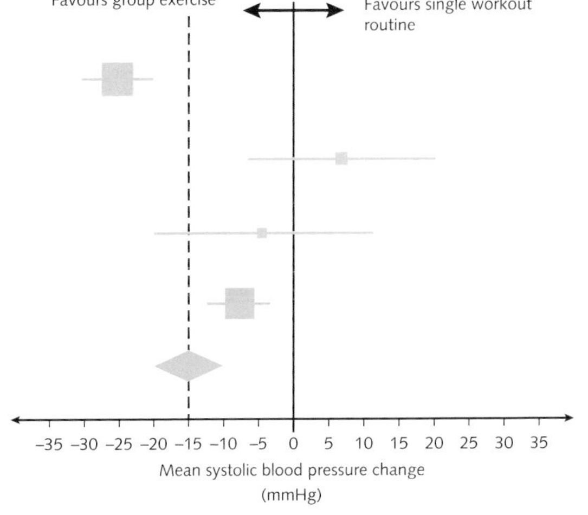

For each of the following questions, select the appropriate answer from the list of options. Each option may be used once, more then once, or not at all.

1. What is the name of the plot shown in the figure?
2. Considering the I^2 statistic calculated showed no evidence of heterogeneity between the studies, what method was used to calculate the pooled estimate?
3. What is the summary effect estimate of the meta-analysis?
4. What type of plot should the research group construct in order to detect any potential publication bias?
5. The investigators feel that two of the trials included in the meta-analysis are of low quality. What type of analysis should the research group perform to determine whether the meta-analysis findings are robust after excluding these low-quality studies?

8. Measures of disease occurrence

A. Analytical cross-sectional study
B. Case–control study
C. 0.025
D. 19.8%
E. 0.25
F. Descriptive cross-sectional study
G. 9.2%
H. 80.2%
I. 0.11
J. 90.8%

Patients registered with a number of GP practices were, with their consent, interviewed by telephone to ascertain whether they were depressed and whether they engaged in online social networking.

		Depression		Total
		Yes	**No**	
Social networking profile	Yes	40	394	434
	No	130	32	162
	Total	170	426	596

For each of the following questions, select the appropriate answer from the list of options. Each option may be used once, more then once or not at all.

1. What study design was used to investigate the burden of depression amongst subjects with and without an online social networking profile?
2. What is the prevalence of depression in subjects who have a social networking profile?

3. What is the prevalence of depression in subjects who don't have a social networking profile?
4. What is the prevalence odds ratio?
5. What is the prevalence ratio?

9. Qualitative studies

A. Snowball sampling
B. Maximum variation sampling
C. Reliability
D. Participant observation
E. Negative sampling
F. Focus group
G. In-depth interview
H. Reflexivity
I. Transferability
J. Quota sampling

For each of the following definitions/statements, select the appropriate title from the list of options. Each option may be used once, more then once, or not at all.

1. Collecting data on naturally occurring behaviours of participants in their usual setting.
2. Using study participants as informants to identify other people who could potentially participate in the study.
3. Searching for unusual or atypical cases.
4. During the design phase of the study, a decision is made on how many people with certain characteristics are to be included as study participants.
5. The researcher reflects on whether his or her values and attributes may have influenced (or biased) any stages of the study.

10. Confounding

A. 3.0
B. Sensitivity analysis
C. Case–control
D. Stratification
E. Cohort
F. Cross-sectional
G. Hip fracture
H. Death
I. 2.01
J. 0.03
K. There is a strong association between bedsores and death.
L. There is a weak association between bedsores and death.
M. There is no association between bedsores and death.

A research group carries out a study investigating whether an association exists between the development of new bedsores and death among patients admitted to the orthopaedic ward with neck of femur fractures. All such admissions were included in the study. The study participants were then followed up during their hospital stay to see whether they survived until discharge. The study results are shown in the table underneath.

		Death		**Total**
		Yes	**No**	
Bed sores	Yes	32	202	234
	No	35	733	768
	Total	67	935	1002

For each of the following questions, select the appropriate answer from the list of options. Each option may be used once, more then once, or not at all.

1. What study design was used to investigate the association between bedsores and death?
2. What is the risk ratio?
3. The research group suspected that those patients with many co-morbidities were more likely to acquire bedsores than those with a few or no co-morbidities. To be considered as a confounding variable, the co-morbidity variable must also be associated with which variable?
4. All patients recruited were categorised into two separate subgroups (medically unwell versus medically well) based on the number/severity of their co-morbid conditions. A table similar to that above was subsequently constructed for each subgroup. What is the name of this type of analysis?
5. The risk ratio for death in the presence of bedsores was 1.02 in the medically unwell subgroup and 1.0 in the medically well subgroup. What conclusion can be reached from the study results?

11. Screening

A. 8813
B. 10 000
C. 99.95%
D. 8809
E. 5%
F. 11.2%
G. 76
H. 63.32%
I. 6.40%
J. 0.05%

Mammography is a common imaging tool used as a first screen for breast cancer. Assume the sensitivity and specificity of mammography in the detection of breast cancer are 95% and 88.8%, respectively. Assume the total number of people being imaged for breast cancer is 10 000 and that the prevalence of breast cancer in the population is 0.8%. The following 2 × 2 table can be used to summarise this information:

		Breast cancer		Total
		Yes	No	
Mammography	Positive	a	b	$a+b$
	Negative	c	d	$c+d$
	Total	$a+c$	$b+d$	10 000

For each of the following questions, select the appropriate answer from the list of options. Each option may be used once, more then once, or not at all.

1. What is the type 1 error of using mammography to detect breast cancer?
2. What is the type 2 error of using mammography to detect breast cancer?
3. What is the value of $(c+d)$ from the table above?
4. What is the positive predictive value?
5. What is the negative predictive value?

12. Calculating the *P*-value

A. Mann–Whitney U test
B. Unpaired *t*-test
C. McNemar's test
D. One-sample *t*-test
E. One-way ANOVA test
F. Chi-squared test
G. Paired *t*-test
H. Repeated measures one-way ANOVA test
I. Kruskal–Wallis test

For each of the following studies, select the appropriate statistical test that should be used to analyse the data from the list of options. Each option may be used once, more then once, or not at all.

1. We have a sample of patients with coronary artery disease. We know that the serum level of triglyceride in healthy individuals has a geometric mean of 1.74 mmol/L. Is the average level in our sample of patients the same as the population value? Assume that the data are sampled from a population that follows a Gaussian (normal) distribution.
2. We carry out a randomised controlled trial investigating the incidence of coronary artery restenosis within 3 months after angioplasty with either a bare metal stent (control group) or drug-eluting stent (intervention group).
3. We carry out a prospective study investigating whether sulfasalazine can reduce ESR levels in patients with active rheumatoid arthritis. The ESR level gives us an indication of how active the rheumatic disease is in the body. ESR levels were measured at baseline (prior to administering sulfasalazine), and again at 3 and 6 months after treatment. The three standard deviations are fairly similar and a statistical test for normality shows that all three groups follow a normal distribution.
4. A random sample of 20 medical students have a mean IQ of 120, with a standard deviation of 8. A random sample of 20 dental students have a mean IQ of 110, with a standard deviation of 8. We want to know whether medical students are significantly more intelligent than dental students. Assume the IQs of both groups are normally distributed.
5. We carry out a study investigating whether the teaching style used (lecture-based versus problem-based) influences the mark (scored from 0 to 100) achieved by final year medical students for the medicine and surgery written exam. All questions asked in the exam are of equal difficulty. Twelve students are randomised to each teaching style and the exam results compared. The data do not follow a Gaussian distribution and the variances between the groups are unequal.

13. Economic evaluation

A. Cost–benefit analysis
B. Cost-utility analysis
C. Cost-minimisation analysis
D. 12.62
E. 14.53
F. 113,200
G. Treatment A is dominant over treatment B.
H. Treatment B is dominant over treatment A.
I. 2657
J. 4543

A research group conducted an economic evaluation alongside a randomised controlled trial comparing two different treatments for a medical condition. The Euro-Qol-5D questionnaire was used to measure the average health state in the 'no treatment', 'treatment A' and 'treatment B' groups. The mean lifetime additional costs for either treatment A or treatment B, compared to having no treatment, were also recorded. Relative to the 'no treatment' group, there was no improvement in the life expectancy in either treatment groups. This information can be summarised in the following table:

Treatment group	Life expectancy	EuroQol-5D health state	Health state score	Cost of treatment	QALYs
No treatment	17 years	33233	0.523	£0	8.89
Treatment A	17 years	11231	0.767	£11 000	13.03
Treatment B	First 12 years	11121	0.837	£16 900	
	Final 5 years	33333	0.516		

For each of the following questions, select the appropriate answer from the list of options. Each option may be used once, more then once, or not at all.

1. Calculate the QALYs gained for treatment B compared to having no treatment.
2. Which treatment is dominant over the other?
3. Calculate the ICER gained for treatment A compared to having no treatment.
4. Assuming that society are willing to pay £30 000 per QALY, calculate the net monetary benefit.
5. What type of economic evaluation study design was employed?

14. Bias

A. Confounding
B. Healthy worker effect bias
C. Berkson's bias
D. Loss-to-follow-up bias
E. Recall bias
F. Random misclassification bias
G. Follow-up bias
H. Non-response bias
I. Interviewer bias
J. Reverse causality

For each of the following scenarios, select the appropriate type of bias implicated from the list of options. Each option may be used once, more then once, or not at all.

1. A case–control study to investigate the association between passive smoking and asthma was conducted. Cases (newly diagnosed individuals with asthma) were compared with controls (random sample of individuals without asthma) with regard to exposure to smoke from smokers over the previous 15 years. What type of bias may occur when collecting these data?
2. A case–control study to investigate the association between smoking and diabetes was conducted. Hospitalised patients with diabetes (cases) were compared to hospitalised patients without diabetes (controls). Considering hospitals contain a higher proportion of smokers than the general population, what type of bias may occur?
3. A cohort study to investigate the association between smoking and hair loss was conducted. To measure the exposure status, subjects were classified into groups based on the number of cigarettes smoked per day. What type of bias may occur when collecting this data?
4. A randomised controlled trial to investigate the effect of a new treatment on hypertension was conducted. The investigator is aware of which treatment arm (intervention versus control) participants were randomised to. What type of bias may occur when the investigator takes blood pressure measurements from the study participants?
5. A randomised controlled trial where participants were randomised to medical or surgical therapy for benign prostatic hyperplasia was conducted. If patients undergoing surgical treatment do well (i.e. the symptoms of benign prostatic hypertrophy, such as intermittent micturition, resolve) and do not return for follow-up, what type of bias may be introduced?

15. Study design

A. Systematic review
B. Randomised controlled trial
C. Retrospective cohort study
D. Qualitative study
E. Ecological study
F. Case–control study
G. Prospective cohort study
H. Meta-analysis
I. Cross-sectional study
J. Case series

For each of the following studies, select the appropriate study design employed from the list of options. Each option may be used once, more then once, or not at all.

1. To determine whether selective serotonin-reuptake inhibitors (SSRIs) are implicated in the aetiology of persistent pulmonary hypertension, infants with the condition were matched with infants without pulmonary hypertension. Rates of past exposure to SSRIs were then recorded.
2. To determine the long-term effectiveness of the influenza vaccine in elderly people, vaccinated and unvaccinated individuals were recruited and followed up over time. Hospitalisation rates for pneumonia or influenza were recorded.

3. The effects of raloxifene on fracture risk in postmenopausal women were studied. Subjects were recruited and randomly allocated to either raloxifene or a placebo drug. The study participants were followed up over 5 years and new cases of vertebral fracture recorded in each group.
4. A retrospective review of the evidence for thrombolytic therapy in the prevention of myocardial infarction was carried out. The results from all studies identified were pooled together and a summary estimate calculated.
5. The relationship between an area measure of socioeconomic status and the density of fast-food outlets was determined. Different areas across England were compared.

SBA answers

1. **C** Using a randomised controlled trial (RCT) study design with effective randomisation and blinding is most useful when assessing the benefits and harms of a treatment. It is this process of randomisation that makes RCTs the most rigorous method for determining a cause–effect relationship between an intervention and outcome, thus placing RCTs at the top of the hierarchy of evidence compared to the other study design options.

2. **D** The sensitivity of the new diagnostic test

$$= \frac{\text{True positive}}{\text{True positive} + \text{False negative}}$$

$$= \frac{567}{567 + 667} = 45.9\%$$

The specificity of the new diagnostic test

$$= \frac{\text{True negative}}{\text{True negative} + \text{False positive}}$$

$$= \frac{1145}{1145 + 89} = 92.8\%$$

The positive predictive value of the new diagnostic test

$$= \frac{\text{True positive}}{\text{True positive} + \text{False positive}}$$

$$= \frac{567}{567 + 89} = 86.4\%$$

The negative predictive value of the new diagnostic test

$$= \frac{\text{True negative}}{\text{True negative} + \text{False negative}}$$

$$= \frac{1145}{1145 + 667} = 63.2\%$$

3. **D** Most case reports and case series cover one of six topics:
   1. Identifying and describing new diseases.
   2. Identifying rare or unique manifestations of known diseases.
   3. Audit, quality improvement and medical education.
   4. Understanding the pathogenesis of a disease.
   5. Detecting new drug side effects, both beneficial and adverse.
   6. Reporting unique therapeutic approaches.

4. **E** All statements are correct. Case series studies are commonly used to report on a consecutive series of patients with a defined disease treated in a similar manner (without a control group).

5. **C** Number needed to treat for benefit or harm

$$= \frac{1}{|\text{Risk difference between two treatment groups}|}$$

$$= \frac{1}{(114/2500) - (61/2500)} = \frac{1}{0.0212} = 47$$

Therefore, 47 patients would need to be treated for *3 years* with the new anti-diabetic drug to cause 1 *extra* myocardial infarction.

6. **C** This study employs a factorial trial design as two interventions (aspirin and beta-carotene) are evaluated *simultaneously* and compared with a control group (one control for each intervention) in the same trial. This type of RCT is commonly used to evaluate interactions between treatments.

   In a cross-over trial, each subject acts as his or her own control, receiving all the treatments in a particular sequence.

   The objective of a superiority trial is to determine whether a new intervention is *better than* the control (e.g. placebo or usual treatment).

   Cluster randomised trials involve groups of patients, clinics or communities, as opposed to individuals. These clusters are randomised to receive the intervention or a control.

   The objective of an equivalence trial is to determine whether a new intervention is *similar* in effectiveness to the usual treatment.

7. **B** The sensitivity and specificity of a test are prevalence-independent. In other words, assuming the performance of the test was rigorously investigated in the high prevalence population, the sensitivity and specificity should be the same in the low prevalence population. However, the predictive values are dependent on the prevalence of the disease in the population being studied. The only situation in which the predictive values are unaffected is when the sensitivity and specificity of the test are both 100%.

The negative predictive value (NPV) can be written as:

$$\text{NPV} = \frac{\text{True negative}}{\text{True negative} + \text{False negative}}$$

As there are more people in the low prevalence population who will not have the disease, more people will have a negative test result and the negative predictive value will slightly increase.

The positive predictive value (PPV) can be written as:

$$\text{PPV} = \frac{\text{True positive}}{\text{True positive} + \text{False positive}}$$

As there are less people in the low prevalence population who have the disease, less people will have a positive test result and the positive predictive value will slightly decrease.

8. **C** It would be sensible to use a case–control study design as:
    - The outcome is rare (a case–control study design involves identifying all cases and controls at the start of the study). Apart from retrospective cohort studies, RCTs and prospective cohort studies are prospective in design and involve waiting for the outcome to occur.
    - There may be a relatively long time lag between the exposure and outcome (no prospective follow-up is required in a case–control study design). Apart from retrospective cohort studies, RCTs and prospective cohort studies are prospective in design and involve waiting for the outcome to occur.
    - Little is known about the aetiology of the disease (a case–control study allows you to investigate whether a large number of exposures may be causing the disease). RCTs, prospective cohort studies and even retrospective cohort studies would not be helpful as little is known about what risk factors or exposures are causing the disease.

    Case reports sit low down on the hierarchy of evidence. A case report usually describes a single unique case or finding of interest. They are generally used to generate hypotheses, rather than test them.
9. **D** Having demonstrated the effectiveness and safety profile of the new drug (using information from pre-clinical trials up to phase III trials), the drug can be subsequently licenced, marketed and made available for all patients. The main objective of phase IV trials is to gather information on:
    - How well the drug works in various populations.
    - The long-term risks and benefits of taking the drug.
    - The side effects and safety of the drug in larger populations.
    - Whether the drug can be used in combination with other treatments (as in this example).
10. **E** The paired *t*-test is used to analyse the data as we are:
    - Comparing two matched (or paired) groups.
    - Analysing the distribution of the before–after differences of interval data (blood pressure is an interval variable).

    We are not told whether the distribution of the before-after differences in blood pressure follows a Gaussian distribution or whether the variances (standard deviations) are constant between the groups. If the distribution is Gaussian and the variances are constant between the two groups, the paired *t*-test should be used. However, if these criteria are not satisfied, the Wilcoxon matched pairs signed-rank test should be used. Considering the Wilcoxon test is not an option, the answer is E, the paired *t*-test. Please refer to Chapter 15 for an overview of which statistical test to use when.
11. **E** If there truly is a difference in blood pressure between the two treatment groups, but the study did not detect this difference, a false negative (or type 2 error) has occurred. The power of the study is the *probability of not committing a type 2 error* and depends on:
    - The significance level (type 1 error) criterion used (i.e. the *P*-value cut-off).
    - The sample size.
    - The effect size.
    - Whether a one- or two-tail statistical test is used.
12. **E** The set of values of a ratio variable have a true zero and are equidistant from each other. Pain scale is an ordinal variable; there is a 'rank-ordered' logical relationship between the categories (1–5). The distance or interval between the categories is not known (please refer to Fig. 2.1).
13. **E** The probability density function of the normal distribution becomes *more* peaked (curve is tall and narrow) as the variance decreases and *flattens* (curve is short and wide) as the variance increases, provided the mean remains fixed.
14. **B** For positively skewed distribution (Fig. 2.18A), e.g. the F-distribution:
    - The mass of the distribution is concentrated on the left.
    - There is a long tail to the right.
    - The mode is lower than the median, which in turn is lower than the mean (mode < median < mean).
15. **E**

$$\text{Mean} = \bar{x} = \frac{\sum_{i=1}^{n} x_i}{n}$$

$$= \frac{6+12+6+2+17+11+6+3+21+5}{10}$$

$$= 8.9 \textit{ days}$$

Mode = most frequently occurring value in the set = 6 days

Range = difference between the largest and smallest values = 21 – 2 = 19 days

Sample variance =

$$s^2 = \frac{\sum(x_i - \bar{x})^2}{n-1}$$

$$= \frac{(6-8.9)^2+(12-8.9)^2+(6-8.9)^2+(2-8.9)^2+(17-8.9)^2+(11-8.9)^2+(6-8.9)^2+(3-8.9)^2+(21-8.9)^2+(5-8.9)^2}{(10-1)}$$

$$= \frac{348.9}{9} = 38.8 \text{ days}^2$$

Sample standard deviation

$$= \sqrt{s^2} = \sqrt{38.8} = 6.2 \text{ days}$$

16. **D**

Incidence rate

$$= \frac{\text{Number of new cases of disease}}{\text{Population at risk(initially disease-free)} \times \text{Time interval}}$$

$$= \frac{39}{4000 \times 3} = 0.00325 \text{ cases per year}$$

= 325 cases per 100 000 person-years

17. **D** For a normally distributed variable, *x*, 95% of the values of *x* lie within 1.96 standard deviations of the mean (mean – [1.96 × standard deviation]) to (mean + [1.96 × standard deviation]). In other words, the probability that a normally distributed variable lies between (mean – [1.96 × standard deviation]) and (mean + [1.96 × standard deviation]) is 0.95. This is known as the 95% reference range.

95% reference range

= (mean – [1.96 × standard deviation]) to (mean + [1.96 × standard deviation])

$= (71.4 - [1.96 \times 9.4])$ *to* $(71.4 + [1.96 \times 9.4])$

$= 53.0 - 89.8$ *kg*

18. **B**

- The I^2 statistic is commonly used when conducting a meta-analysis as part of a systematic review.
- It provides an estimate of the proportion of the total variation in effect estimates that is due to heterogeneity between studies. In other words, it indicates the percentage of the observed variation in effect estimates that is due to real differences in effect size.
- The I^2 statistic is based on the Q statistic and ranges from 0 to 100%.
- The more heterogeneity, the larger the I^2 statistic.

19. **C** The fixed effects meta-analysis is used when there is no evidence of (statistical) heterogeneity between the studies.

The analysis:

- Assumes that different studies are estimating the *same* true population exposure effects.
- Assumes that there is a single underlying 'true' effect that each study is estimating.
- Assumes that the only reason for variation in estimates between studies is sampling error (within-study variability).
- Gives more weight to the bigger studies.
- Calculates the weight using the inverse of the variance of the exposure effect estimate (variance = (standard error)^2).

20. **A** A sensitivity analysis determines whether the findings of the meta-analysis are robust to the methodology used to obtain them. It involves comparing the results of two or more meta-analyses, which are calculated using different assumptions. In this example, the assumption involves omitting low-quality studies.

21. **B** Publication bias in meta-analyses is usually explored graphically using 'funnel plots'. These are scatter plots, with:

- The relative measure of exposure effect (risk ratio or odds ratio) on the horizontal axis.
- The standard error of the exposure effect (which represents the study size) on the vertical axis.

In the absence of publication bias, the plot will resemble a symmetrical inverted funnel.

22. **E** Referring to Fig. 5.4, a randomised controlled trial (RCT) is the most appropriate study design for investigating this research question as:

- We are comparing two interventions.
- There is no evidence that one intervention is more (or less effective) than the other. We therefore have clinical equipoise.
- Confounding of the intervention and prognosis will be minimised. This is because study pariticipants are randomised to the alternative procedures.

23. **C** Let's work our way down the hierarchy of evidence (Fig. 1.5). When considering the effects of smoking, it would be unethical to randomise study participants to smoke or not to smoke and then follow them up to determine who develops bloodophilia. It would therefore be impossible to carry out a randomised controlled trial. As the disease in question is rare, a cohort study would be too large and costly to identify a sufficient number of study participants who develop the disease. A case–control study would therefore be the most feasible option to investigate the research hypothesis. A sufficient number of cases and controls would be identified at the start of the study.

24. **A** The biggest scientific issue in cohort studies is the loss of patients over time. Subjects, who are followed-up until the outcome occurs or the study ends, may lose contact with the investigators, move out of the area, die, etc. Loss-to-follow-up bias may be an issue if the reasons why patients are lost to follow-up are associated with *both the exposure and outcome*, e.g. associated with exposed cases.

There are no interventions in cohort studies as they are observational. Confounding is less of an issue than in case–control studies. In general, cohort studies are less expensive than randomised controlled trials.

25. **B** Randomisation ensures that those patient characteristics which may affect the outcome measure are distributed evenly between the groups. With this in mind, provided the trial is reasonably large, any observed differences between the study arms are due to differences in the treatment alone and not due to the effects of confounding factors (known or unknown) or selection bias.

26. **C** As long as data are available, a study with a long time lag between exposure and outcome is best carried out using a retrospective cohort study design.

27. **B** The differences in BMI between the two groups would have occurred by chance (despite randomisation). BMI may be a confounding factor as there were differences in the BMI between the two treatment groups at the start of the trial and BMI may be related to blood pressure. As the trial is complete, confounding can be controlled for during the analysis phase of the study. It is important not to lose any information from the data when analysing the results, so excluding all patients in both groups with a BMI greater than 30 would be incorrect.

28. **C** The chi-squared test should be used to analyse the data as we are:

- Comparing two independent (or unpaired) groups.
- Analysing nominal data.

29. **B**

- Option A refers to 'reversibility': removing the exposure should reduce or prevent the disease outcome.
- Option B refers to 'biological gradient (dose–response)': as in this example, there seems to be a direct relationship between the level of exposure and the risk of disease.
- Option C refers to 'consistency': numerous studies should be carried out before a statement can be made about the causal relationship between two variables.
- Option D refers to 'biological plausibility': the apparent cause and effect must be plausible in the light of current knowledge.
- Option E refers to 'temporal sequence': the exposure *must* always precede the outcome.

30. **C** Healthy worker effect bias leads to an underestimation of the morbidity/mortality related to occupational exposures. In general, working individuals are healthier than the general population, which includes people who are unemployed because they are too sick to work.

31. **C** The odds ratio indicates the increased (or decreased) odds of the disease being associated with the exposure of interest. The odds ratio can take any value between 0 and infinity. If the odds ratio is 0.87, the exposure of interest reduces the odds of disease by 13%. If the odds ratio was 1.87, the exposure of interest increases the odds of disease by 87 times.

32. **D** Selecting up to four controls per case may improve the statistical power of the study to detect a difference between cases and controls. Including more than four controls per case does *not* generally increase the power of the study much further.

33. **A** When the disease is not rare, the odds ratio can *overestimate* the risk ratio.

34. **E** The situation described is known as incidence–prevalence bias (also known as survival bias or Neyman bias), which is a type of ascertainment bias, where the patients included in the study do not represent the cases arising in the target population. In incidence–prevalence bias, the sample of cases enrolled has a distorted frequency of exposure if the exposure itself determines the prognosis (i.e. mortality) of the outcome (i.e. myocardial infarction).

It is also important to understand the difference between bias and confounding. In general, bias involves error in the measurement of a variable while confounding involves error in the interpretation of what may be an accurate measurement.

35. **B**

$$\text{Incidence risk} = \frac{\text{Number of new cases of the disease in a given time period}}{\text{Population at risk (initially disease-free)}}$$

$$= \frac{300}{30\,000} = 0.01 = 1.0\%$$

36. **D**

- A cross-sectional study is a form of observational study that involves collecting data from a target population at a single point in time.
- This methodology is particularly useful for assessing the true burden of a disease or the health needs of a population. Cross-sectional studies are therefore useful for planning the provision and allocation of health resources. Most government surveys conducted by the National Centre for Health Statistics are cross-sectional studies.

37. **E** It has been recognised that the decision for individuals in the study population to take part (or not take part) in a study is not random. A *lower* (not higher) socioeconomic status is associated with a low response rate.

38. **E** Higher cholesterol levels are associated with a lower stroke mortality rate. However, at an individual level, there is still a positive association between these two variables. This is referred to as a reversal of association.

39. **D** Effect modification may be an issue when the rate difference for the exposure effect varies across groups. Effect modification is different from confounding as instead of 'competing' with the exposure (alcohol) as an aetiological factor for the disease (liver disease), the effect modifier (smoking) identifies subpopulations (or subgroups) that are particularly susceptible to the exposure of interest. Effect modifiers are therefore not in the causal pathway of the disease process. If smoking status was a confounding factor, the stratum specific risk ratio of liver disease amongst bartenders who drink alcohol would be identical or very similar in smokers and non-smokers.

40. **D** In purposive sampling, sample sizes are often determined by the saturation point. This is the point in data collection where interviewing new people will no longer bring additional insights to the research question. This theoretical saturation point can only be determined if data review and analysis are done in conjunction with data collection. This process is known as iteration, i.e. moving back and forth between sampling and analysis.

41. **B** Negative sampling (also known as deviant case sampling) involves searching for unusual or atypical cases of the research topic of interest.

42. **D** In qualitative research, the researcher should reflect on whether his or her values and attributes may have influenced (or biased) any stages of the study. This is often referred to as 'reflexivity'.

43. **A** Current clinical practice should be compared to a defined set of explicit criteria that reflect *best* practice.

44. **C** The results are only specific to the local patient group audited. This limits the generalisability of the findings.

45. **B** The majority of the medical errors in healthcare practice are due to faulty systems and processes, not because of individual errors or mistakes.

46. **D** A process measure asks whether the steps in the system are performing as originally planned. When investigating access to out-patient appointments, it is important to determine whether the doctors running the clinics are allocating a certain number of hours for these appointments, as stated on their contract.

47. **A** Outcome measures help determine whether the desired patient goal is being achieved. They inform us whether any changes made (i.e. educating the junior doctors on good prescribing practice) have led to an improvement in the outcome we are ultimately trying to improve (i.e. a reduction in the number of adverse drug events per 100 doses).

48. **B** Despite there being evidence that the changes were effective at East Hospital, the quality improvement project should be repeated at West Hospital in order to:
- Evaluate the related costs and compromises at the new setting.
- Increase the reigistrar's belief, as well as the belief of his colleagues, that the change will lead to an improvement at the new setting.
- Minimise the amount of resistance from the organisation when implementing the change on a larger scale, if proven to be effective at the new setting.

49. **C** An international group of experienced authors have published guidance for authors to assist them in the reporting of systematic reviews and meta-analyses. This guidance, known as the PRISMA (Preferred Reporting Items for Systematic reviews and Meta-Analyses) statement, consists of a 27-item checklist and a four-phase flow diagram.

Clinical trials should be reported according to the CONSORT (Consolidated Standards of Reporting Trials) guidelines.

50. **D** The sensitivity and specificity describe the properties of the diagnostic test and are not dependent on the clinical sample (or target population). The sensitivity and specificity of a test are prevalence-independent. On the other hand, positive predictive values (and negative predictive values) are dependent on the population being studied (and therefore provide more clinically useful information). The positive predictive value increases (and the negative predictive value decreases) with increasing disease prevalence.

51. **B** The answer to this question involves calculating the number needed to treat (NNT).

$$\text{NNT} = \frac{1}{\text{Risk difference between two treatment groups}}$$

The difference in outcome between the two groups, as denoted by the denominator of the formula above, is given as 25%.

$$\text{NNT} = \frac{100}{25} = 4$$

You therefore need to treat four patients with the new drug to prevent one hospital admission due to an acute exacerbation of asthma.

52. **E**

$$\text{Cost-effectiveness ratio} = \frac{\text{Cost of intervention}}{\text{Health effect outcome}} = \frac{\pounds 13\,000}{80 \text{ weeks}} = \pounds 162.50/\text{week}$$

53. **E**

$$\text{ICER} = \frac{\text{Cost of drug B} - \text{Cost of drug A}}{\text{Health effects of drug B} - \text{Health effects of drug A}}$$

$$= \frac{£13\,000 - £7\,000}{80 \text{ weeks} - 70 \text{ weeks}}$$

$$= £600 \text{ per additional week free of depression}$$

54. **B** Economical costs incorporate not only the financial cost of resources but also the time, energy and effort involved for which there may be no associated financial payment. 'Opportunity cost' is what is lost when an alternative service is not provided because resources are directed elsewhere. The concept of opportunity cost highlights the struggle that policy-makers are faced with when deciding how resources are allocated to various competing services/drugs.

55. **B** Option A refers to spectrum bias.

Option B is correct: Partial verification bias (also known as work-up bias) occurs when the decision to perform the reference (gold standard) test on an individual is based on the results of the diagnostic study test.

Option C is incorrect: Partial verification bias may be avoided if the *reference test* is always performed *prior to the study test.*

Option D refers to differential verification bias.

Option E is incorrect: Partial verification bias cannot always be prevented. While it is possible to blind the investigator between the study test and reference test results, blinding may not always be possible. For example, you wouldn't perform surgery (reference test) prior to imaging (study test)!

56. **D**

$$\text{Sensitivity} = \frac{\text{True positive}}{\text{True positive} + \text{False negative}}$$

$$= \frac{44}{44 + 9} = 83.0\%$$

57. **A**

$$\text{Specificity} = \frac{\text{True negative}}{\text{True negative} + \text{False positive}}$$

$$= \frac{307}{307 + 140} = 68.7\%$$

58. **B** The pre-test probability is 0.10 or 10%

$$\text{Pre-test odds} = \frac{\text{Pre-test probability}}{1 - \text{pre-test probability}}$$

$$= \frac{0.10}{1 - 0.10} = 0.11$$

The likelihood ratio of depression if the two-question screening test is positive is:

$$\frac{\text{Sensitivity}}{1 - \text{Specificity}} = \frac{0.83}{1 - 0.687} = 2.65$$

The post-test odds in a person with a positive result are:

Post-test odds

$$= \text{Pre-test odds} \times \text{Positive likelihood ratio}$$

$$= 0.11 \times 2.65 = 0.29$$

The post-test odds can be converted back into a probability:

$$\text{Post-test probability} = \frac{\text{Post-test odds}}{\text{Post-test odds} + 1}$$

$$= \frac{0.29}{0.29 + 1} = 0.225 = 22.5\%$$

59. **B** Referring to Figs. 15.4 and 15.5, the expected frequency for the number of patients randomised to the bare metal stent who had restenosis within 3 months after angioplasty is:

$$\frac{(a + c) \times (c + d)}{(a + b + c + d)} = \frac{(124 + 155) \times (155 + 270)}{850}$$

$$= 139.5$$

60. **C** Option A is incorrect: When the sample size of a study is small, parametric tests are *not very robust* when analysing data that do not follow a Gaussian distribution.

Option B is incorrect: When the sample size of a study is small, normality tests have *little power* to detect whether a sample comes from a Gaussian distribution.

Option C is correct: When the sample size of a study is small, non-parametric tests have little power to detect a significant difference.

Option D is incorrect: When the sample size is large, non-parametric tests almost have *as much power* as parametric tests when analysing data that follow a Gaussian distribution.

Option E is incorrect: When dealing with large sample sizes, the decision to choose a parametric or non-parametric test *matters less*.

EMQ answers

1. Describing the frequency distribution

1. C 'Mu' (μ) is often used to denote the population mean, while x-bar ($\bar{x}$) refers to the mean of a sample.
2. A If there are an odd number of observations, *n*, there will be an equal number of values both above and below the median value.
3. G Quantifies how accurately you know the true population mean. The standard error measures the precision of the sample mean as an estimate of the population mean. It takes into account the sample size and the value of the standard deviation.
4. E The inter-quartile range is bounded by the lower and upper quartiles (25% of the values lie below the lower limit and 25% lie above the upper limit). In other words, it is the difference between the upper quartile and the lower quartile.
5. F Quantifies scatter. The standard deviation measures the amount of variability in the population. It informs us how far an individual observation is likely to be from the true population mean.

2. Randomised controlled trials

1. E This definition specifically describes the process of allocation concealment. Having generated a random allocation sequence, the second part of randomisation involves ensuring that the sequence is concealed. The allocation sequence can always be concealed at the time of recruitment in an RCT.
2. B Blinding may not be possible if the RCT involves a technology, e.g. surgery versus chemotherapy, or a programme of care, e.g. exercise therapy versus medication.
3. C There must be no evidence that the new intervention is better, worse or the same as any of the treatments currently being used in clinical practice or the placebo treatment, if used. If these criteria are satisfied, the trial has 'clinical equipoise'.
4. F The statement describes loss-to-follow-up bias (or attrition bias), which is a type of selection bias. It refers to systematic differences between the treatment groups in terms of the number of subjects lost. Loss-to-follow-up bias may also occur if there are differences between those not adhering to the study protocol and those who remain in the study.
5. A A cluster trial is appropriate when evaluating interventions that are likely to have a group effect. Such interventions include preventative health services (e.g. smoking cessation programmes or vaccines).

3. Types of variables

1. J Gender is a dichotomous variable (a type of nominal variable). This variable only takes one of two values, i.e. male or female.
2. I In addition to having all the characteristics of nominal and ordinal variables, an interval variable is one where the distance (or interval) between any two categories is the same and constant. For example, the difference between the beginning of day 1 and the beginning of day 2 is 24 hours, just as it is between day 2 and day 3.
3. G When a 'rank-ordered' logical relationship exists among the categories, the variable is only then known as an ordinal variable. For disease staging, the categories may be ranked in order of magnitude, i.e. none, mild, moderate and severe.
4. D In addition to having all the characteristics of interval variables, a ratio variable also has a natural zero point. Other examples of interval variables include weight and the incidence of disease.
5. F If there are three or more categories for a variable, the data collected are multinomial (a type of nominal variable).

4. Calculating the strength of an association

A contingency table should be constructed to help you with your calculations:

	Myocardial infarction	No myocardial infarction	Total
Statstatin	60	390	450
Simvastatin	103	362	465
Total	163	752	915

1. F 60/390 = 0.154
2. C 60/450 = 0.133
3. A

$$\frac{\text{Odds of myocardial infarction in statstatin group}}{\text{Odds of myocardial infarction in simvastatin group}}$$

$$= \frac{0.154}{103/362} = 0.541$$

4. H

$$\frac{\text{Risk of myocardial infarction in statstatin group}}{\text{Risk of myocardial infarction in simvastatin group}}$$

$$= \frac{0.133}{103/465} = 0.602$$

5. I The number needed to treat for benefit

$$= \frac{1}{|\text{Risk difference}|} = \frac{1}{|0.133 - 0.222|}$$

$$= \frac{1}{0.089} = 11.2$$

Therefore, for every 11 patients treated with statstatin instead of simvastatin, we would prevent one case of myocardial infarction.

5. Extrapolating from sample to population – working with proportions

To help make sense of the data, it is useful to first calculate the percentage (or proportion) of cases of myocardial infarction in both treatment groups:

	Myocardial infarction	No myocardial infarction	Total
Statstatin	60 (**13.3%**)	390 (**86.7%**)	450
Simvastatin	103 (**22.2%**)	362 (**77.8%**)	465
Total	163	752	915

1. E

$$SE(p) = \sqrt{\frac{p \times (1-p)}{n}} = \sqrt{\frac{0.133 \times (0.867)}{450}}$$

$$= 0.0160 = 1.60\%$$

The 95% confidence interval is therefore:

$$13.3 - (1.96 \times 1.60) \text{ to } 13.3 + (1.96 \times 1.60)$$
$$= 10.2 \text{ to } 16.4\%$$

2. B

$$SE(p) = \sqrt{\frac{p \times (1-p)}{n}} = \sqrt{\frac{0.222 \times (0.778)}{465}}$$

$$= 0.0193 = 1.93\%$$

The 95% confidence interval is therefore:

$$22.2 - (1.96 \times 1.93) \text{ to } 22.2 + (1.96 \times 1.93)$$
$$= 18.4 \text{ to } 26.0\%$$

3. F

% of cases in statstatin group
−% of cases in simvastatin group
$= 13.3\% - 22.2\% = -8.9\%$

4. C

$$SE(p_1 - p_0) = \sqrt{[SE(p_1)]^2 + SE[(p_0)]^2}$$
$$= \sqrt{[0.0160]^2 + [0.0193]^2} = 0.0250 = 2.5\%$$

The 95% confidence interval of the difference in the percentage of cases of myocardial infarction in the two treatment groups

$$= -8.9 - (1.96 \times 2.5) \text{ to } -8.9 + (1.96 \times 2.5)$$
$$= -13.8 \text{ to } -4.0\%$$

Therefore, with 95% confidence, treating patients with high cholesterol using statstatin rather than simvastatin leads to a 5-year reduction in the rate of myocardial infarction by as large as 13.8% or as small as 4.0%.

5. I We are comparing unpaired (or independent) groups (i.e. simvastatin versus statstatin). The data recorded are nominal and the expected value in each of the four cells of the contingency table will be ≥5. We therefore use a chi-squared test to compare our data.

6. Extrapolating from sample to population – working with means

1. C

$$\frac{SD}{\sqrt{n}} = \frac{0.24}{\sqrt{450}} = 0.0113$$

2. B

$$\frac{SD}{\sqrt{n}} = \frac{0.49}{\sqrt{465}} = 0.0227$$

3. A

Mean cholesterol level in statstatin group −
Mean cholesterol level in simvastatin group
= 3.6 − 4.2 mmol/L = −0.6 mmol/L

4. F

$$SE(\bar{x}_1 - \bar{x}_0) = \sqrt{[SE(\bar{x}_1)]^2 + [SE(\bar{x}_0)]^2}$$
$$= \sqrt{[0.0113]^2 + [0.0227]^2} = 0.0254$$

The 95% confidence interval for the difference in the mean cholesterol level in the two treatment groups

$$= -0.6 - (1.96 \times 0.0254) \text{ to } -0.6 + (1.96 \times 0.0254)$$
$$= -0.65 \text{ to } -0.55 \text{ mmol/L}$$

Therefore, with 95% confidence, treating patients with high cholesterol using statstatin rather than simvastatin leads to a 5-year reduction in mean cholesterol level by as large as 0.65 mmol/L or as small as 0.55 mmol/L.

5. J We are comparing unpaired (or independent) groups (i.e. simvastatin versus statstatin). The cholesterol level is a ratio variable and we are told that the data follow a normal distribution. We therefore use the unpaired *t*-test to compare our data.

7. Meta-analyses

1. B The results of meta-analyses are often presented in a standard way known as a 'forest plot'.
2. E The fixed effects analysis is used when there is no evidence of (statistical) heterogeneity between the studies. It assumes that different studies are estimating the *same* true population exposure effects and that the only reason for variation in estimates between studies is due to sampling error (within-study variability).
3. C The centre of the diamond (and broken vertical line) represents the summary effect estimate of the meta-analysis.
4. F Publication bias in meta-analyses is usually explored graphically using 'funnel plots', which are a type of scatter plot. In the absence of publication bias, the plot will resemble a symmetrical inverted funnel.
5. J A sensitivity analysis determines whether the findings of the meta-analysis are robust to the methodology used to obtain them. It involves carrying out a meta-analysis with and without the assumption (i.e. omitting low-quality studies, studies which appear to be outliers, etc.) and comparing the two results for statistical significance.

8. Measures of disease occurrence

1. A Analytical cross-sectional studies are used to investigate the interrelationship between any variables of interest. For example, a target population could be sampled to determine the characteristics (age, sex, ethnicity, etc.) of people with ischaemic heart disease.
2. G

$$\frac{\text{Number of cases of depression in subjects with a social networking profile}}{\text{Total number of subjects with a social networking profile}}$$

$$= \frac{40}{434} = 9.2\%$$

3. H

$$\frac{\text{Number of } \textit{cases} \text{ of depression in subjects without a social networking profile}}{\text{Total number of subjects without a social networking profile}}$$

$$= \frac{130}{162} = 80.2\%$$

4. C

$$\frac{\text{Odds of depression amongst subjects with a social networking profile at a single point in time}}{\text{Odds of depression amongst subjects without a social networking profile at a single point in time}}$$

$$= \frac{40/394}{130/32} = 0.025$$

5. I

$$\frac{\text{Probability of depression amongst subjects with a social networking profile at a single point in time}}{\text{Probability of depression amongst subjects without a social networking profile at a single point in time}}$$

$$= \frac{40/434}{130/162} = 0.11$$

9. Qualitative studies

1. D Participant observation is based on traditional ethnographic research, whose objective is to understand perspectives held by study populations. It involves understanding the life and customs of people living in various cultures.
2. A The study participants, with whom contact has already been made, use their social networks to identify groups not easily accessible to researchers, such as the homeless.
3. E Negative sampling (also known as deviant case sampling) involves searching for unusual or atypical cases of the research topic of interest.
4. J Quota sampling initially involves choosing which characteristics (i.e. age, socioeconomic class, profession, etc.) you are trying to identify in potential subjects. The characteristics chosen are to identify people most likely to have insight or have experienced the research topic. Individuals from the community are then recruited until the pre-defined quota is satisfied.
5. H The values and attributes considered when assessing for reflexivity may include ethnicity, gender, age, whether the researcher has the same condition as the one being investigated, etc.

10. Confounding

1. E This is a (prospective) cohort study. Subjects were selected on the basis of their exposure status (bedsores versus no bedsores). The outcome data (death) was collected prospectively.
2. A

$$\frac{\text{Risk of death in bedsores group}}{\text{Risk of death in no bedsores group}} = \frac{32/234}{35/768} = 3.0$$

3. H Confounding occurs when the association between an exposure and disease outcome is distorted by a third variable, which is known as a confounder. In this example, people with many co-morbidities may be more likely to acquire bedsores than those with a few or no co-morbidities. Furthermore, people with many co-morbidities may have a higher death rate.

4. D We can estimate the association between the exposure and disease outcome separately for different levels (strata) of the confounding variable. In this example, the two strata are medically unwell and medically well.
5. M The association seen between bedsores and death (risk ratio 3) does *not* persist in the strata of the confounder. Consequently, the level (number/severity) of co-morbid conditions seems to explain the observed association seen in the unadjusted risk ratio. As the risk ratio in both strata is 1.0, the confounder seems to explain *all* of the observed association.

11. Screening

All five questions can be easily answered if you fill in the missing values in the table:

- As the prevalence of breast cancer in the population is 0.8%, $(a+c)$ must equal $0.008 \times 10\,000 = 80$
- Sensitivity $= 0.95 = [a/(a+c)]$

$$0.95 = a/80$$
$$a = 0.95 \times 80 = 76$$

- $c = [(a+c) - a]$

$$c = 80 - 76 = 4$$

- Specificity $= 0.888 = [d/(b+d)]$

$$(b+d) = \text{Total} - (a+c)$$
$$(b+d) = 10000 - 80 = 9920$$

Therefore, $0.888 = d/9920$

$$d = 8809$$

- $b = (b+d) - d$

$$b = 9920 - 8809 = 1111$$

- $a+b+c+d = 76 + 1111 + 4 + 8809 = 10000$

In summary:

		Breast cancer		Total
		Yes	No	
Mammography	Positive	76	1111	1187
	Negative	4	8809	8813
	Total	80	9920	10000

1. F Type 1 error represents the false-positive rate, which answers the question 'What proportion of those who do not have the disease will have a positive test?' It is calculated as $b/(b+d)$. In this example it is $1111/9920 = 11.2\%$
2. E Type 2 error represents the false-negative rate, which answers the question 'What proportion of those with the disease will have a negative test?' It is calculated as $c/(a+c)$. In this example it is $4/80 = 5\%$.
3. A
4. I Positive predictive value (PPV): Among those who test positive, what fraction actually have breast cancer?

$$\text{PPV} = a/(a+b) = 76/1187 = 6.40\%$$

Therefore only 6.4% of those who test positive actually have breast cancer.

5. C Negative predictive value (NPV): Among those who test negative, what fraction actually don't have breast cancer?

$$\text{NPV} = d/(c+d) = 8809/8813 = 99.95\%$$

Therefore 99.95% of those who test negative actually don't have breast cancer.

12. Calculating the *P*-value

1. D The one-sample *t*-test is used to analyse the data as we are:
   - Comparing one group to a hypothetical value (1.74 mmol/L).
   - Analysing numerical (specifically ratio) data (serum triglyceride level) with a Gaussian distribution.
2. F The chi-squared test is used to analyse the data as we are:
   - Comparing two independent (or unpaired) groups (control vs intervention).
   - Analysing nominal data, specifically binomial data (there are two possible outcomes, coronary artery restenosis or no coronary artery restenosis).
3. H The one-way repeated measures ANOVA is used to analyse the data as we are:
   - Comparing three matched groups (ESR levels are measured in the same subjects at three time points).
   - Analysing the differences of numerical (specifically ratio) data (ESR level) across time categories. We are also told that the data follow a Gaussian distribution and that the variances (standard deviations) are constant between the groups.
4. B The unpaired *t*-test is used to analyse the data as we are:
   - Comparing two independent (or unpaired) groups (medical students vs dental students).
   - Analysing numerical (specifically interval) data (IQ), which follow a Gaussian distribution and have equal variances (standard deviations). IQ is an interval variable as there is no such thing as zero IQ. Furthermore, 120 IQ is not twice as intelligent as 60 IQ.

5. A The Mann–Whitney U test (or the Wilcoxon two-sample signed rank test) is used to analyse the data as we are:
    - Comparing two independent (or unpaired) groups (lecture-based vs problem-based).
    - Analysing numerical (specifically ratio) data (exam results) that do not follow a Gaussian distribution. The variances of the variable are also unequal between the two groups.

   The 'test mark' variable is a ratio variable as:
    - It includes a zero value, i.e. if all answers in the test are wrong.
    - The questions are of equal difficulty. This means if someone has 60 correct answers, he has twice as many correct answers as someone with 30 correct answers (and he is twice as good in the module examined).

13. Economic evaluation

1. D QALYs for treatment B $= (12 \times 0.837) + (5 \times 0.516) = 12.62$ QALYs.
2. G It is important to understand that the higher the EQ-5D health state score, the better the health. Intervention A is 'dominant' over intervention B, as the former is more effective and less expensive for each additional unit of health effect.
3. I

$$\text{ICER} = \frac{\text{Cost of treatment A} - \text{Cost of no treatment}}{\text{Number of QALYs for treatment A} - \text{Number of QALYs for no treatment}}$$

$$= \frac{11\,000 - 0}{13.03 - 8.89} = £2657 \text{ per QALY}$$

4. F

$$\text{NMB} = [(\text{Number of QALYs for intervention A} - \text{Number of QALYs for no intervention}) \times \lambda] - (\text{Cost of intervention A} - \text{Cost of no intervention})$$

We are told that $\lambda = £30\,000$.

$$\text{NMB} = [(13.03 - 8.89) \times 30\,000] - (11\,000 - 0) = £113\,200$$

5. B Utility measurements were combined with survival estimates to generate quality-adjusted life years (QALYs), which were used in a cost-utility analysis of competing healthcare interventions (treatment A vs treatment B).

14. Bias

1. E When a history of exposure to passive smoke is recalled by subjects who know their disease status, those with the disease (cases) may put in extra effort (ruminate) into recalling their exposure status. In other words, subjects with asthma may have greater incentive, due to their concern, to recall past exposures compared to controls without asthma. This type of recall bias is known as rumination bias.
2. C Considering hospitalised patients are more likely to suffer from many illnesses and engage in less healthy behaviours, they are probably not representative of the target population. Berkson's bias, one form of hospital admission bias, may be an issue if controls are selected from the same hospital from which cases were recruited.
3. F Random misclassification bias (also known as non-differential misclassification bias) can occur when either the exposure or outcome is classified incorrectly (with equal probability) into different groups. In our case, the misclassification is random as the errors in exposure classification have occurred independent of the disease outcome. When assessing smoking status, subjects were classified into groups based only on the number of cigarettes smoked per day. In order to avoid random misclassification bias, it would have been important to also ask about:
    - Cigarette brand (and therefore nicotine content).
    - Whether they normally take deep breaths whilst smoking.
    - Whether each cigarette is smoked to the end.
4. I This is a type of interviewer (or observer) bias. As the investigator is not 'blind' to the exposure status (i.e. treatment allocation) when taking blood pressure measurements, he may underestimate the blood pressure in those who have been treated with the new intervention and overestimate it in those in the control group. In general, interviewer bias may be minimised if the investigator is 'blind' to the exposure status when gathering data on disease outcome.
5. D This is an example of loss-to-follow-up bias. In this case, the reason why patients are lost to follow-up (improvement in symptoms of benign prostatic hypertrophy) is associated with *both the exposure and outcome*. If the proportion of subjects lost is substantial (e.g. 20% lost to follow-up), this will affect the validity of the study, can lead to data misinterpretation and limit the generalisability of the study.

15. Study design

1. F Subjects with the outcome (infants with persistent pulmonary hypertension) and without the outcome (infants without persistent pulmonary hypertension) are selected and data on previous exposure to SSRIs are collected retrospectively in both groups.
2. G A prospective cohort study is a form of observational study that aims to investigate whether exposure of subjects to a certain factor (influenza vaccine) will affect the incidence of a disease (pneumonia or influenza) in the future.
3. B A randomised controlled trial is an interventional study in which study participants are randomised to different treatment options. In this example, the treatment options were raloxifene or a placebo drug.
4. H A meta-analysis is a statistical procedure of integrating the results of several independent studies considered to be 'combinable'.
5. E An ecological study is an observational study in which the unit of observation (density of fast food outlets and socioeconomic status) and analysis is at a group level, rather than at an individual level.

Further reading

Chapter 1

Lefebvre, C., Manheimer, E., Glanville, J., 2011. Searching for studies. In: Higgins, J.P.T., Green, S. (Eds.), Cochrane Handbook for Systematic Reviews of Interventions. Version 5.1.0 (updated March 2011). The Cochrane Collaboration.

National Institute for Health and Clinical Excellence, March 2012. The Guidelines Manual. National Institute for Health and Clinical Excellence, London. Available from:http://www.nice.org.uk.

Sackett, D.L., Rosenberg, W.M.C., 1995. The need for evidence based medicine. J. R. Soc. Med. 88, 620–624.

Sackett, D.L., Rosenberg, W.M.C., Gray, J.A.M., Haynes, R.B., Richardson, W.S., 1996. Evidence based medicine: What it is and what it isn't. BMJ 312, 71–72.

Sackett, D.L., Straus, S., Richardson, S., Rosenberg, W., Haynes, R.B., 2000. Evidence-Based Medicine: How to Practice and Teach EBM, second ed. Churchill-Livingstone, London.

Straus, S.E., McAlister, F.A., 2000. Evidence-based medicine: A commentary on common criticisms. CMAJ 163, 837–841.

Chapter 2

Bland, M., 2000. An Introduction to Medical Statistics, third ed. Oxford University Press, Oxford.

Chapter 3

Bland, M., 2000. An Introduction to Medical Statistics, third ed. Oxford University Press, Oxford.

Motulsky, H.J., 2007. Prism 5 Statistics Guide. GraphPad Software Inc., San Diego CA. http://www.graphpad.com.

Schervish, M.J., 1996. P Values: What They Are and What They Are Not. The American Statistician 50 (3), 203–206.

Sterne, J.A.C., Smith, G.D., 2001. Sifting the evidence – what's wrong with significance tests? BMJ 322 (7280), 226–231.

Chapter 4

Altman, D.G., Smith, G.D., Egger, M., 2001. Systematic Reviews in Health Care: Meta-analysis in Context, second ed. BMJ.

Cochrane, A.L., 1972. Effectiveness and efficiency: Random Reflections on Health Services. Nuffield Provincial Hospitals Trust, London (Republished jointly with *British Medical Journal*, 1989).

Cochrane, A.L., 1979. 1931–1971: A critical review, with particular reference to the medical profession. In: :Medicines for the Year 2000. Office of Health Economics, London.

Greenhalgh, T., 1997. How to read a paper: Papers that summarise other papers (systematic reviews and meta-analysis). BMJ 315, 672–675.

Liberati, A., Altman, D.G., Tetzlaff, J., Mulrow, C., Gøtzsche, P.C., Ioannidis, J.P.A., et al., 2009. The PRISMA statement for reporting systematic reviews and meta-analyses of studies that evaluate health care interventions: Explanation and elaboration. BMJ 339, b2700.

Moher, D., Liberati, A., Tetzlaff, J., Altman, D.G., The PRISMA Group, 2009. Preferred reporting items for systematic reviews and meta-analyses: The PRISMA statement. BMJ 339, b2535.

The Cochrane Collaboration, http://www.cochrane-net.org.

Chapter 5

Goodman, N.W., Edwards, M.B., 1997. Medical Writing: A Prescription for Clarity. Cambridge University Press, Cambridge.

Hall, G. (Ed.), 1996. How to Write a Paper. BMJ Books, London.

Wager, E., Godlee, F., Jefferson, T., 2002. How to Survive Peer Review. BMJ Books, London.

Chapter 6

Altman, D.G., 1996. Better reporting of randomised controlled trials: the CONSORT statement. BMJ 313 (7057), 570–571.

Hennekens, C.H., Buring, J.E., 1987. Epidemiology in Medicine. Lippincott Williams & Wilkins, Philadelphia.

Kendall, J.M., 2003. Designing a research project: Randomised Controlled trials and their principles. Emerg Med J. 20 (2), 164–168.

Moher D, Hopewell S, Schulz KF, Montori V, Gøtzsche PC, Devereaux PJ, Elbourne D, Egger M, Altman DG, for the CONSORT Group. (2010) CONSORT, 2010. Explanation and Elaboration: updated guidelines for reporting parallel group randomised trial. BMJ c869, 340.

Schulz KF, Altman DG, Moher D, for the CONSORT Group. (2010) CONSORT, 2010. Statement: updated guidelines for reporting parallel group randomised trials. Ann Int Med 152.

Sibbald, B., Roland, M., 1998. Understanding controlled trials: Why are randomised controlled trials important? BMJ. 316, 201.

The CONSORT Statement, http://www.consort-statement.org.

Chapter 7

Grimes, D.A., Schulz, K.F., 2002. Cohort studies: marching towards outcomes. Lancet 359 (9303), 341–345.

Chapter 8

Rothman, K.J., Greenland, S., 1998. Case-control studies. In: Rothman, K.J., Greenland, S. (Eds.), Modern Epidemiology, second ed. Lippincott-Raven, Philadelphia.

Schlesselman, J.J., 1982. Case-Control Studies: Design, Conduct, Analysis. Oxford University Press, New York.

Chapter 9

Levin, K.A., 2006. Study Design III: cross-sectional studies. Evid. Based Dent. 7, 24–25.

Chapter 10

Morgenstern, H., 1995. Ecologic studies in epidemiology: Concepts, principles, and methods. Annu. Rev. Public Health 16, 61–81.

Chapter 11

Albrecht, J., Meves, A., Bigby, M., 2005. Case reports and case series from Lancet had significant impact on medical literature. J. Clin. Epidemiol. 58, 1227–1232.

Cohen, H., 2006. How to write a case report. Am. J. Health Syst. Pharm. 63, 1888–1892.

Vandenbroucke, J.P., 2001. In defence of case reports and case series. Ann. Intern. Med. 134, 330–334.

Chapter 12

Barbour, R., 2001. Checklists for improving rigour in qualitative research: A case of the tail wagging the dog? BMJ 322, 1115–1117.

Glaser, B.G., Strauss, A.L., 1967. The Discovery of Grounded Theory: Strategies for Qualitative Research. Aldine, Chicago.

Mack, N., Woodsong, C., MacQueen, K.M., Guest, G., Namey, E., 2005. Qualitative Research Methods: A Data Collector's Field Guide. Family Health International, Research Triangle Park, NC.

Chapter 13

Mamdani, M., Sykora, K., Li, P., Normand, S.L.T., Streiner, D.L., Austin, P.C., et al., 2005. Reader's guide to critical appraisal of cohort studies: 2. Assessing potential for confounding. BMJ 330, 960–962.

Normand, S.L.T., Sykora, K., Li, P., Mamdani, M., Rochon, P.A., Anderson, G.M., 2005. Readers guide to critical appraisal of cohort studies: 3. Analytical strategies to reduce confounding. BMJ 330, 1021–1023.

Chapter 14

Akobeng, A.K., 2007. Understanding diagnostic tests 2: likelihood ratios, pre- and post-test probabilities and their use in clinical practice. Acta Paediatr. 96 (4), 487–491.

Fagan, T.J., 1975. Letter: Nomogram for Bayes theorem. N. Engl. J. Med. 293 (5), 257.

Laupacis, A., Wells, G., Richardson, S., Tugwell, P., 1994. Users guides to the medical literature. V. How to use an article about prognosis. JAMA 272, 234–237.

McGee, S., 2002. Simplifying likelihood ratios. J. Gen. Intern. Med. 17 (8), 646–649.

Chapter 15

Bland, M., 2000. An Introduction to Medical Statistics, third ed. Oxford University Press, Oxford.

Motulsky, H.J., 2007. Prism 5 Statistics Guide. GraphPad Software Inc., San Diego CA. http://www.graphpad.com.

Motulsky, H.J., 2010. Intuitive biostatistics, second ed. Oxford University Press, Oxford.

Chapter 16

Clinical Governance Support Team, 2004. A Practical Handbook for Clinical Audit. UK National Health Service.

National Institute for Health and Clinical Excellence, 2002. Principles for Best Practice in Clinical Audit. Radcliffe Medical Press, Oxford.

Chapter 17

Institute for Healthcare Improvement, http://www.ihi.org.

Institute of Medicine, 1999. To Err is Human: Building a Safer Health System (L. Kohn, J. Corrigan, M. Donaldson, Eds.). National Academies Press, Washington, DC.

Langley, G.J., Nolan, K.M., Nolan, T.W., Norman, C.L., Provost, L.P., 1996. The Improvement Guide. Jossey-Bass, San Francisco.

Langley, G.L., Nolan, K.M., Nolan, T.W., Norman, C.L., Provost, L.P., 2009. The Improvement Guide: A Practical Approach to Enhancing Organizational Performance, second ed. Jossey-Bass, San Francisco.

Chapter 18

Briggs, A., Claxton, K., Sculpher, M.J., 2006. Decision Modelling for Health Economic Evaluation. Oxford University Press, Oxford.

Drummond, M.F., Jefferson, T.O., 1996. Guideline for authors and peer reviewers of economic submissions to the BMJ. The BMJ Economic Evaluation Working Party. BMJ 313, 275–283.

Drummond, M.F., Sculpher, M.J., Torrance, G.W., O'Brein, B.J., Stoddart, G.L., 2005. Methods for the Economic Evaluation of Health Care Programmes, third ed. Oxford University Press, Oxford.

National Institute for Health and Clinical Excellence, Guide to the methods of technology appraisal. Available at: http://www.nice.org.uk/niceMedia/pdf/TAP_Methods.pdf (accessed 14.05.12.).

Phillips, C., Thompson, G., 1998. What is a QALY? Hayward Medical Communications, London.

Philips, C.J., 2005. Health Economics: An Introduction for Health Professionals. Blackwell Publishing, Oxford.

Chapter 19

Delgado-Rodríguez, M., Llorca, J., 2004. Bias. J. Epidemiol. Community Health 58, 635–641.

Greenhalgh, T., 2010. How to Read a Paper: The Basics of Evidence Based Medicine, fourth ed. Wiley-Blackwell/BMJ Books, London. The electronic copy of this book is also available online: http://www.bmj.com/about-bmj/resources-readers/publications/how-read-paper.

Chapter 21

Modernising Medical Careers and the UK Clinical Research Collaboration, 2005. Medically- and dentally-qualified academic staff: Recommendations for training the researchers and educators of the future. pp. 1–34.

Modernising Medical Careers, http://www.mmc.nhs.uk.

The Academy of Medical Sciences, http://www.acmedsci.ac.uk.

The Academy's academic medicine site: http://www.academicmedicine.ac.uk.

UK Clinical Research Collaboration, http://www.ukcrc.org.

Glossary

Accuracy is the closeness of the data to the true value.

Audit, or rather **clinical audit**, is a technique used to examine clinical practice to determine the degree to which it meets agreed standards.

Bias or systematic error refers to the phenomenon where a statistic is calculated in a way that makes the result systematically different from the true result. Bias can be divided into selection bias and measurement bias.

Blinding refers to patients and investigators (including those involved in recruitment and assessing the outcome) having no knowledge of treatment allocation.

Case–control study is a study in which patients with a certain condition (cases) are identified, along with similar patients without the condition (controls). Both groups are then assessed with the aim of identifying one or more factors which might account for the fact that cases have developed the condition and controls have not.

Case series is a series of cases with a certain condition, with no controls.

Cluster randomised controlled trial is one in which the intervention is randomly allocated to groups of patients (e.g. patients of one practice) rather than to individuals.

Cohort study is a study in which patients who have been exposed to something (a possible cause of disease, or a drug) are compared to a similar group who were not exposed. It is usually prospective (subjects are followed up to see who develops the disease) but it can be retrospective (subjects' past histories are examined).

Confidence interval (CI), or confidence limits, describes a range of values. The 95% CI is the range within which there is a 95% chance that the true value for the population lies. The 95% confidence interval is roughly equal to two standard deviations about the mean.

Confounding occurs when the association between an exposure and disease outcome is distorted by a third variable, which is known as a confounder. For instance, a study appears to show that standing in the street outside a public space causes lung cancer. Smoking is the confounder which makes smokers stand in the street and which causes lung cancer.

Cost–benefit analysis measures the cost of an intervention and the benefit that ensues, both being measured in the same units (usually financial).

Cost–consequence analysis measures the cost of the intervention and includes the non-health consequences.

Cost-effectiveness analysis measures the costs and benefits of an intervention without describing them both in monetary terms.

Cost-effectiveness ratio (CER) is the cost divided by the health outcome. **The incremental cost-effectiveness ratio (ICER)** is the difference in cost between two interventions divided by the difference in health effects.

Cost-minimisation analysis measures only the costs of alternative treatments. The benefits are assumed to be the same.

Cost-utility analysis measures the benefits of an intervention in terms of personal preferences and describes the benefit in terms of what it costs to achieve a certain quality of gain, usually as the cost per quality-adjusted life year, QALY.

Cross-over study analyses two or more groups, all of whom are exposed to all the interventions being tested, in turn.

Cross-sectional study is an examination, at one point in time, of a sample, looking for the presence of variables (exposures, diseases, test results) which may be associated with each other.

Ecological studies survey populations rather than individuals, looking for relationships between exposures and diseases. It can be at one point in time, or several points in time, comparing changes in the different populations.

Effectiveness indicates whether the intervention works in practice.

Efficacy indicates whether the intervention could work in practice if ideal conditions were met; for instance, that every patient completes the treatment.

Heterogeneity is the word used in systematic reviews to describe the fact that different studies give different findings, suggesting that the results of each study are context-specific. This means the results should not be combined.

Incidence is the number of new cases of a certain disease occurring in a specified time.

Incidence rate is the incidence risk in a specified unit of time e.g. 100 person-years.

Incidence risk is the number of new cases divided by the number in the population-at-risk.

Intention to treat analysis is where the subjects of the study are analysed in the groups into which they were initially randomised. For instance, a subject randomised to treatment A is analysed in group A even if clinical necessity meant that the subject was changed to treatment B or left the trial all together.

Likelihood ratio indicates how many times more likely it is that there will be a certain test result in a patient with the disease compared to a patient without the disease. **The likelihood ratio for a positive result (LR+)** is the proportion of people with the disease who have a positive test, divided by the proportion without the disease with a positive test. It is sensitivity divided by 1 – specificity, i.e. the true-positive rate over the false-positive rate. **The likelihood ratio for a negative result (LR–)** is the proportion of people with the disease who have a negative test divided by the proportion without the disease with a negative test. It is 1 – sensitivity divided by specificity, i.e. the false-negative rate over the true-negative rate.

Matching is the technique of ensuring that, for every case, there are one or more controls who have the same characteristics e.g. sex, age, smoking status.

Mean is the arithmetic mean, which is the sum of all the values divided by the number of values. The geometric mean is the mean calculated using log-transformed values.

Measurement bias occurs when the information collected for the exposure and/or outcome variables is inaccurate. Measurement bias can be divided into random or non-random misclassification bias.

Meta-analysis is a systematic review that summarises the results of all eligible studies in a single figure.

Non-parametric statistics does not assume that the data are normally distributed.

Non-random misclassification bias (also known as differential misclassification bias) can lead to the effect of the exposure on the disease outcome being biased in either direction. This type of misclassification occurs only when the exposure measurement is related to the disease outcome status or vice versa.

Normal distribution, also called Gaussian distribution, is one in which the different values are distributed symmetrically in a bell-shaped curve. Technically, it means that the mean = the median = the mode.

Number needed to treat (NNT), or number needed to treat for benefit (NNTB) is the number who need to be treated for one of them to achieve the benefit in question. It is 1 divided by the risk difference.

Number needed to harm (NNH) or number needed to treat for harm (NNTH) is the number who need to be treated for one of them to be harmed by the adverse effect in question. It is 1 divided by the risk difference, which is the percentage of subjects with that harm after the intervention minus the percentage of controls with that harm.

Odds are the ratio of the probability of an event divided by the probability of no event. Where p = the probability, the odds are p divided by $1 - p$.

Odds ratio is the odds of an event in cases divided by the odds of the event in controls.

Opportunity costs are what is lost when resources are allocated to one intervention or service and not elsewhere.

Participant observation is based on traditional ethnographic research, whose objective is to understand perspectives held by study populations. Ethnographic research methods may include both observing people/processes and participating, to various degrees, in the day-to-day activities in the community setting.

Post-test odds are the odds that the patient has the condition or disease after you know the result of the diagnostic test. It is the pre-test odds times the likelihood ratio.

Post-test probability is the likelihood that the patient has the condition or disease after you know the result of the diagnostic test. It is the post-test odds divided by 1 + post-test odds.

Power refers to the ability of a study to detect a difference if there is one. If the study has sufficient power then a negative result can be taken to mean that there is no effect from the intervention.

Precision is the degree to which similar results are obtained on each testing. It is independent of accuracy.

Predictive values are estimates of how likely it is that a patient has, or does not have, the disease. **The positive predictive value** is the probability that the patient has the disease if the test is positive. **The negative predictive value** is the probability that the patient does not have the disease if the test is negative.

Pre-test odds are the odds that the patient has the condition or disease before you know the result of the diagnostic test. It is the pre-test probability divided by 1 – pre-test probability.

Pre-test probability is the likelihood that the patient has the condition or disease before you know the result of the diagnostic test.

Prevalence is the proportion of people with the disorder in the population at the specified point in time.

Probability value (P) is the probability that a result has arisen by chance. It is the same as the significance level. $P = < 0.05$ means that the probability that the result has arisen by chance is less than 5%.

Purposive sampling is the technique of choosing the subjects of research with a purpose in mind rather than as a random sample.

QALY is the quality-adjusted life year: a measure of the utility of an intervention that takes into account the length of life gained and the patient's assessment of the quality of that life.

Qualitative research is research in which the outcome cannot be expressed numerically. It is usually designed to answer a general, rather than a specific, research question.

Random misclassification bias (also known as non-differential misclassification bias) can occur when either the exposure or outcome is classified incorrectly (with equal probability) into different groups. The misclassification is random if the errors in exposure classification have occurred independent of the disease outcome.

Regression analysis is a technique for estimating the relationship between variables, which shows how the dependent variable (the outcome) changes when one of the independent variables is changed.

Relative risk reduction (RRR) is the reduction in risk where that person's risk was previously 1 or 100%. An RRR of 40% means that the person's risk is reduced to 60% of what it was. **Absolute risk reduction (ARR)** is that person's actual risk (of dying, for instance) after the intervention. If the risk of dying was 1%, an intervention with an RRR of 40% reduces that risk to 0.6%, which is an ARR of 0.4%.

Reliable means that the same results are likely to be found if the study is repeated.

Risk is a measure of the probability (between 0 and 1) of developing a particular disease in a stated time period.

Risk difference describes the absolute change in risk that is attributable to the exposure of interest and can take any value between −1 and +1. It is the same as the 'absolute risk reduction' (ARR).

Risk ratio or relative risk indicates the increased (or decreased) risk of disease associated with the exposure of interest.

Selection bias occurs when the association between an exposure and disease is different for those who complete the study, compared with those who are in the target population. Selection bias may exist when procedures for subject selection or factors that influence subject participation affect the outcome of the study.

Sensitivity is the ability of a test to detect people who do have the disease. It is the true positive rate.

Sensitivity analysis is an analysis of a study to see whether the assumptions made during the design of the study have led to a biased result. For instance, if certain people have been excluded from the study, would their inclusion alter the results?

Significance may be **statistical**, meaning the degree to which the result is unlikely to be due to chance, or **clinical**, meaning the degree to which the benefit or harm of a treatment is meaningful to the patient.

Specificity is the ability of a test to detect people who do not have the disease. It is the true negative rate.

Standard deviation is a measure of how far values are scattered around the mean. The lower the standard deviation, the closer values are to the mean. It is the square root of the variance.

Standard error of the mean is a measure of how close the sample mean is to the true population mean. It is the standard deviation divided by the square root of the sample size.

Stratification refers to the separation of subjects into groups, or strata, such that members of each group share the same characteristic, e.g. smoking status. This permits an analysis of each group separately, thus removing the effect of a possible confounder.

Systematic review is a study of all detectable literature on a topic which has been searched for, assessed and combined according to pre-determined standards.

Transferable (or generalisable) means that the results of the study can be applied to other populations and other settings.

Triangulation is a term used especially in qualitative research to describe the technique of using several different research methods to see whether they point to the same result.

Validity refers to whether a research study measures what it intends to measure. Internal validity means that the results are likely to be true for those who participated in the study. The three main threats to internal validity are bias, confounding and causality. External validity means that the results are likely to be generalisable (or transferable) to the population of interest.

Variables may be numerical (described by numbers) or categorical (described by categories). Categorical variables can be nominal (just names), ordinal (names that can be ranked in order), interval (ranked names with a constant interval between each one and the next) and ratio (interval variables with a natural zero).

Variance is a measure of the scatter of values around the mean (see standard deviation). It is the sum of the square of each individual deviation from the mean, divided by the number of observations.

Index

Notes: *vs.* indicates a comparison or differential diagnosis
To save space in the index, the following abbreviations have been used.
PICO - Patient Intervention Comparison Outcome
RCT - randomised controlled trial

Page numbers followed by *f* indicate figures and *b* indicate boxes.

A

B

C

D

Q

R

S

T

U

V

W